Global Bioethics and Human Rights

Contemporary Perspectives

Second Edition

EDITED BY

Wanda Teays

Mount Saint Mary's University, Los Angeles

and

Alison Dundes Renteln

University of Southern California

ROWMAN & LITTLEFIELD
Lanham • Boulder • New York • London

Executive Editor: Natalie Mandziuk
Editorial Assistant: Michael Tan

Published by Rowman & Littlefield
An imprint of The Rowman & Littlefield Publishing Group, Inc.
4501 Forbes Boulevard, Suite 200, Lanham, Maryland 20706
www.rowman.com

6 Tinworth Street, London SE11 5AL, United Kingdom

British Library Cataloguing in Publication Information Available

Library of Congress Cataloging-in-Publication Data

Names: Teays, Wanda, editor. | Renteln, Alison Dundes, editor.
Title: Global bioethics and human rights : contemporary perspectives /
   edited by Wanda Teays and Alison Dundes Renteln.
Description: Second edition. | Lanham : Rowman & Littlefield Publishers, 2020. |
   Includes bibliographical references. | Summary: "The ethical issues we face in
   healthcare, justice, and human rights extend beyond national boundaries—they are
   global and cross-cultural in scope. The second edition of this interdisciplinary and
   international collection features new essays on gender identity, vaccines, stem cells,
   bioterror, and other pressing contemporary concerns"—Provided by publisher.
Identifiers: LCCN 2019048497 (print) | LCCN 2019048498 (ebook) |
   ISBN 9781538123744 (cloth) | ISBN 9781538123751 (paperback) |
   ISBN 9781538123768 (epub)
Subjects: LCSH: Bioethics. | Human rights.
Classification: LCC QH332 .G5626 2020 (print) | LCC QH332 (ebook) |
   DDC 174.2—dc23
LC record available at https://lccn.loc.gov/2019048497
LC ebook record available at https://lccn.loc.gov/2019048498

We dedicate this volume to all those working to protect
human rights and challenge global injustice

Contents

PART III: Life and Death

PART IV: Public Health

ADDITIONAL RESOURCES

Acknowledgments

We are grateful to Rowman & Littlefield for greenlighting a second edition of *Global Bioethics and Human Rights* and the opportunity to expand the text. The new chapters have made for wider coverage of the issues.

We are also grateful to our editor, Natalie Mandziuk, whose guidance helped shape the direction of this new edition. We so appreciate your insights and encouragement.

We thank our contributors—ethicists from around the world. Your excellent essays will be most appreciated by readers of this second edition.

And thanks to all of you whose interest in global bioethics and human rights makes this volume possible.

Introduction to the Text

Every seeking gets guided beforehand by what is sought.

—Martin Heidegger

To convince someone of the truth, it is not enough to state it, but rather one must find the path from error to truth.

—Ludwig Wittgenstein

Wherever we turn, we confront ethical dilemmas. Some are personal—our own issues to resolve. Should I stop eating animals? How honest should I be with my ailing mother? Should I turn in my friend who cheated on the exam?

Some are those facing friends, family, or acquaintances seeking our advice, for example, about dropping out of school, choosing chemo over radiation, joining a political protest group, or becoming a subject in a pesticide experiment to make some extra cash.

Some dilemmas face people far removed from our own lives, but whose decisions reverberate, setting a precedent for others to follow—or to contest. For instance, is it wrong of doctors to refuse to perform an abortion or treat a child suffering from monkey pox, a relative of smallpox? Is it right of rich patients to buy a kidney from a poor person? Should doctors participate in lethal injections?

The issues range all over the map in terms of diversity and complexity. Take the man, identity unknown, who has been on life support for nearly 17 years, going in and out of consciousness. No one knows whether he has a family looking for him and what sort of care they would want him to receive. What do we owe him?

Then, there's the detainee held at a CIA black site who may or may not know anything useful to his interrogators. Should it be permissible to slam his head into a wall or confine him to a box with holes drilled in it for air? Are there exceptions to professional duties, regulations, and principles?

Consider also the dilemma facing a victim of an IVF mistake resulting in a pregnancy with the wrong embryos—and whose genetic parents want "their" baby. What should she do? Decisions, decisions—few are easy and the factors brought to bear are shaped by the context in which they arise and the values rooted in a culture or religion.

Heidegger's advice that we be guided by what is sought requires setting goals and keeping our perspectives in mind. Those goals and perspectives lay the groundwork for a truly *global* bioethics. And we need to take heed of Wittgenstein's observation—and recommendation— that we can't just assert truisms. We must show the way from error to truth and from moral shortcomings to virtue. To accomplish that goal, the boots have to be on the ground, as they say. Abstract principles—truisms—can be inspiring. But effecting change means *doing* something, tackling ethical issues head-on and trying to make our way to defensible decisions— ones that are just and fair.

We are pleased to have a second edition of this work and the opportunity to expand the coverage of the volume. Readers will appreciate the new chapters—which include such topics as medical tourism, abortion, euthanasia, surrogacy, mental health, institutional review boards, solitary confinement, long-term care for the elderly, vaccination programs, and the ways bioethics intersects with environmental ethics.

As with the first edition, we have incorporated a diverse range of perspectives—ones that underscore the significance and influence of values and beliefs. The various readings show how bioethics issues raise justice concerns—concerns that extend across the globe, with communities responding differently to these challenges. Western conceptions and normative standards are then called into question (Airhihenbuwa 1995). We see this with the Western emphasis on patient autonomy—at odds with family-centered decision-making that health caregivers often face.

And with more frequent migration, medical professionals are confronted with moral and cultural conflicts that are frequently unfamiliar or multilayered. This requires us to delve into policies and differing worldviews, leading us to ask how many, if any, ethical principles are universal. Authors in Part I tackle this issue and examine the ways theoretical perspectives frame the inquiry and lay the groundwork for a global bioethics.

The perspective taken can make all the difference. This is the case both in the framing of problems and the very concepts that are used. We see this, for example, with the interpretation of truth-telling. When an individual is diagnosed with a health problem, it is generally thought that medical professionals must inform the patient regarding treatment options. However, that presumption is not shared worldwide, as some cultures leave the patient out of the equation, particularly if the prognosis is grim.

As the chapters in Part II indicate, bioethics is fundamentally about human rights and the fiduciary duties of medical personnel and researchers. This includes such issues as patient rights, disability rights, informed consent, the rights of human subjects, the right not to be tortured, and protections against exploitation and invasive procedures.

Another focus of bioethics concerns such life-and-death issues as abortion, euthanasia, and the appropriate use of reproductive technology. We need only look at the fertility market. It is international in scope—from Southern California's high-tech fertility centers to India's low-cost in vitro fertilization and surrogacy brothels. What is permitted prior to conception, much less afterward, has generated numerous ethical conflicts—many ongoing and unsettled.

A major concern is the boundary of personal autonomy, as seen when others are asked to play a role in the "right" of personal liberty. That the procreation market includes those who sell their own gametes to those who gestate the genetic children of others merits our scrutiny. Moreover, both reproductive autonomy and patient autonomy at the end of life put self-determination at center stage. What duties do others have in ensuring personal autonomy is upheld? Can I ask you—or pay you—to give birth to my genetic child? Can I ask you to take my life when I want to die? What are the limits of self-determination when others are asked to play a part?

The ethical concerns go beyond what we do to our own bodies to how others are used to accomplish our ends. For instance, author Cecilia Wee discusses active and passive euthanasia from the perspective of Confucianism. Her explication helps us see how morality, culture, and religion can intersect and impact attitudes regarding killing versus letting die.

The range of public health concerns is both deep and wide. Bioethics is inherently about health—our bodies, procreation and birth, disease and suffering, pain and death. It is about access to health care, the allocation of resources, and just versus unjust medical practices. It is about vulnerable populations used in research and experimentation, as sources of human organs, or as "gestational carriers" bearing children for others.

We are not immune to its reach. Just one traveler from China brought SARS to the West. Health is a basic good, and so it is vital that we give thought to different perspectives on the concept of "health" and look at the way it is understood across nations. The chapters in this book show how often health issues are human rights issues.

As the essays in Part IV demonstrate, we cannot ignore health inequities. As a result, questions of justice in health care deserve our attention. Throughout this book, we see that is the case. In the Preamble to the Constitution of the World Health Organization (WHO), health is defined as "a state of complete physical, mental and social well-being, and not merely the absence of disease or infirmity." WHO further asserts that governments are responsible for providing "adequate health and social measures."

We might ask whether access to health care is a fundamental right. A great deal follows from the answer to that question. WHO's definition of health has brought with it considerable debate, given its social and ethical implications. In addition, it provides neither a discussion of the nature of mental or social well-being nor guidelines as to how they might be achieved. The very generality of the definition, as Daniel Callahan (1973) observes, has resulted in a concept that may be too broad. Callahan's recommendation is to pull in the reins. Thus, he offers the following definition: "Health is a state of physical well-being." That state need not be "complete," he argues, but it must be adequate.

When looking at public health on the global scale, it is easy to see why WHO suggested a broader approach to health. In many cases, physical well-being, mental well-being, and social well-being are intertwined. Assumptions, culture, traditions, and values, as well as biases and prejudices, transform what each person considers good health. They also affect who has moral standing or whose health concerns are considered most pressing. This can result in disparities regarding access to resources and personnel, treatment options, decision-making, and policy considerations.

The valuable insights gathered in this anthology help broaden our understanding of bioethics and deepen our appreciation for the global impact of the issues examined.

ORGANIZATION OF THIS BOOK

This book is set out in four parts. They are as follows:

Part I: Theoretical Perspectives

This first unit presents key approaches to bioethics, starting with the question of whether there can be a global ethical framework. This leads to the issue of whether a universal morality is compatible with multiculturalism. A central issue has to do with truth-telling and what sort of assumptions and principles should guide us. Another theoretical concern dealt with here—one typically overlooked in bioethics—is the interplay between bioethics and environmental ethics. The last perspective discussed in Part I links back to the opening question; namely, does a global bioethics require a global moral language?

Part II: Human Rights

This second unit turns to human rights and its importance in bioethics. We begin with a historical overview that grounds the discussion and shows how widespread are the concerns. The next three chapters illustrate the ways bioethics puts human rights under the spotlight—as shown in torture, disability rights, and medical tourism. Each issue asks us to consider the right to be treated with dignity and respect, and what we owe to one another in protecting that right. The remaining chapters in Part II focus on human experimentation. They look at the role of institutional review boards, the vulnerability of human subjects, particularly in third world countries, and concerns and recommendations regarding aboriginal research.

Part III: Life and Death

The third unit focuses on life and death. The opening chapter looks at pediatric genomics, zeroing in on adolescents' participation in decision-making. Their engagement and power to decide about genomic testing has been limited—thus calling for a reconsideration of who decides what in treatment issues and control of genomic data. We then turn to reproductive freedom, starting with one of the most controversial issues in all of ethics—abortion. The debate rages on, making it clear that the issue warrants examination and resolution. Another concern around reproduction is whether it is morally permissible to allow the use and trade in gestational surrogacy. Is it exploiting an underclass of needy women or a legitimate vocational activity? The next three chapters turn to euthanasia—another crucial life-and-death issue. As these chapters demonstrate, the perspective and underlying values can make all the difference. The final chapter in Part III examines lethal injection in China and, with that, whether harvesting organs should be permissible.

Part IV: Public Health

The fourth and last unit of the text examines issues in public health care and related systemic concerns. We start with an overview of global health ethics and key issues raised about justice. The next two chapters look at global mental health and then feminist perspectives on global aging.

Neither topic has received much attention from bioethicists—making these essays all the more important. The fourth chapter focuses on virginity restoration surgery—which asks us to weigh in cultural traditions and the role of self-determination. The next two essays raise issues around human rights and the right to health care for people out of the reach of public scrutiny. The fifth chapter looks at those held in immigration detention and, in the sixth chapter, those in solitary confinement. The last essay of Part IV and of the text examines vaccination programs—all too relevant in an age where pandemics are a vital global matter.

KEY FEATURES OF THIS BOOK

- International perspectives and cases offer a wider and deeper understanding of bioethics
- Emphasis on human rights puts justice in the foreground
- High-quality original essays by experts in the field offer vital insights for both health care professionals and academics
- Essays and exercises that help develop students' and other readers' critical thinking and moral reasoning skills
- Thoughtful pieces for professional development that remind us of our obligations and duties as ethicists, professors, and medical caregivers to those who depend on us for guidance
- Accessible chapters that will inspire students to reflect on moral dilemmas and the relevance of ethics to their lives
- Real-world cases and interesting discussion topics for each unit of the book—perfect for classroom activities, group projects, or essay assignments
- Additional resources, including essay questions, case analyses, and recommended bioethics in the movies
- Essays that widen the playing field beyond Western assumptions and values by recognizing other cultures, values, and religions
- Suitable for both graduate and undergraduate classes
- The inclusion of voices not often heard, resulting in a broader range of readings than commonly found in bioethics texts
- Chapters and units that work together but are independent of one another, giving faculty flexibility in setting out the course

NEW TO THIS EDITION

We have reshaped the second edition and expanded the coverage of issues with 10 new or updated readings. These include

- Robert Baker's reply to Bernard Gert and Tom L. Beauchamp
- Peter Tagore Tan's argument that bioethics is fundamentally about environmental ethics
- Virginia L. Warren's essay on medical tourism
- Wanda Teays's two chapters—one on torture and one on solitary confinement
- Alison Dundes Renteln's two chapters—one on institutional review boards and the other on virginity restoration surgery
- Maya Sabatello's examination of pediatric genomics

- Michael Boylan's analysis of the abortion debate
- Sharmin Islam, Rusli Bin Nordin, Ab Rani Bin Shamsuddin, Hanapi Bin Mohd Nor, and Abu Kholdun Al-Mahmood's study of surrogacy from the perspectives of Western secular and Islamic bioethics
- Carlos Verdugo Serna's focus on whether there is a medical duty regarding euthanasia
- Udo Schüklenk's overview of issues in global health ethics
- Zenon Culverhouse's chapter on global mental health
- Rosemarie Tong on feminist perspectives on global aging
- Keymanthri Moodley, Kate Hardie, Michael J. Selgelid, Ronald J. Waldman, Peter Strebel, Helen Rees, and David N. Durrheim's ethical inquiry into vaccination programs

As you can see from the list of new chapters, this second edition goes far beyond a minor revision. The additions, combined with the excellent readings from the first edition, make this book a most appealing resource—as a reference book, a supplementary anthology, or a primary text for a bioethics class.

WORKS CITED

Airhihenbuwa, Collins O. 1995. *Health and Culture: Beyond the Western Paradigm*. Thousand Oaks: Sage Publications.

Callahan, Daniel. 1973. "The WHO Definition of 'Health.'" *The Hastings Center Studies* 1, no. 3: 77–78.

Part I

THEORETICAL PERSPECTIVES

1

A Global Ethical Framework for Bioethics

Bernard Gert

ABSTRACT

Although morality is universal, it allows for some significant variations because of cultural differences. Bioethics is morality applied to medicine and medical research, so a global bioethics should be thought of as an application of the common moral system to medicine and medical research that allows for significant variations in different cultures or societies. Common morality has rules that prohibit killing, causing pain or disability, deceiving and breaking promises, but there is some variation in the interpretation of these rules, as well as in what counts as an adequate justification for violating them. Different societies also have some significant differences in their laws and in the duties that they regard physicians as having. There are also differences in whom they hold as fully protected by the moral rules. These societal variations have significant effects on what morality encourages, prohibits, and requires physicians to do.

INTRODUCTION[1]

Different cultures give different answers to some of the questions with which bioethics is concerned. This much seems obvious, and it has led many to conclude that there is no universal morality, while leading others to conclude that where there is disagreement one of the disagreeing cultures must be mistaken. In this article I describe what I believe is the universal moral system and explain how its universality is consistent with limited but true moral disagreement.

To begin, I distinguish the claim that morality is universal both from the claim that it always provides a unique correct solution and from the claim that it is explicitly recognized by every (or any) culture. As with grammatical rules, the moral system is normally followed without conscious reflection.

I next present the ten moral rules that I believe constitute the core of the universal moral system. One source of moral disagreement arises from different interpretations of these rules themselves. For instance, although the rule prohibiting killing is universal and cultures normally agree on when an action is a killing, certain actions (removing from a ventilator) may constitute killings in some cultures but not in others.

In every culture, violations of the moral rules require moral justification; thus, universal morality includes not only rules but also a procedure for justifying violations of these rules. I next introduce a two-step procedure for justifying violations of moral rules and consider how, using the identical procedure, members of different cultures can come to different conclusions about whether a particular violation is morally permissible.

In the last section, I discuss moral disagreements arising from differences of opinion regarding who or what is fully protected by this moral system, an issue the system itself cannot resolve. In all cultures, moral agents must be treated morally, but some cultures include others within morality's sphere of protection as well. And, finally, I note that, although a certain amount of disagreement is consistent with our universal morality, that morality itself puts substantial limits on the permissible ways of resolving the disagreements it sanctions.

MORALITY OR THE MORAL SYSTEM

Morality is a public system that is known by all those who are held responsible for their actions (i.e., all moral agents). A public system is a system that has the following two characteristics. In normal circumstances, (1) all persons to whom it applies (i.e., those whose behavior is to be guided and judged by that system) understand it (i.e., know what behavior the system prohibits, requires, discourages, encourages, and allows), and (2) it is not irrational for any of these persons to accept being guided and judged by that system.

The clearest example of a public system is a game, such as bridge or football. A game has an inherent goal and a set of rules that form a system that is understood by all of the players (i.e., they all know what kind of behavior is prohibited, required, discouraged, encouraged, and allowed by the game), and it is not irrational for all players to use the goal and the rules of the game to guide their own behavior and to judge the behavior of other players by them. Although a game is a public system, it applies only to those playing the game, and, if one does not want to abide by the rules, one can quit playing the game. No one can quit being governed by morality. Morality is a public system that applies to all people who understand it and can guide their behavior accordingly. Moral agents are subject to moral judgments simply by virtue of being rational persons who are responsible for their actions.

Although there is general agreement about who is subject to moral judgment, there is considerable disagreement about who is protected by morality. Some, for example, Kant, hold that only moral agents are fully protected, whereas others, for example, Bentham, hold that all beings who can suffer pain are protected. Morality has the inherent goal of lessening the amount of harm suffered by those included in the protected group, either all moral agents or a more inclusive group.

It contains rules that prohibit some kinds of actions, such as killing, and require other kinds, such as keeping promises, and moral ideals that encourage certain kinds of actions, such as relieving pain. It also contains a procedure for determining when it is justified to violate a moral rule, such as when a moral rule and a moral ideal conflict. Morality does not provide unique answers to every question; rather, it sets the limits to legitimate moral disagreement. It is important to realize that unresolvable moral disagreement on some important issues, such as abortion, is compatible with total agreement in the overwhelming number of situations where moral judgments are made.

A useful analogy to morality or the moral system is the grammar or grammatical system used by all competent speakers of a language. Almost no competent speaker can explicitly describe the grammatical system that she uses, yet all competent speakers know the grammar of their language in the sense that they use it when speaking and in interpreting the speech of others. If presented with an explicit account of the grammatical system, competent speakers have the final word on its accuracy.

They should not accept any description of the grammatical system if it rules out speaking in a way that they regard as acceptable or allows speaking in way that they regard as completely unacceptable. Morality or the moral system requires consistency in a way that grammar does not; so moral agents should not accept any description of morality if it conflicts with the overwhelming set of their considered moral decisions or judgments that are consistent.

There is such overwhelming agreement in most moral matters that we do not even make conscious moral judgments about them, for example, causing pain to someone simply because one feels like doing it. But morality involves one's emotions and interests far more than grammar, so people sometimes make moral decisions and judgments that are inconsistent with the vast majority of their considered moral judgments because they are distorted by their emotions or interests. This has the result that sometimes even competent moral agents can be shown that some of their moral decisions or judgments are mistaken.

COMMON MORALITY[2]

When some people claim that there is a common morality, they sometimes mean that there is a universal moral system that provides a unique correct answer to every moral question. Those who deny that there is a common morality sometimes mean that there is not a unique correct answer to any moral problem.

Not surprisingly, both of these extreme views are mistaken. To claim that there is a common morality is to claim that there is a universal moral system that provides a global framework for all acceptable moral decisions and judgments, but it does not mean that there is a unique correct solution to every moral problem.

There are, of course, unique correct answers to many moral questions, but these are usually moral questions that no one ever asks, such as "Is it morally acceptable to torture someone because I enjoy seeing someone in pain?" Even in most situations where one might be tempted to do an immoral action, no one consciously deliberates about what is the morally right thing to do, such as keeping an important promise that it is inconvenient for one to keep. Similarly, in most situations, no one consciously makes a judgment about someone who does not do a morally wrong action, for example, refrains from cheating in a game.

Bioethics is a field in which people often do consciously deliberate about what is the morally right thing to do, such as whether to perform an abortion. Physicians also sometimes consciously make judgments about someone who does not give in to the temptation to do the morally wrong action, for example, does not give an unnecessary antibiotic to a patient who requests it. In what follows, I shall provide a brief description of the common morality that provides a global framework for bioethics, but I shall also show that, even when there is complete agreement on the facts, including probabilities of future harms and benefits, there can be unresolvable differences in the decisions and judgments that people make.[3]

MORAL RULES

There is universal agreement that actions such as killing, causing pain or disability, and depriving of freedom or pleasure are immoral unless one has an adequate justification. Similarly, there is universal agreement that deceiving, breaking a promise, cheating, violating the law, and neglecting one's duties also need justification in order not to be immoral.

When I say that all societies have moral rules that prohibit such actions, all I mean is that doing these kinds of actions are immoral unless one has an adequate justification for doing them. Although there are alternative ways of formulating the moral rules, following is a list of moral rules that includes all of the kinds of action that need justification. Although these rules are subject to some variation in interpretation, they can be understood by all those who are held responsible for their actions.

1. Do not kill.
2. Do not deceive.
3. Do not cause pain.
4. Keep your promises.
5. Do not disable.
6. Do not cheat.
7. Do not deprive of freedom.
8. Obey the law.
9. Do not deprive of pleasure.
10. Do your duty.

The rule prohibiting causing pain prohibits causing not only physical pain but also mental pain, the rule prohibiting causing disabilities prohibits causing not only physical disabilities but also mental and volitional disabilities, the rule prohibiting depriving of freedom includes prohibiting depriving of opportunities and resources, and the rule prohibiting depriving of pleasure includes prohibiting depriving of future pleasure as well as present pleasure. The rule prohibiting deceiving can be broken by withholding information, as well as by lying, and the rule requiring one to keep one's promises requires keeping informal agreements, as well as formal contracts.

Finally, "duty," in the rule requiring one to do one's duty, is meant in its everyday sense, where duties are determined by one's social role, job or profession, or special circumstances. Someone who takes a job is often told what duties are involved. "Duty" is not used as philosophers customarily misuse it, to mean whatever one morally ought to do. We are morally required to obey all of the moral rules unless we have an adequate justification for not doing so, but in the everyday sense of "duty" it is a misuse to say we have a duty to obey these rules (e.g., not to kill) or to do our duties.

Duties in this everyday sense are not derived from our common morality, but in each society duties develop from social roles and from the history and practice of the professions in that society. Knowing about social roles and the practices of a field or profession in a particular society is not only necessary for understanding what duties people have in that society, but it is sometimes also necessary for understanding the interpretation of the moral rules in that society.

In many societies, these rules are understood to prohibit not only actual violations but also attempts to violate them, even if the attempt is unsuccessful. They are also often understood to prohibit not only intentional violations but also violations done knowingly but not intentionally. They can even be understood to prohibit some unknowing violations if the person should have known that his action was a violation of a moral rule or that he was likely to cause harm to someone. But what it means "to cause harm to someone" is not as simple and straightforward as it initially seems. Although one can take "Do not kill" to mean "Do not cause death," causing death, like causing pain or disability, does not mean simply doing an intentional act that you know will result in a person's death, pain, or disability.

Consider a physician who is deciding whether to comply with a competent ventilator-dependent patient's refusal to stay on the ventilator. If the physician does decide to disconnect the patient from the ventilator, does that count as killing him or even as assisting his suicide? For most people in American society, complying with a competent patient's refusal to stay on the ventilator when one knows that disconnecting the patient from the ventilator will result in the patient's death does not count as either killing the patient or even as assisting his suicide.

This is also the legal view in this society. In every state of the United States, physicians are legally required to take a competent patient off of the respirator if the patient refuses to be on it any longer, yet in every state physicians are prohibited from killing patients, even competent patients who have requested to be killed. Further, although all states require complying with a competent patient's refusal to continue on a ventilator, almost all states do not even allow physician-assisted suicide.

However, some religious people in the United States regard taking a competent patient off of a respirator, even if the patient refuses to be on it any longer, as interfering with the will of God and hence as killing the patient, and they do not sanction it. This may also be the view of those societies in which religion has a greater influence on the interpretation of the moral rules than is the case in the United States.

Although no society denies that when physicians comply with a terminal patient's request to be given a lethal injection, they are killing that patient, some more secular societies, such as the Netherlands, consider it morally justified for a physician to kill a patient in these circumstances. Thus, societies can differ from one another not only in their interpretation of the rule prohibiting killing; they can also differ from each other in what they consider to be morally justified cases of killing. These differences do not conflict with all societies accepting that violating the moral rule that prohibits killing needs moral justification.

Like "cause," "deprive" is also not as simple as it initially seems. "Do not deprive of freedom" does not mean simply do not intentionally do any act that you know will have the result that someone does not have the freedom or opportunity to do something he would have had if you had not done that act. For example, in every country with automobiles and parking lots, if, in the normal course of affairs, you arrive at a parking lot before another person, you do not deprive him of the opportunity to park in that lot if you take the last parking place. You do not even need to justify parking in the last space. Further, no one in any country holds that someone who wins a race fairly has deprived the other runners of the pleasure of winning the race.

However, there may be societal differences concerning whether a teacher who grades a student's exam fairly and gives it a very bad grade has broken the rule prohibiting causing pain. Some might say that she has broken the rule but that she is justified in doing so because it is her duty to grade exams fairly, but others might say that she has not broken the rule at all. Similarly, some might claim that a physician who tells a patient about his very poor prognosis, even if she does so in a very compassionate manner, is still violating the rule against causing pain.

However, similar to what some would say about the teacher, some might claim that the physician is justified in violating the rule because it is her duty to tell her patient the truth about his prognosis, while others might claim that telling the patient the truth does not even violate the rules against causing pain and so does not need to be justified at all. But in some societies, doctors do not regard it as necessary to tell a patient the unpleasant truth in order to proceed with treatment. If the physician only has a duty to tell a member of the patient's family, she is not justified in causing pain to the patient.

Deciding whether to tell a patient bad news can also be influenced by a society's interpretation of the rule prohibiting deceiving. Although every society regards a physician lying to a patient as deceiving, one society may also regard a physician as deceiving a patient if she withholds unpleasant information about the patient's medical condition because doctors have a duty to tell their competent patients about their diagnosis and prognosis.

However another society, which does not regard a doctor as having a duty to tell patients bad news, such as Russia, may not regard withholding unpleasant information as deceiving at all. Given this wide variation in the interpretation of the rules, some based on the differences in the duties doctors have in that society, it may seem as if talking about a common morality or a global framework for bioethics is a sham. However, that is because we are discussing interesting cases, where there are legitimate differences in the interpretation of a moral rule. However, most cases are not interesting. In the overwhelming majority of cases, all societies agree when a given moral rule has been violated and also agree on whether the violation is justified.

DISAGREEMENTS BASED ON DIFFERENT INTERPRETATIONS OF A MORAL RULE

Different interpretations of a moral rule can lead to unresolvable moral disagreement not only between different societies but also within a given society. I include in the category of disagreements based on different interpretations of the rules only those different interpretations that do not involve deciding who is impartially protected by the moral rules.

Even when there is no doubt that all involved are impartially protected by the moral rules, there is sometimes disagreement on what counts as breaking the rule (e.g., what counts as killing or deceiving). Even people who agree that complying with a competent patient's refusal to continue on the respirator is not killing sometimes disagree on whether discontinuing food and fluids counts as killing. In addition to the disagreement about whether withholding information counts as deceiving, there is also disagreement about whether dying one's hair counts as breaking that rule.

Some of these disagreements can be resolved, but some cannot. And often some institution will have to make a decision that settles the matter for the people governed by that institution. Hospitals may adopt rules determining when it is allowed to discontinue life-sustaining treatments, and those physicians that follow those rules are not regarded as having killed their patients but only as having allowed them to die.

Because different societies have different legal systems and impose different duties on physicians, the moral rules prohibiting violating the law and neglecting one's duties will differ in the actions that they prohibit and require. For example, in the United States, doctors have a duty to tell their competent patients about their diagnosis and prognosis, but, in many countries in South America, Israel, and Russia, doctors may tell family members rather than the patient. A universal morality allows for significant cultural or societal variation.

Although there is overwhelming agreement on the moral status of the vast majority of actions, these kinds of actions are those about which no one consciously makes moral decisions and judgments. Normally, we consciously make moral decisions and judgments only on actions about which there is some controversy. With regard to these kinds of situations, morality often does not provide a unique solution to every moral problem, even within a particular society.

Moreover, because their legal systems differ and different duties are assigned, societies may differ in the judgments that are made about particular actions even when these judgments are uncontroversial within each society. But the differences in laws and duties do not affect the universality of morality any more than the fact that people make different promises affects the universality of morality. And just as promises can sometimes be justifiably broken, so laws can sometimes be justifiably violated and duties can be justifiably not performed. Morality places significant limits on legitimate moral variation between societies, as well as within societies.

MORALLY RELEVANT FEATURES AND THE TWO-STEP PROCEDURE FOR JUSTIFYING VIOLATIONS

In addition to the agreement about the kinds of actions that need moral justification, there is general agreement about the way in which violations of moral rules can be justified. There is overwhelming agreement that what counts as an adequate justification for one person must be an adequate justification for anyone else in the same situation. However, since no two situations are exactly alike in all respects, each society must have some way of determining what counts as the same situation.

When it is said that morality requires impartiality, what should be meant is that the same situation does not change simply because the identity of the persons involved in that situation changes. This does not mean that everyone must agree about whether a violation of a moral rule is justified. Impartiality does not require uniformity; impartiality is compatible with disagreement about what counts as an adequate moral justification for any particular violation (e.g., killing or deceiving).

For the same reason, the judges on the US Supreme Court can agree completely on the facts, be impartial, and yet come to different conclusions. It is also important to realize that morality requires impartiality only when one is concerned with the violation of a moral rule; morality does not require impartiality when following a moral ideal (i.e., doing something morally good, such as aiding the needy or relieving pain). Morality allows people to give to whatever charity they prefer; morality does not require impartiality when giving to charities.

One of the most important differences between moral rules and moral ideals is that it is possible for moral rules to be impartially obeyed all of the time. That is why, unless they have an adequate justification for not doing so, people can be required to obey the moral rules all of the time. People are only encouraged, not required, to follow the moral ideals, and no one can even favor following moral ideals all of the time because it is humanly impossible to do so. The moral rules set constraints on one's behavior regardless of what one's goals are, and it is possible for these constraints to be obeyed all of the time. The moral ideals provide goals for one's behavior, but there is a limit on how much time it is possible to spend trying to achieve these goals. Nonetheless, moral ideals express the point of morality more clearly than moral rules, for following them is directly acting to achieve the goal of morality, which is the lessening of suffering harm by all those protected by morality.

Although obeying the moral rules is required and following the moral ideals is only encouraged, when following a moral ideal conflicts with obeying a moral rule, it is sometimes justified to violate the moral rule in order to follow the moral ideal. When there is a conflict between two moral rules or between obeying a moral rule and following a moral ideal, there is a two-step procedure for deciding what one morally ought to do.

This two-step procedure is employed in all societies, though usually not consciously, to determine whether a violation of a moral rule is justified. As stated above, when we are talking about impartiality, everyone agrees that what counts as an adequate justification for one person must be an adequate justification for anyone else in the same situation. But for this statement to serve any purpose or have any force, there must be a specification of what counts in the same situation.

For the purposes of justifying a violation of a moral rule, two situations count as the same situation when all of their morally relevant features are the same. A morally relevant feature is a feature such that, if it changes, it can change whether a rational person would regard that violation of a moral rule as justified. In ordinary circumstances, the day of the week, the time of the day, and the season of the year are not morally relevant features. Unless the day, time, or season are related to some other feature, a change in them cannot change whether a violation of a moral rule is justified.

I have compiled a list of ten questions, the answers to which are morally relevant features. I do not claim that any change in any of these features would lead a rational person to change his position concerning whether a particular violation is justified. I do claim that, for a rational person who does not use any idiosyncratic beliefs (i.e., beliefs that are not shared by all rational persons), only a change in these features can change whether that person regards the violation as justified.

Two violations count as being in the same circumstances or as the same kind of violation if all of the following questions have the same answers. The answers to these questions are the morally relevant features of the violation.

1. What kind of act is it (i.e., what moral rule is it a violation of)?
2. What harms are caused, avoided (not caused), and prevented?
3. What are the relevant beliefs and desires of the person harmed?
4. What is the relationship between the parties?
5. What goods are being gained?
6. Is a violation of a moral rule being prevented?
7. Is a violation of a moral rule being punished?
8. Are there alternative actions that will not violate a moral rule or cause less harm?
9. Is the action being done intentionally or only knowingly?
10. Is the situation an emergency?

When serving on the ethics committee of a hospital, I found that, if one did not recognize all of these morally relevant features, one was quite likely to make a moral judgment that no one, including oneself, would accept. For example, an unacceptable moral judgment could result from a failure to recognize that it is a morally relevant feature that two situations differ in that in one situation there is an alternative action that would result in less harm. Similarly, a seriously mistaken moral judgment may result from a failure to recognize that it is a morally relevant feature if two situations differ in that one situation is an emergency situation. I cannot show that all of the morally relevant features are answers to just these 10 questions.

Perhaps in some other society, or even in my society, some other morally relevant features may be discovered. But, in each society, there must be some way of identifying what counts as the same situation or the same kind of violation. Describing a situation in terms of its morally relevant features is the first step in the two-step procedure that all people in all societies must employ to guarantee that what counts as an adequate justification for one person counts as an adequate justification for anyone else in the same situation.

The second step in the two-step procedure is estimating the results of everyone knowing that they are allowed to violate the rule in these circumstances. If one estimates that *less* harm would result from everyone knowing that they are allowed to violate the rule in these circumstances than from everyone knowing that they are *not* allowed to violate the rule in these circumstances, then one is acting impartially in violating that rule. If everyone would make the same estimate, then the violation is strongly justified; if not everyone would make the same estimate, then the violation is only weakly justified. Weakly justified violations involve serious moral disagreement.

If everyone would estimate that *more* harm would result from everyone knowing that they are allowed to violate the rule in these circumstances than everyone knowing that they are *not* allowed to violate the rule in these circumstances, then the violation is unjustified. What one estimates about the harms and benefits of everyone knowing that violating a rule in the specified situation is allowed is shown by whether one would favor everyone knowing that they are allowed to violate the rule in these circumstances. This has a superficial resemblance to Kant's categorical imperative, but both its foundation and its results are significantly different.

DISAGREEMENTS BASED ON DIFFERENCES ABOUT WHEN A VIOLATION OF A MORAL RULE IS JUSTIFIED

In addition to the unresolvable disagreements that arise from differences in the interpretation of the moral rules, there are two other kinds of differences that can lead to unresolvable disagreements between different societies, or even between persons in the same society, about whether a violation of a moral rule is justified. The first is a difference in the ranking of the harms and benefits, although not in what counts as harms. Everyone agrees on what the harms are (i.e., death, pain, disability, loss of freedom, and loss of pleasure). All rational persons try to avoid these harms unless they have an adequate reason for not avoiding them (e.g., to avoid what they take to be a greater harm or to gain a compensating benefit for themselves or someone else).

This may not be obvious because sometimes one may not appreciate the benefit involved (e.g., some cultures require suffering pain in order to gain the status necessary for being a full member of the society, a practice not unlike fraternity hazing). Also, for some religious people, the harm they will avoid is based on religious belief. For example, a Jehovah's Witness may refuse a blood transfusion that will save his life because he believes that having a blood transfusion violates the biblical prohibition against eating blood and so will result in the loss of eternal bliss.

Although there is universal agreement on what counts as harms, people do not all agree on the ranking of these harms. Further, pain, disability, loss of freedom, and loss of pleasure have degrees, and even death occurs at very different ages so that there is no agreement that one of these harms is always worse than the others. Some people rank dying several months earlier as worse than a specified amount of pain and suffering while other people rank that same amount of pain and suffering as worse. Thus, for most terminally ill patients, it is rationally allowed either to refuse death-delaying treatments or to consent to them.

Most actual moral disagreements (e.g., whether to discontinue treatment of a terminally ill incompetent patient) are based on disagreements about the facts of the case (e.g., how painful the disease is, how painful the treatment is, and how long the treatment would prolong the patient's life). Differences in the rankings of the harms account for much of the rest of the moral disagreements (e.g., how much pain and suffering it is worth to prolong life for three months).

Often, the factual disagreements about prognoses are so closely combined with different rankings of the harms involved that they cannot be distinguished. Further complicating the matter, the probability of suffering any of the harms can vary from very low to almost certain, and people can differ in the way that they rank a given probability of one harm against a different probability of another harm. Disagreement about involuntary commitment of people with mental disorders that make them dangerous to themselves involves a disagreement about both what percentage of these people would die if not committed and whether a significant probability of death within one week (e.g., 2 percent) compensates for a 100 percent probability of three to five days of a very serious loss of freedom and a 30 percent probability of long-term mental suffering.

Actual cases usually involve much more uncertainty about outcomes, as well as the rankings of many more harms. Thus, complete agreement on what counts as a harm or evil is compatible with considerable disagreement on what counts as the lesser evil or greater harm in any particular case. It should be apparent that there is also considerable disagreement concerning the rankings of the benefits or goods (i.e., consciousness, abilities, freedom, and pleasure), but the rankings of the benefits play a much smaller role in justifying violations of moral rules than the rankings of harms.

Obviously, if people rank the harms differently, even when they agree on all of the facts, they will disagree in their estimates of whether more harm would result from everyone knowing that they are allowed to violate the rule in these circumstances than from everyone knowing that they are not allowed to violate the rule. Hence, they will differ in whether they favor everyone knowing that they are allowed to violate the rule in these circumstances. Suppose that two people agree that legalizing active euthanasia will result in the same reduction in the amount of pain and suffering of terminally ill patients and that they also agree that, due to mistakes and pressure, it will result in the same increase in people dying somewhat earlier than they might want to die. If they rank pain and death differently, they may disagree about whether one should legalize active euthanasia. One may hold that death is such a serious evil that avoiding quite a large amount of pain and suffering does not justify any significant increase in the number of earlier deaths, wanted or unwanted, whereas another may hold that death for a terminally ill patient is not as serious as the pain and suffering that results from living longer. Different societies may differ in the rankings that most of their members hold, and many different rankings seem acceptable.

But even if they rank the reduction of pain and suffering and the increase in somewhat earlier deaths exactly the same, they may still disagree because of their differing views of human nature. This difference may be most marked when one is considering people in different societies. People in a relatively homogeneous society may have a different estimate concerning what would be the result of everyone knowing that they can violate the rule against killing terminally ill patients in clearly specified circumstances than people living in a quite heterogeneous society like the United States. People in a homogeneous society may believe that there will be relatively few cases of unwanted earlier deaths due to mistakes and pressure, whereas those in a heterogeneous society may believe that there will be far more unwanted earlier deaths due to mistakes and pressure.

But, even within a particular society, people can have different views about what would happen if everyone knows that they are allowed to break a moral rule in the same circumstances. For example, some people hold that, when asked about how you like someone's clothes or hair, it is justifiable to deceive them in order to avoid hurting their feelings. They would favor allowing deception in this kind of situation because they believe that everyone knowing that this kind of violation is allowed would result in significant harm being avoided with only a minimal loss of trust. Others would not favor allowing deception in this kind of situation because they believe that the loss of trust would be significant and would outweigh the amount of harm avoided.

This ideological difference concerning human nature may also involve a different ranking of the harms involved, and there may be no way to decide which of these estimates is correct. It may be that one estimate is shared by most in one society and another by most in another society, but there may be no way to decide which of these estimates is correct even in a particular society.

DISAGREEMENTS BASED ON DIFFERENCES REGARDING WHO IS IMPARTIALLY PROTECTED BY THE MORAL RULES

The debates about abortion and animal rights are best understood as debates about who is included in the group that is impartially protected by the moral rules. However, there is no way to resolve this issue, for it makes sense to talk of impartiality only when the group toward which one is supposed to be impartial has been specified. Fully informed rational persons who hold that animals are not protected as strongly as moral agents can disagree about how much they should be protected (i.e., they can disagree about how strong a reason has to be to be an adequate reason to justify killing or causing pain to an animal). People can also disagree about whether fetuses are protected as strongly as moral agents and, if they are not, how much they are protected. They may even disagree about whether a fetus is protected to the same degree at all stages or whether the fetus deserves more protection as it develops. Some societies do not even hold that neonates are protected as strongly as moral agents and so allow infanticide with no justification or much less than is needed to justify killing a moral agent.

That there is no unique correct answer to the question about who is protected as strongly as moral agents is why discussions of abortion and animal rights are so emotionally charged and often involve violence. Morality, however, does set limits to the morally allowable ways of settling unresolvable moral disagreements. These ways cannot involve violence or other unjustified violations of the moral rules but must be settled peacefully. Indeed, one of the proper functions of a democratic government is to settle unresolvable moral disagreements by peaceful means.

As mentioned at the beginning of this article, some maintain that morality is only, or primarily, concerned with the suffering of harm by moral agents while others maintain that the harms (e.g., death, pain, and loss of freedom) suffered by of those who are not moral agents is as important, or almost so, as the harms suffered by moral agents. But, even if one regards animals as not included in the group impartially protected by the moral rules, this does not mean that one must hold they should receive no protection. There is a wide range of morally acceptable options concerning the amount of protection that should be provided to those that are not included in the group toward which morality requires impartiality.

Many hold that, although the reasons that are adequate to justify killing or causing pain to animals do not have to be as strong as the reasons that are adequate to justify killing or causing pain to moral agents, some reasons are needed. Few hold that it is morally justifiable to cause pain to animals just because one feels like doing so. Many states have laws prohibiting cruelty to animals to enforce this moral position. Yet many hold it is justifiable to use animals in painful medical experiments that will help provide treatments for important human maladies. Many also hold that it is justifiable to kill animals for food, even when alternative vegetarian alternatives are available. Many also hold that it is justifiable to deprive animals of their freedom so that people can enjoy seeing them in zoos, but many now feel that they should be put in larger more comfortable surroundings than the small cages that were commonly used.

Regardless of the cultural variations in morality, the similarity in the content of morality is sufficiently great that there is general agreement that the world would be a better place if everyone acted morally and that it gets worse as more people act immorally more often. This explains why we teach children to act morally and why every society has laws that prohibit serious immoral actions. A complete account of morality would discuss the moral virtues, but, simply from the account of morality presented, it is obvious why the moral virtues connected with the second five rules, truthfulness, trustworthiness, fairness, honesty, and dependability, are those traits of character that all rational people want others to have and at least pretend to have themselves.

Rational persons favor others acquiring the moral virtues in order to lessen their own risk of suffering harm and, since they know that other rational persons also want them to act morally, they must, at least, pretend to cultivate these virtues in themselves. This explains the truth of La Rochefoucauld's saying, "Hypocrisy is the homage that vice pays to virtue."

CONCLUSION

In conclusion, the fact of disagreement between cultures over issues in bioethics does not force us to choose between the idea that one party to any disagreement must always be acting immorally and the idea that there is no universal morality. For the reasons I have given, a universal moral system does not mean universal agreement. But it does limit legitimate disagreement.

Where a culture allows the violation of moral rules in such a way that, even by its own lights, it would not do to have everyone know that actions with the same morally relevant features are permissible, that culture permits actions that are immoral. Thus, for instance, no culture could allow everyone to know that actions with the same morally relevant features as Nazi medical experiments were permissible. No one in any culture could want everyone to know that it was generally permissible to cause death, terrible pain, and disability to many persons to satisfy the curiosity and sadistic impulses of a few. Nor, I expect, could any society accept the consequences of everyone knowing that actions with the same morally relevant features as assisting in involuntary female circumcision were permissible.

Nonetheless, as in some of the examples discussed above, there are times when each party to a disagreement can present a sound moral argument for its own moral position. Recognition and careful application of this distinction between morally defensible disagreement and indefensible disagreement certainly has implications for how practitioners should engage with those with whom they disagree. When the other side advocates what is clearly in conflict with morality, sanctioning their customs may be inappropriate.

In other cases, however, cases where we must admit that morality itself makes no distinction between our own position and the position of those with whom we disagree, nothing more forceful than discussion, or perhaps a vote, is an appropriate way of resolving the disagreement. We may also find that an understanding of how legitimate moral disagreement is possible makes it easier, in appropriate circumstances, to truly respect moral positions that are contrary to our own.

NOTES

1. The editors would like to thank Heather Gert, the author's daughter, for graciously supplying this introduction and conclusion after his untimely death.

2. The phrase "common morality" is explicitly used by Tom Beauchamp and James Childress in later editions of their text, *Principles of Biomedical Ethics*. In that book, they contrast their understanding of common morality with the one presented in this article. However, in a recent paper, Tom Beauchamp acknowledges that the account of common morality presented here is superior to the account provided in *The Theory of Morality* by Alan Donagan, which they used to support their four principles.

3. For a full account of this common moral system, see *Morality: Its Nature and Justification*, revised edition, 2005, Oxford University Press. For a shorter account, see *Common Morality: Deciding What to Do*, paperback edition, 2007, Oxford University Press. For applications of the common moral system to bioethics, see *Bioethics: A Systematic Approach*, Bernard Gert, Charles M. Culver, and K. Danner Clouser, 2006, Oxford University Press.

2

The Compatibility of Universal Morality, Particular Moralities, and Multiculturalism

Tom L. Beauchamp

ABSTRACT

Topics addressed in this chapter are moral relativism, the objectives of morality, universal morality, particular moralities, multiculturalist theory, and cultural moral imperialism. I argue that cultural relativism is an untenable theory and that a universal common morality transcends all cultural standards. The norms of universal morality are not thick in moral content, but they afford a starting framework that we can use to construct thick, action-guiding norms. The common morality allows for moral disagreement and legitimate differences of opinion about how to best specify universal norms, and thus it supports the development of particular moralities that differ from other particular moralities. However, the common morality does not allow for the so-called multicultural world, which some writers in ethics take to mean a world void of universal moral norms. However, their views misrepresent even the commitments of multiculturalist theory. Multiculturalism is the theory that respect is owed to cultural traditions because morality itself demands this form of respect. Multiculturalism asserts that, universally, it is morally wrong to not acknowledge the moral rights of persons merely because their beliefs descend from different cultural histories.

Do all moral beliefs derive from cultural standards, or are there moral standards that transcend cultures and conventions? In one type of theory, morality is relative to cultural arrangements and aspirations. The notion of an objective principle or universal morality has no place in this theory. In another type of theory, universal moral standards, such as human rights and basic moral rules, are independent of particular cultures, nations, and organizations. I will present a version of the second type of theory. In addressing this problem, I will consider the subjects of moral relativism, the objectives of morality, universal morality, particular moralities, multiculturalism, and cultural moral imperialism. I will argue both in opposition to a relativism of basic moral standards and in support of a universally valid common morality.

THE UNTENABILITY OF CULTURAL RELATIVISMS

Moral relativism is an ancient problem about cultural differences that remains vibrant today. Two types of relativism are examined in this section: descriptive cultural relativism and normative cultural relativism. There are many species of relativism, but these are the two most prominent forms.

Descriptive Cultural Relativism

Defenders of descriptive relativism regard many discoveries in the social sciences as constituting evidence of an extensive diversity of moral practices across cultures. This work has cataloged and described many cultural differences, but these differences do not demonstrate that morally committed people in diverse cultures disagree about universal moral standards that underlie and justify their particular moral beliefs and practices. Simple examples are principles of honesty and truth-telling, virtues of caring and trustworthiness, and ideals of charity and friendliness.

Consider the vast similarity, in virtually every nation, in codes and regulations governing research involving human subjects. There are understandable and justifiable differences from country to country, but the differences pale in comparison to the sea of similarity in the norms governing how this research can and cannot be conducted. A few dozen principles are globally accepted as canonical for research ethics. Here are a few (steeply abridged) examples:

- Disclose all material information to subjects in medical research.
- Obtain an individual, voluntary, informed consent to biomedical interventions.
- Maintain secure safeguards for keeping personal information about subjects private and confidential.
- Receive surrogate consent from a legally authorized representative for incompetent subjects.
- Protect subjects in research against excessive risk.
- Ethics review committees must scrutinize and approve research protocols.
- Research cannot be conducted unless its risks and intended benefits are reasonably balanced and risks are minimized.
- Special justification is required if proposed research subjects are vulnerable persons.

Several global organizations and many governments have officially supported these norms in codes and regulations, but the force and authority of the norms themselves are not contingent on any particular form of agreement. As the World Medical Association says of its "Declaration of Helsinki" and as the US government says of its *Belmont Report*, the "ethical principles" governing research involving human subjects are valid independently of any state of cultural belief or law.[1] Scandals in the history of research involving human subjects have occurred precisely when people in cultures neglected these principles in their laws and practices.

True cultural relativists reject these claims. They subscribe to the thesis that no moral principles of any sort, general or particular, are valid independent of the cultural contexts in which they have arisen and shaped to their present form. Relativists regard the relevant social science data as indicating that moral rightness and wrongness vary from place to place and that there are no absolute or universal moral standards that apply across all societies. Even the concepts of rightness and wrongness themselves are meaningless apart from the specific cultural contexts in which they arise, and patterns of culture can be understood only as unique wholes. In a much quoted statement, anthropologist Ruth Benedict once expressed the thesis as being that the term "morality" *means* "socially approved habits" and that the expression "It is morally good" is *synonymous* with "It is habitual."[2]

There is no need to question the anthropological reports on which cultural relativism is erected. Many are informative, solid scientific studies. However, these studies do not show that there are no basic universal moral principles. More importantly, these descriptive reports of what people in fact believe do not support any normative position about what is right and wrong or about what any person or culture ought to believe. This takes me to the second type of relativism.

Normative Cultural Relativism

Though descriptive cultural relativism contains no normative content about how one ought to behave, the theory can be altered and given normative content. In this theory the statement "What is right at one place or time may be wrong at another" is interpreted to mean that *it is right* in one context to act in a way that *it is wrong* to act in another context. According to cultural normative relativism, one ought to behave in the ways one's culture determines to be correct and not behave in ways one's culture determines to be incorrect.

Cultural normative relativism is usually expressed as a theory based on cultural group beliefs and institutions, not merely on beliefs that appear only within the borders of nation-states. Accordingly, normative relativism does not merely say that when one is in Japan one should act as the Japanese do or when in the United States as the Americans do. It is a cultural, not a geographic theory about the source of moral correctness.

Normative group relativists hold both that there is no criterion independent of one's culture for making a judgment that a practice is right or wrong or to assess whether the standards of one's social group are the standards one ought to uphold. More generally, normative relativism is the theory that a form of moral conduct is right or wrong for persons if and only if their culture holds that it is right or wrong.

One weakness in this theory is that it is often difficult to determine which group, society, or institution constitutes the culture that should be followed. For example, in pre-Taliban Afghanistan women were often well educated and worked in professions, but under the Taliban-imposed culture they were not allowed to work or to seek an education beyond the age of eight. Should we say that women should be governed by either of these conflicting sets of norms? Can one ever be bound by a coercively imposed culture? What from a moral point of view are one's obligations under these circumstances? Do any of the series of controlling groups in Afghanistan give any of its citizens the normatively correct set of beliefs and action guides? This is not a problem about Afghanistan and its history. Determining how to identify an appropriate cultural group is a serious theoretical problem for normative relativism.

A bigger problem is that, however precisely formulated, normative relativism has no justification for its view that a norm is acceptable merely because the members of a cultural group believe it in a certain way—or because individuals or the members of a religious group believe it in a certain way. This commitment to being morally bound by group norms is at the heart of the theory of normative cultural relativism and cannot be eliminated without abandoning the theory. But the idea that the slave trade, sexual harassment under a severe threat by a superior, excluding women from training as physicians, and denying human rights to "foreigners" ought to be practiced merely because a group believes in the practice has no moral justification or credibility. It is no more than a justification of tradition by appeal to tradition (or of culture by appeal to culture), a clear case of begging the question of moral justification.

Normative relativism has other problems as well. If right and wrong are entirely relative to a culture's standards, no person could ever maintain that his or her culture's standards are wrong or seek any kind of reform. Rejection by individuals of the culture's standards is wrong in this theory, no matter what the standards are. Similarly, if there are no moral norms about exposing research subjects to high risks, about coercion and exploitation of nursing home populations, about unacceptable occupational risks to health, or about unethical billing for health reimbursements, then normative relativism implausibly maintains that the absence of such standards is morally normative in these situations. No reasonable person would accept such a view.

The unacceptability of descriptive cultural relativism and normative cultural relativism does not mean that a multicultural theory is unacceptable. I will later argue that multiculturalism is no relativism at all and is actually an important defense of universal morality and human rights.

THE OBJECTIVE OF MORALITY

I now turn to a thesis about what I will call the objective of morality.[3] This objective is that of promoting human flourishing by counteracting human circumstances in interactions with others that cause the quality of people's lives to worsen. The objective is to prevent or limit problems of indifference, conflict, suffering, hostility, scarce resources, limited information, and the like. This thesis has notable similarities to, though it is broader than, what Bernard Gert, in chapter 1 in this volume, described as the goal of morality: "Morality has the inherent goal of lessening the amount of harm suffered by those included in the protected group."

Following in the path of Thomas Hobbes and David Hume, I accept the following as the background circumstance of morality: from centuries of experience we have learned that the human condition tends to deteriorate into misery, confusion, violence, and distrust unless certain norms are enforced through a public system of norms.[4] When complied with, these norms lessen human misery and foster cooperation. These norms may not be necessary for the *survival* of a society, as some have maintained,[5] but they are necessary to ameliorate or counteract the tendency for the quality of people's lives to worsen and for social relationships to disintegrate. In every well-functioning society, norms are in place to prohibit lying, breaking promises, causing bodily harm, stealing, fraud, the taking of life, the neglect of children, and failures to keep contracts. These norms, when socially enforced, achieve the objective of morality.

Many philosophers with different conceptions than the one I just presented nonetheless do not significantly disagree about the general norms that comprise morality. That is, philosophers from many different theoretical standpoints converge on the principles, virtues, rights, and responsibilities that are central to morality and in doing so converge on essential conditions of any system of belief that deserves to be called morality.[6] They also agree on paradigm cases such as the judgment that rules legitimating the slave trade are morally unacceptable no matter what a culture might think about the legitimacy of these rules.

The universal character of the human experience and of social responses to threatening conditions (by formulating norms that are suitable for the moral life) helps *explain* why there is a common morality, but it does not *justify* the norms.[7] What justifies the norms of the common morality, in the pragmatic theory I accept, is that they are the norms best suited to achieve the objectives of morality. Once the objective(s) of morality have been identified, a set of standards is pragmatically justified if and only if it is the best means to the end identified when all factors—including human limitations, shortcomings, and vulnerabilities—are taken into consideration. If one set of norms will better serve the objective of morality than a set currently in place, then the former should displace the latter.

This account is my own preferred strategy for the justification of moral norms, but I appreciate that others prefer a different justification, such as a contractarian one or the full account and justification of morality found in Gert's *Morality: Its Nature and Justification*.[8] However, I will not further pursue these theoretical matters because they would make no difference to the arguments I provide hereafter.

THE COMMON MORALITY AS UNIVERSAL MORALITY

What are the principal cross-cultural norms of the common morality?[9] The common morality comprises *rules*, *virtues*, *ideals*, and *rights*—each of which I briefly discuss in this section.

Gert and I both understand the common morality as universal morality. It is not relative to cultures or individuals and is to be distinguished from norms that bind only members of particular groups. Gert views the nature and number of the moral rules in the common morality as precisely determinable,[10] whereas I regard these matters as less cleanly demarcated. I will not address this issue here, but I emphasize that it is of the highest importance in the interpretation of both Gert's theory in chapter 1 of this volume and my account that the focus not be exclusively on moral principles or rules of obligation. "Common morality" references the entire "moral system," to use Gert's preferred language. I will now outline what I see as the main constituent elements in the system (elements that Gert and I catalog somewhat differently, but not in a way that compromises the core of the common morality).

Universal Rules of Obligation

Here are a few examples (not a complete catalog) of rules of obligation in the common morality: (1) Do not kill; (2) do not cause pain or suffering to others; (3) prevent evil or harm from occurring; (4) rescue persons in danger; (5) tell the truth; (6) nurture the young and dependent; (7) keep your promises; (8) do not steal; (9) do not punish the innocent; and (10) obey the law. These norms have been justified in various ways by various philosophical theories, but I will not treat this problem of justification here. These cross-cultural norms obviously are implemented in different ways in different cultural or group settings, a matter I will later discuss when treating the topic of specification.

Universal Virtues

The common morality also contains standards that are *moral character traits*, or virtues. Here are a few examples: (1) honesty; (2) integrity; (3) nonmalevolence; (4) conscientiousness; (5) trustworthiness; (6) fidelity; (7) gratitude; (8) truthfulness; (9) lovingness; and (10) kindness. These virtues are universally admired traits,[11] and a person is deficient in moral character if he or she lacks these traits. Negative traits amounting to the opposite of the virtues are *vices* (malevolence, dishonesty, lack of integrity, cruelty, etc.). They are substantial moral defects, universally so recognized by persons committed to morality.

Universal Ideals

Moral ideals such as charitable goals, community service, dedication to one's job that exceeds obligatory levels, and service to the poor are also a part of the common morality. These aspirations are not *required* of persons, but they are universally *admired* and *praised* in persons who accept and act on them.[12] Here are four examples that can be interpreted both as ideals of virtuous character and ideals of action: (1) exceptional forgiveness; (2) exceptional generosity; (3) exceptional compassion; and (4) exceptional thoughtfulness.

Universal Rights

In addition to the basic obligations, virtues, and ideals just mentioned, human rights form an important dimension of universal morality. Rights in general are justified claims to something that individuals or groups can legitimately assert against other individuals or groups. Human rights in particular are those that all humans possess.[13]

Many philosophers, political activists, lawyers, and framers of political declarations now regard rights theory as the most important type of theory for expressing a universal moral point of view. Human rights language easily crosses national boundaries and supports international law and policy statements by international agencies and associations. Although human rights are, for this reason, often interpreted as legal rights, this interpretation does not properly capture their status. They are universally valid moral claims, and they have been so understood at least since early modern theories of rights were developed in the seventeenth century.[14]

The point of human rights language is to provide standards that transcend norms and practices, in particular, cultures that conflict with human rights. However, as James Griffin has rightly pointed out, we are sometimes satisfied that a basic human right exists, yet we are uncertain about what precisely the basic right gives us a right to.[15] This problem should be handled through what I will refer to in the next section as *specification*—the process of reducing the indeterminate character of abstract norms and giving them specific action-guiding content, often in the context of what I will call particular moralities.

PARTICULAR MORALITIES

It might be thought, given my emphasis on universal morality, that I do not allow for any form of pluralism or for local moral viewpoints—as if morality were a monolithic whole that does not permit disagreements and differences of approach. However, this is a misunderstanding of the connection between universal morality and the many moral norms that are particular to cultures, groups, and even individuals. Unlike the common morality, with its notably abstract and therefore content-thin norms, particular moralities present concrete, nonuniversal, and content-rich norms.

Particular moralities include the many responsibilities, ideals, attitudes, and sensitivities found in, for example, cultural, religious, and professional guidelines. Nonetheless—and this is a key matter in understanding why relativism is an unacceptable theory—*all justified particular moralities share the norms of the common morality with all other justified particular moralities.*

In order to have a practical, action-guiding morality, the norms of the common morality must be made specific in content. We cannot erect policies and practices on vague notions such as "respect for persons." All abstract norms must be carefully defined and then carefully fashioned as specific, well-crafted norms that give specific guidance to actions such as truthful disclosure, maintenance of confidentiality, obtaining an informed consent, providing access to medical care, and the like. These more concrete norms often must be made more concrete still for certain contexts. For example, the requirement of obtaining informed consent will be fashioned somewhat differently for contexts of research and contexts of medical practice.

Consider an example of a rule that sharpens the requirements of a more general norm of avoiding conflicts of interest. The rule to be specified is, "Avoid conflicts of interest in making treatment recommendations" (which itself is a specification of a more general principle of avoiding conflicts of interest). This rule might be specified as follows: "When physicians prescribe pharmaceutical products, they must avoid favoring products in which they have a financial relationship if this financial interest influences their judgment." The initial norm of avoiding conflicts endures, even though it is now a more specific rule.

Specification is a process of reducing the indeterminate character of abstract norms and generating more specific norms.[16] Specifying the norms with which one starts, whether those in the common morality or norms from a source such as a professional code, is accomplished by *narrowing the scope* of the norms, not by explaining what the general norms *mean*. As Henry Richardson puts it, specification occurs by "spelling out where, when, why, how, by what means, to whom, or by whom the action is to be done or avoided."[17] All norms are subject to specification, and many already specified rules will need further specification to handle new circumstances of conflict. Progressive specification can continue indefinitely.

To illustrate progressive specification, consider an additional specification that can be made to the rule already specified above, namely, "When physicians prescribe pharmaceutical products they must avoid favoring products in which they have a financial relationship if this financial interest influences their judgment." To this proscription we can add the following words shown in italic type: "When physicians prescribe pharmaceutical products they must avoid favoring products in which they have a financial relationship if this financial interest influences their judgment *and they must avoid prescribing products if their judgment is influenced by a personal relationship they have with a representative of a company that distributes the product(s)*." These specified rules can be indefinitely specified and turned into a whole policy governing this type of conflict of interest.

Very commonly, more than one line of specification is available when confronting practical problems and moral disagreements, and different persons or groups will offer conflicting specifications. For any moral problem several competing specifications may be offered by thoughtful and fair-minded parties, and thereby many different provisions in particular moralities are coherent ways to specify the common morality. This latitude must be permitted in practical moral thinking. We cannot demand more of people than that they faithfully specify norms with an eye to the overall coherence of the resulting particular morality while ensuring that their specifications do not violate the norms of universal morality.

Good examples of particular moralities that contain at least some specifications are *professional moralities* in biomedical research, medical practice, nursing practice, veterinary practice, and the like. These moral codes, declarations, and standards of practice often legitimately vary from other moralities in the ways they handle justice in access to health care, human rights, justified waivers of informed consent, government oversight of research involving human subjects, privacy provisions, and the like.

MULTICULTURALISM AS A UNIVERSALISTIC THEORY

It is an undisputed fact that multiple cultures have constructed unique particular moralities. This fact suggests to several writers in ethics that it is likewise an undisputed fact that morals are relative to cultures, or "pluralistic," the word now commonly heard in bioethics. Some writers in bioethics insist that we live in a multicultural world in which many moral cultures can live together peacefully, without need for the outmoded notion of universal, basic norms.

This characterization has matters upside down. In this section, I argue that multiculturalism requires and insists on universal norms. Multiculturalism is not a pluralism or relativism. Multiculturalism is a universalistic theory to the effect that particular moralities are owed respect because morality itself demands it. The term "multicultural world" has been hijacked by various writers in bioethics to suggest the reverse, and especially to suggest that there is no universal morality and no commonly held morality.[18]

THE UNIVERSAL NORMS IN MULTICULTURALISM

The term *multiculturalism* refers to theories that support the moral principle that cultural or group traditions, institutions, perspectives, and practices should be respected and should not be violated or oppressed as long as they do not themselves violate the standards of universal morality. The objective of multiculturalism is to provide a theory of the norms that should guide the protection of vulnerable cultural groups when threatened with marginalization and oppression caused by one or more dominant cultures.

Resistance to forceful dominance and cultural oppression drive multiculturalist theory, which holds that respect is owed to people of dissimilar but peaceful cultural traditions because it is unjust and disrespectful to marginalize, oppress, or dominate persons merely because they are of an unlike culture or subculture. The moral notions at work in this account are universal theses about rights, justice, respect, and nonoppression.[19]

The major demand in multiculturalism is that people of one culture are morally obligated to tolerate and not interfere with the views of those in other cultures (as long as those views are themselves not in violation of universal moral norms). This universally valid demand is independent of any particular culture's values and is not valid *because* a culture accepts it.[20] These are matters of human rights, not of human contracts or cultural arrangements or the current state of national or international law. Without universal norms of toleration, respect, restraint, and the like, a multiculturalist could neither explain nor justify multiculturalism.

In short, the moral obligation to respect the views of people from other cultures is not confined to people in cultures that *recognize* this obligation. By design of multiculturalism as a moral theory, moral obligations of respect and tolerance apply to all cultures whether or not they recognize these norms. Harvey Siegel puts it accurately when he says "multiculturalism is itself a culturally transcendent or universal moral, educational, and social ideal in the sense that it is applicable to all cultures . . . and rests upon other equally transcendent, moral imperatives and values."[21]

CULTURAL IMPERIALISM

Some seem to think that my support of transcendent, universal moral standards is merely a disguised form of cultural imperialism. Persons outside of a given culture who press for recognition within that culture of the human rights of women, minorities, children, the ill, the disabled, the oppressed, the marginalized, the economically disadvantaged, and other vulnerable groups have been denounced in some literatures as cultural imperialists who incorporate "Western values" that are uncritically assumed to be universally valid, but that—beneath the veneer of fairness, equity, and respect—simply camouflage the continuance of Western dominance.

These charges of cultural imperialism have understandable roots in hundreds of years of colonial political and economic domination. Despite this perplexing history, threats of "cultural imperialism" today have nothing to do with so-called Western values or with any history of moral imperialism emanating from the Western world or from any history of imperialism from any particular region of the world. Virtually every region of the world has a horrid history of imperialistic control extending from one people to another.

Numerous cultural traditions, past and present, and in all parts of the world, have held that their cultural values are universal values to which everyone should conform. This claim might be correct in the sense that one culture might have understood and insisted on universal norms not recognized by some other culture(s). However, the concern here is the *imposition* of norms by one culture on another.

THE PRACTICAL IMPORTANCE OF CONTROLLING CULTURAL OPPRESSION BY UNIVERSAL NORMS

There is today a convergence of global opinion that cultural differences must not be allowed to obscure the conditions of injustice and oppression that are presented by despotic rulers as nothing more than ways of protecting a culture's traditional values.[22] There are no more important human rights than rights against oppression—a broad category, but today the most consequential form of human rights violation.

Even the governments of many nations that are signatories to the UN Universal Declaration of Human Rights do not protect the basic human rights of women and children, or at least they have an unduly narrow vision of what those rights are. When complaints and resistance movements arise, governments often claim that they are treating women and children in accordance with *their* cultural traditions, but here is a true case in which forms of oppression are being disguised by dominant powers that have no respect for universal values.

Susan Okin has justly argued that conflict between traditional cultural practices and persons subordinated to those practices cannot be resolved by the theory that regional control, based on some tradition, may legitimately be asserted over persons in the local region who do not come from or follow the dominant tradition. She argues that, when these conflicts arise, they ought always to be resolved in terms of the rights of the oppressed, never resolved merely in terms of cultural practices or some kind of balancing of competing interests. Neither tradition nor a balancing of interests should be given priority when there are serious human rights violations. The enforcement of human rights that override even long-standing traditional values ought, in this account, to be the primary consideration.[23]

We are often told in writings in ethics that there are important East–West moral differences and that Western values should not be imposed on Eastern nations. However, these alleged differences are virtually never explained in detail and documented. The available empirical literature on the subject often does not support the claims. Amartya Sen points out that the idea of "Asia as a unit" with a set of Asian values different from those of the West makes no sense despite its frequent mention. He notes that about 60 percent of the world lives in Asia, with virtually nothing to solidify it as a uniform moral culture (other than universal morality, which simply solidifies it with the rest of the world): "There are no quintessential values that apply to this immensely large and heterogeneous population, that differentiate Asians as a group from people in the rest of the world."

Sen notes that violations of basic rights of freedom occur routinely in many parts of Asia and that dictatorial heads of state use the excuse that "Asian nations" do not accord the same value to personal autonomy and political freedom as do Western countries; therefore, the human rights to freedom extolled in the West are either irrelevant or objectionable. Sen rightly sees such claims as morally unacceptable while noting an interesting piece of history: The idea of "Asian values" and "the Orient" were originally the products of a Eurocentric perspective that regarded the whole of the Asian region as united by a body of non-Western standards. Sen briskly criticizes Western governments, including those in the United States and European nations, for indirectly backing this unfounded idea of Eastern values and allowing such a specious conception to serve as an excuse for not giving primacy to human rights.[24]

CONCLUSION

The arguments in this chapter all move to the conclusion that a universal set of moral norms comprises the common morality. Although these norms are thin in their abstract moral content, they are far from empty, and they afford a starting point for the specification of action-guiding norms, in particular, moralities and practical ethics. They constitute a wall of moral standards that cannot justifiably be violated in any culture or by any group or individual.

NOTES

1. See the 2008 revision of the World Medical Association's "Declaration of Helsinki: Ethical Principles for Medical Research Involving Human Subjects," Part B, "Basic Principles for all Medical Research" (first adopted 1964); *The Belmont Report: Ethical Guidelines for the Protection of Human Subjects of Research* (Washington, DC: DHEW Publication OS 78-0012, 1978). It first appeared in the *Federal Register* on April 18, 1979.

2. Ruth Benedict, "Relativism and Patterns of Culture," in *Value and Obligation*, ed. Richard B. Brandt (New York: Harcourt Brace and World, 1961), 457.

3. The term and much of my understanding of the issues derive from G. J. Warnock's similar language in *The Object of Morality* (London: Methuen & Co., 1971), esp. 15–26.

4. Cf. Bernard Gert, *Morality: Its Nature and Justification*, revised ed. (New York: Oxford University Press, 2005), 11–14.

5. See the sources referenced in Sissela Bok, *Common Values* (Columbia, MO: University of Missouri Press, 1995), 13–23, 50–59 (citing several influential writers on the subject).

6. Cf. Tom L. Beauchamp and James F. Childress, *Principles of Biomedical Ethics*, sixth ed. (New York: Oxford University Press, 2009), 260–61, 361–63.

7. John Mackie, *Ethics: Inventing Right and Wrong* (London: Penguin, 1977), 22–23, 107ff.

8. Gert, *Morality: Its Nature and Justification*.

9. Although there is only one universal common morality, there is more than one *theory* of the common morality. For the theories pertinent to this volume, see Bernard Gert, *Common Morality: Deciding What to Do* (New York: Oxford University Press, 2004, paperback edition, 2007); and Tom L. Beauchamp and James F. Childress, *Principles of Biomedical Ethics*, sixth ed. (New York: Oxford University Press, 2009), chaps. 1, 10.

10. See, in the present volume, Gert's list of 10 moral rules. Gert readily acknowledges that there is disagreement among philosophers on the matter and says that there is not even "complete agreement concerning what counts as a moral rule." Gert, *Morality: Its Nature and Justification*, 13.

11. See Martha Nussbaum's assessment that, in Aristotelian philosophy, certain "nonrelative virtues" are objective and universal: "Non-relative Virtues: An Aristotelian Approach," in *Ethical Theory, Character, and Virtue*, ed. Peter French et al. (Notre Dame, IN: University of Notre Dame Press, 1988), 32–53, esp. 33–34, 46–50.

12. See Gert, *Common Morality: Deciding What to Do*, 20–26, 76–77; Richard B. Brandt, "Morality and Its Critics," in *Morality, Utilitarianism, and Rights* (Cambridge: Cambridge University Press, 1992), chap. 5.

13. Cf. Joel Feinberg, *Rights, Justice, and the Bounds of Liberty* (Princeton, NJ: Princeton University Press, 1980), esp. 139–41, 149–55, 159–60, 187. See also Alan Gewirth, *The Community of Rights* (Chicago: University of Chicago Press, 1996), 8–9.

14. Pioneering theories of international rights and natural rights—now generally restyled as *human rights*—first prospered in philosophy through the social and political theories of Hugo Grotius, Thomas Hobbes, and John Locke. See Anthony Pagden, "Human Rights, Natural Rights, and Europe's Imperial Legacy," *Political Theory* 31 (2003): 171–99.

15. James Griffin, *On Human Rights* (Oxford: Oxford University Press, 2008), 97, 110.

16. Henry S. Richardson, "Specifying Norms as a Way to Resolve Concrete Ethical Problems," *Philosophy and Public Affairs* 19 (Fall 1990): 279–310; and "Specifying, Balancing, and Interpreting Bioethical Principles," in *Belmont Revisited: Ethical Principles for Research with Human Subjects*, ed. James F. Childress, Eric M. Meslin, and Harold T. Shapiro (Washington, DC: Georgetown University Press, 2005), 205–227.

17. Richardson, "Specifying, Balancing, and Interpreting Bioethical Principles," 289.

18. Examples are H. Tristram Engelhardt Jr., *The Foundations of Bioethics*, second ed. (New York: Oxford University Press, 1996); Robert Baker, "A Theory of International Bioethics: Multiculturalism, Postmodernism, and the Bankruptcy of Fundamentalism," *Kennedy Institute of Ethics Journal* 8 (1998): 201–31; Leigh Turner, "Bioethics in a Multicultural World: Medicine and Morality in Pluralistic Settings," *Health Care Analysis* 11 (2003): 99–117.

19. Compare the arguments in the essays in Robert K. Fullinwider, ed., *Public Education in a Multicultural Society* (Cambridge: Cambridge University Press, 1996).

20. See the essays by Charles Taylor, Amy Gutmann, Steven C. Rockefeller, Michael Walzer, and Susan Wolf, in *Multiculturalism and "The Politics of Recognition,"* ed. Amy Gutmann (Princeton, NJ: Princeton University Press, 1992).

21. Harvey Siegel, "Multiculturalism and the Possibility of Transcultural Educational and Philosophical Ideals," *Philosophy* 74 (1999): 387–409.

22. See Martha Nussbaum and Jonathan Glover, eds., *Women, Culture, and Development* (Oxford: Oxford University Press, 1995); and Marcia Angell, "The Ethics of Clinical Research in the Third World," *New England Journal of Medicine* 337 (1997): 847–49.

23. Susan Moller Okin, "Is Multiculturalism Bad for Women?" in *Is Multiculturalism Bad for Women?*, published as an anthology, ed. Joshua Cohen, Matthew Howard, and Martha C. Nussbaum (Princeton: Princeton University Press, 1999), 20–24.

24. Amartya Sen, *Human Rights and Asian Values* (New York: Carnegie Council, 1997). The quote is on page 13.

3

Reply to Gert and Beauchamp

Robert Baker

As I argued in the first edition of *Global Bioethics* (see Part II, chapter 2), the singular virtue of grounding bioethics in human rights is that, in principle, it offers a globally recognized discourse and standard of morality that all member states of the United Nations are committed to respecting. Drawing on this shared vocabulary and related concepts in biomedical ethics, different societies can more readily articulate a global ethics that addresses diverse societies' common interest in fighting infectious diseases, in providing health care to our peoples, and in ensuring that our peoples are not exploited by unscrupulous researchers. Rights-based bioethics can thus provide a common starting point for developing a form of global bioethics that is sensitive to cultural and society diversity.

In the opening chapters of this book, however, Bernard Gert and Tom Beauchamp insist that global bioethics requires more than a common vocabulary, shared concerns, and over-lapping interests; it requires, to quote Gert, "a universal moral system," accepted across cultures despite some points of "moral disagreement."[1] Furthermore, Beauchamp emphasizes, "common morality, as universal morality . . . is not relative to culture or individuals and is to be distinguished from norms that bind only members of particular groups."[2]

I believe that the possibility of a culturally independent set of universal standards "not relative to culture" is merely wishful thinking. Worse yet, I fear that it is more likely to facili-tate disruptive claims of cultural imperialism than to provide foundations for a commonly accepted global bioethics. In point of historically based fact, whatever ideals intellectuals from a given society may claim to be universal, objective, or self-evidently true, whether penned in the eighteenth century or inputted from keyboards of the twenty-first century, they are more likely to reflect the ideals of their own era and culture than ideals universally shared across all cultures or for all time periods.

As anyone perusing the history of morality will quickly discover—and as both Beauchamp and Gert acknowledge—people in the past conceptualized morality differently. They drew on different concepts to formalize their conceptions of morality, drew on different paradigms of virtue and vice, and made different judgments about what is good or bad, right or wrong, virtuous or vicious. For example, the ancient Greek founders of the Western moral philo-sophical tradition, Plato and Aristotle, deemed slavery and infanticide morally acceptable.[3]

Yet Western societies today would condemn both. It follows that insofar as Aristotle and Plato lauded as virtuous actions that we would today condemn as immoral, and praised as morally right what we condemn as morally wrong, we do not share a substantive common morality with the founding figures of Western moral philosophy. Moving from the past to the present, we in the English-speaking cultural sphere do not share many important bioethical concepts with contemporary continental Europeans.

They have a robust moral concept of "solidarity": a nonsexist ideal of "fraternity," of all for one and one for all. They draw on this concept to justify, among other things, societal support for national health insurance systems. The concept of solidarity is among those used in the 2005 UNESCO Declaration on Bioethics and Human Rights,[4] but it is notably absent from Anglo-American discussions of bioethics and moral philosophy, including those of Beauchamp and Gert, who appeal to a different set of moral concepts.

I understand and admire those who, like Beauchamp and Gert, thirst for some set of universally absolute common moral truths because, like Alonso Quixano himself, they thirst for justice and moral order in a world that all too frequently lacks either. Yet, like Quixote, I believe they are tilting at windmills, failing to recognize that the concept of "common morality" is either a misleading misnomer or, worse yet, a dangerous fiction. It is, I believe, a misleading misnomer for the metaethical observation that, by virtue of a common goal of all moralities—facilitating cooperation and minimizing conflict—successful moralities commonly place constraints on killing. It is undoubtedly true that every morality (or, more accurately, every moral system that I have examined) places constraints on some forms of killing. However, except for Jainism,[5] every morality also permits killing fellow humans—albeit, not in the same circumstances.

Some communities believe that fellow humans may be killed to exterminate unbelievers or heretics, or to prevent a person from suffering (euthanasia, medically assisted dying), or in defense of honor (as in duels and other honor killings); other communities believe that humans may be sacrificed to ideals of retributive justice (*lex talionis*, capital punishment), or to honor personal autonomy (physician-assisted suicide). On the other hand, many communities believe it wrong to kill unbelievers and heretics, or to practice capital punishment, euthanasia, medically assisted dying, or physician assisted suicide. Communities both constrain and permit killing, but they do not share one substantive common or universal moral standard with respect to which or when fellow humans may or may not be killed.

The point to appreciate from these observations is that to conflate common moral constraints on killing with a substantively common universal morality is to conflate an observation about areas of regulation with substantively common content in regulations. Societies commonly regulate the flow of traffic in their cities, but that does not mean that we all drive on the same side of the road. To confuse the generic with the specific in this way is the type of confusion philosophers refer to as a "category mistake."[6]

I also believe that to fail to recognize the virtue inherent in our diversity of moral concepts, moral virtues, and moral norms in the name of some singular ideal of a substantive universal morality would be to reify a static conception of morality, fettering our moral development to current conceptions of a good moral life or ethical biomedical practice. If adopted, such a fixed conception of morality or biomedical ethics would naturally inhibit our communities' ability to respond to morally disruptive ecological, socioeconomic, and technological change. Fettering a society or an ethic to a single set of paradigms, concepts, norms, and laws—such as those favored by twentieth-century American bioethicists—would undermine the natural processes of moral reform and moral revolution that enable societies and cultures to adapt their paradigms, concepts, norms, and laws to morally disruptive challenges. In morality, as in law and the sciences, the "absolute," "ideal," "true," "universal," and "self-evident" are by their nature inflexible, and so, to paraphrase Voltaire, "presumptively universal truths become the enemy of all that is new."[7]

Worse yet, despite the good intentions of its proponents, the notion of a universally common morality is not only predicated on metaethical error; it is also likely to cloak an implicit form of cultural imperialism since to designate any one community's morality as ideal, common, or universal is to imply that all other moralities must in some way measure up to, or be reconciled with, this ideal, universal, common morality—or be condemned as, in some sense, deficient. As Beauchamp forthrightly admits, "If one set of norms will better serve the objective of morality than a set currently in place then the former should displace the latter," assuming the costs of transition do not outweigh the benefits achieved.[8]

The history of societies that embrace absolute truths is as bleak in morality as it is in the sciences. Such societies imprisoned their scientific and moral discontents, from Giordano Bruno and Galileo to feminist reformers like Alice Paul and Margaret Sanger. The historical evidence is that deeming any one conception of morality as "true" or "universal" invites intolerance, irrespective of whether the believers are Buddhists, Christians, communists, Comstockians, fascists, Islamists, progressives, socialists—or bioethicists. Given the common problems posed by morally disruptive biomedical technologies and discoveries, given our common concerns to facilitate the ethical delivery of health care to our peoples and to protect our peoples against exploitive research, I believe that we should recognize and respect differences in our conceptions of morality, even as we strive for a cross-cultural global consensus on basic issues of bioethics and human rights.[9]

NOTES

1. Bernard Gert, "A Global Ethical Framework for Bioethics," this volume, 9.

2. Tom L. Beauchamp, "The Compatibility of Universal Morality, Particular Moralities, and Multiculturalism," this volume, 26.

3. According to classicist Cynthia Patterson, ordinary citizens of ancient Greece and their philosophers, Aristotle and Plato, distinguish "infanticide" (i.e., killing a child), which they called *paidoktoneo*, from exposing a newborn, a practice that they called *ektithemi*. The distinction turns on whether an infant was killed before induction into a family, which they called *ektithemi*, or after it had been inducted into a family and recognized by the community. Recognition involved a special ceremony, the *Amphidromia*, at which children received their name. Killing after induction into a family would be *paidoktoneo*—or, as we would put it, infanticide. If, during the pre-induction period, a newborn appeared disfigured, weak, illegitimate, or otherwise unworthy of family membership—or if it was a female born to a family that could not afford to provide a suitable dowry—it could be excluded from the family and thus exposed (*ektithemi*). The family's conscience was salved by the fact that *ektithemi* at a ceremonial site was not necessarily a death sentence since childless couples, or anyone seeking to rear slaves, could adopt exposed newborns—for the most part, however, *ektithemi* was fatal. Cynthia Patterson, "Not Worth the Rearing": The Causes of Infant Exposure in Ancient Greece," *Transactions of the American Philological Association* 115 (1985): 103–23. Other cultures had similar practices. From the seventeenth to the early twentieth century, for example, Japanese midwives practiced *mabiki*, a gardening term for thinning or pruning that involved suffocating newborns, to provide better care for those children already born. See Fabian Drixler, *Mabiki: Infanticide and Population Growth in Eastern Japan, 1660–1950* (Berkeley: University of California Press, 2013).

4. UNESCO, *Universal Declaration on Bioethics and Human Rights* (2005), http://portal.unesco.org/en/ev.phpURL_ID=31058&URL_DO=DO_TOPIC&URL_SECTION=201.html (accessed June 30, 2018).

5. One of the core moral concepts of the Jains is *ahimsa*, noninterference or nonviolence. Gandhi made this concept integral to nonviolent protest. On Jain morality, see Paul Dundas, *The Jains* (New York: Routledge, 2002), 160.

6. Common morality theorists also have a "reconciliation" problem. Beauchamp and other common morality theorists recognize that, in addition to the common morality, there are also "Particular moralities . . . religious and professional guidelines . . . [but] . . . all justified particular moralities share the norms of common morality with all other justified particular moralities" (Beauchamp, "The Compatibility of Universal Morality," 27). Yet it will be challenging to reconcile common and particular moralities. For example, as noted above, common morality prohibits killing fellow humans, yet, in Belgium, Canada, and the Netherlands, physicians are permitted to kill their patients (i.e., to perform acts of medically assisted dying at their patients' request), and physicians in California, Oregon, Vermont, and Washington may lawfully assist their patients in suiciding (i.e., aid their patients in killing themselves). Insofar as these acts appear incompatible with common morality, Beauchamp and other theorists must reconcile these aspects of particular morality with common morality—or condemn medically assisted dying and physician-assisted suicides of suffering patients as immoral contraventions of common morality.

7. Voltaire [1770, 1772]. Voltaire's *bon mot* is more accurately translated as the "Perfect is the enemy of the good" in *Wikipedia* (revised February 26, 2018), https://en.wikipedia.org/wiki/Perfect_is_the_enemy_of_good (accessed April 1, 2018).

8. Beauchamp, "The Compatibility of Universal Morality," 25.

9. For a more fleshed out analysis of the position sketched in this paper, see Robert Baker, *The Structure of Moral Revolutions: Studies of Changes in the Morality of Abortion, Death, and the Bioethics Revolution* (Cambridge, MA: MIT University Press, forthcoming).

4

Culture and Ethical Aspects of Truth-Telling in a Value Pluralistic Society[1]

Ilhan Ilkilic

ABSTRACT

Advances in medical science and technology offer us not only new diagnostic measures and possibilities but also allow us to make better prognoses in terminal disease stages. As a consequence, physicians can work out more precise diagnoses, enabling them to inform their patients about the expected future course of their condition. Under these circumstances, truth-telling as a classical issue of medical ethics remains a highly charged problem. The concept of truth-telling has become controversial in multicultural societies because of the differences in attitude toward this practice, based on diverse cultural value systems and preferences. The demographic changes effected by migrant groups, especially in western European countries, mean that truth-telling will be an ever more common problem in everyday medical practice, posing serious challenges for health care professionals.

This chapter describes some arguments pertinent to this issue and discusses a real case history recorded at a German hospital. Telling the truth about a diagnosis in an intercultural setting and the participation of family members in the decision-making process in a multicultural society are identified as the key ethical points of this case. It also discusses some metaethical issues, such as the universal applicability of the ethical principle of "respect for autonomy" with regard to truth-telling. Some practical suggestions for everyday medical practice in a multicultural society are developed, and, in the conclusion, some ethical theses are proposed.

INTRODUCTION

Rapid developments in medicine enable us not only to produce better diagnoses but also to make more accurate predictions about the future development of illnesses. As a result of these developments, unfavorable diagnoses, such as malignant cancer, are made more frequently, and infaust (dire) prognoses are to be communicated to patients. Thus, the standard question of medical ethics concerning the morally correct way of handling the disclosure of unfavorable diagnoses and prognoses persists. It is even more complicated given the existence of different values among patients and caregivers. Ethical questions in medical practice have increased as a consequence of pluralistic value systems and demographic changes associated with new migrants in western European countries.

The first part of this chapter discusses arguments in the context of the communication of an unfavorable diagnosis and prognosis. The second part provides a concrete case in an intercultural setting recorded in a German hospital, involving a patient and his family coming from a Muslim country. The central problems included the demand of family members to be involved in the decision-making process, identifying the appropriate mode of communication, and the general search for an ethically acceptable way of dealing with a patient from a foreign culture. Because the patient and his family were Muslims, I consider Islamic principles relevant to truth-telling. The third part discusses two ethical approaches associated with possible options for action in such a conflict situation and evaluates them. Finally, I offer practical recommendations for dealing with such conflicts in a pluralistic society in an ethically appropriate way.

PART 1: ARGUMENTS IN THE CONTEXT OF COMMUNICATING AN UNFAVORABLE DIAGNOSIS AND PROGNOSIS

In industrial countries, well into the 1960s, the disclosure of an unfavorable diagnosis and infaust prognosis to patients was considered to contravene the Hippocratic principle of "doing no damage" (*nil nocere*). Empirical studies from the early 1960s made in the United States show that 90 percent of doctors were against informing their patients of a diagnosis of cancer (Oken 1961). Physicians, on their own, chose to withhold information from patients ostensibly to save them from fear and desperation so as not to weaken their powers of recovery (Van de Loo 2000).

This attitude changed somewhat in the 1970s when the self-determination and responsibility of the patient in the relationship between doctor and patient were deemed more important (Steinhart 2002). In another study from the United States, conducted in 1977, only 2 percent of American doctors spoke out against informing a patient of an unfavorable diagnosis and prognosis (Novack et al. 1979). Eventually, informing the patient about the diagnosis, therapy options, and prognosis became an integral part of a doctor's responsibilities (Brown 1995). The historical analysis of this development, in particular in the European and Western world, indicates that the moral assessment of this practice is closely tied to the value placed on the autonomy of the patient (Faden and Beauchamp 1986, Tuckett 2004, Surbone 2006).

Truthfulness in conversations with a patient is crucial for establishing a relationship of trust between patient and doctor. It represents the indispensable basis for any ethically acceptable medical intervention and cannot be established without honesty on the part of the doctor. This implies being informed of any illness, even if it is difficult or impossible to cure (Jameton 1995, Van de Loo 2000, Salomon 2003).

In addition to the issue of truthfulness, there are other substantial arguments in favor of communicating a negative prognosis (Sullivan et al. 2001). Rapid developments in biomedicine have created new diagnostic and therapeutic measures allowing for better treatments and sometimes even healing diseases previously considered incurable. There are also increasingly more options for treating an illness with various impacts on a patient's quality of life. For this reason, being informed enables patients to weigh their options, according to their values and preferences, thereby being involved in determining their own futures (Jameton 1995).

Receiving information about a serious illness allows the patient to contemplate the serious side effects of, for example, chemotherapy, on an adequate informational basis—while one cannot expect a patient left with the impression that he or she has only a harmless illness to agree to a therapy with serious side effects (Salomon 2003). The patient can evaluate such a therapy appropriately only if he or she is in a position to perceive the benefits offered and to decide about them on the basis of the required information. Only if the danger of a disease becomes more evident is one prepared to undergo a long and unpleasant therapy. Communicating the gravity of a condition can thus support patient compliance.

Besides the ethical arguments, there are also legal norms that determine the framework for medical decision-making and action. In the German legal system, every medical intervention for diagnostic and therapeutic purposes is seen as a potential personal injury and can be legitimated only by gaining the patient's informed consent (Walter 2000). The validity of such consent presupposes the patient's ability to understand the planned intervention and thus his or her being appropriately informed by the doctor. It follows from these premises that the doctor is obligated, in all but a few exceptional cases, to communicate unfavorable diagnoses to the patient. These legal regulations and the guidelines of professional institutions in Germany are based on specific ethical norms, including the concepts of human well-being and human dignity. A contravention of these regulations and guidelines leads to sanctions or criminal proceedings (Ulsenheimer 2008).

Despite these arguments, one can imagine situations in which withholding an unfavorable diagnosis would be legitimate and even ethically desirable. The central paradigm "respect for the autonomous decision of the patient" implies not only the right to know but also the right not to know (Macklin 1999, 100; Chadwick 1997). Consequently, withholding medical information could be ethically allowed if the patient wants to make use of his or her negative rights and refuses to receive relevant information.

In addition, withholding information can also be ethically justified if the information to be communicated would harm the patient seriously without benefiting him or her in any way. In this case, the doctor, not the patient, decides because of the professional scientific expertise and experience with the procedure. A perceived risk of suicide or a serious depression after being informed of the diagnosis can legitimate such medical decisions. For good reason, this procedure requires a very sensitive investigation of the situation and a critical approach to the case on the part of the doctor in charge (Brody 1997).

Withholding an unfavorable diagnosis does, however, bring up numerous ethical problems. Regardless of whether this withholding of information has been requested by the patient or contemplated by the doctor, it must not lead to refusing therapy, as a patient might refuse to hear the true diagnosis ("right not to know") but nevertheless wants an appropriate therapy. But this poses a problem: how can necessary chemotherapy with its serious side effects be carried out legitimately without the patient suspecting a cancer diagnosis? In a case like this, one wonders if it is reasonable to expect a desirable degree of compliance at all.

The communication of such information is also *lege artis* of central importance. A quiet place without time pressure or the presence of others is certainly more appropriate for the communication of a negative diagnosis and prognosis than a crowded ward (Pilchmaier 1999, Salomon 2003). It is desirable to create suitable circumstances for answering patients' questions. The use of easy-to-understand language and an appropriate tone of voice is bound to have a positive effect on the communication. Providing for professional psychological counseling of the patient following the conversation is equally important.

PART 2: TRUTH-TELLING IN AN INTERCULTURAL CONTEXT

In a multicultural society characterized by the existence of different cultures and value systems, truth-telling gives rise to several ethical questions. First, it may be difficult for the physician to understand the values of a patient from another culture (or family members' attempts to influence the doctor's procedure in communicating an unfavorable diagnosis and prognosis), which can cause ethical conflicts. Legal regulations, codes of conduct established by professional institutions, and procedural conventions can limit the options for dealing with actual problems. As an example, let us consider some ethical problems that arose in an actual case in a German hospital. My colleagues Prof. Dr. Abdullah Takim and Assoc. Prof. Dr. Rainer Brömer informed me about this case.

> A 23-year-old Turkish man was diagnosed with malignant cancer. Several cycles of chemotherapy achieved no success in treatment. The patient's state of health deteriorated progressively, making his imminent death more and more likely. The patient was transferred to a palliative ward. Both the patient and his parents had only rudimentary knowledge of the German language, which did not allow for an adequate communication with the medical team. With the help of an interpreter, who was a member of their wider family, the doctor in charge informed the parents about their son's hopeless situation; the son was also partly involved in this talk.
>
> A nurse of Turkish descent happened to overhear the conversation and later informed the doctors that the interpreter had not passed on to the patient the information about his expected imminent death, probably on the request of his parents. The doctors considered this a clear contravention of the patient's "right to know." With the help of a different interpreter, they arranged another conversation with the patient during which he was informed of the possibility that he might soon die. Two days later the patient passed away. The parents later accused the doctors of being responsible for their son's death: they had contributed to the worsening of his condition and thus hastened his demise.

Here, there is a conflict of opinion between the patient's parents and the medical team regarding disclosure to the patient of an unfavorable diagnosis and prognosis. In this ethical conflict, the medical team believes that the patient himself should decide whether he wants to receive the full information about his condition. The balance between the *right to know* and the right *not to know* should be made by the patient himself, out of respect for the patient's autonomous decision-making. Among the other norms, autonomy is accorded the highest priority in the medical team's decision-making process. As an adult and autonomous human being, the patient should decide, through an individual evaluation of his various options. Withholding requisite information would mean disenfranchising the patient and violating his right to self-determination.

The starting point for the parents' decision and attitude is, however, a different one. Their approach may be described as caring and consequentialist. In their decision-making process, patient autonomy does not play a central role. For the parents, the issue is primarily whether the disclosure of the infaust prognosis will affect their son's well-being. They expect that the medical team's course of action will upset their son and thus weaken his regenerative powers. This approach is regarded as harmful in preference to one of withholding the diagnosis and prognosis. In this case, the patient died two days after receiving the information. His parents therefore felt that their decision had been vindicated, and they accused the medical team of having acted wrongly.

Communication and Dealing with the Family

Communication difficulties often play a decisive role in the processes leading up to clinical–ethical conflicts in medical practice. Linguistic and cultural barriers in an intercultural setting increase those difficulties, further complicating the conflict (Ilkilic 2002, 2007; Hancock et al. 2007). Since the solution of such conflicts initially requires the clarification of the conflict parties' different interests, overcoming these barriers is of central importance (Krakauer et al. 2002; Valente 2004; Volker 2005). In an intercultural context, a linguistic understanding of the patient's wishes and preferences is necessary but often not sufficient to guarantee an ethically appropriate way of dealing with a given problem. Rather, the significance and sometimes the background of these wishes in a given culture should be clarified in writing, as well as verbally (Kagawa-Singer and Blackhall 2001). Only then can one hope for an appropriate ethical evaluation of goods.

In the case described above, it is striking to observe that no conversation took place between the two conflicting parties after the patient's death, that is, the medical team and the parents. Neither party really knew why the other acted the way it did, nor did they grasp the different sets of values brought to bear on the decision-making. The medical team probably saw in the family's position a clear violation of the patient's autonomy and self-determination and considered it to be ethically unacceptable. The family members, on the other hand, believed that the patient must be protected at all costs from the damage that his being informed about his unfavorable diagnosis would presumably cause. They did not understand why the medical team would want to harm him in such a way.

In this case, it would have been sensible for the responsible doctor to take the initiative in a conversation with the parents. Such a conversation could have provided both parties more information about the backgrounds of the other's position, opening a broader access to the culturally alien motivation, possibly enabling a reflective attitude to their own positions. A better understanding of one another based on such a conversation, even though it cannot guarantee consensus in such cases, seems to be an indispensable instrument—particularly in an intercultural setting.

In such a conversation, the family members could have informed the medical team from their own cultural perspective about the normative meaning of withholding an unfavorable diagnosis and prognosis, to be understood, in their culture, as a moral imperative based on the conviction that the communication of such information directly harms the affected person and is therefore to be avoided. Disclosure would also destroy the hope of healing, which would create, according to this anthropology, an unacceptable situation. In addition, this knowledge would be a burden for the patient and thus decrease his quality of life. Not to know about one's imminent death is considered beneficial for the patient's well-being and is therefore a desirable condition.

On the other hand, the medical team could have informed the family about the legal constraints of which they probably were unaware. This information would have given the family a better idea of the range of options for decision-making and action available to the medical team and thus perhaps created a basis for understanding the chosen action. Further, ethical arguments and their backgrounds could have been presented, including the conviction that a person as a self-determined and thus responsible being has a right to make decisions about his current state. This presupposes, further, the doctor's responsibility to provide information about the medical conditions of this state (Van de Loo 2000, 284).

In medical ethical terms, the communication of an unfavorable diagnosis and infaust prognosis is not to be viewed as direct harm. Such harm arises only through the perception and reflection of the affected person. From this understanding, the wishes and preferences of the family members cannot be allowed to guide the attitude of the doctors—unless, that is, they can provide information about the presumed will of the patient. This aspect is, however, irrelevant in this case, since the patient himself was competent to express his own opinion and make his own decisions.

Even though it is not to be expected that this comprehensive exchange of views will lead directly to consensus, it would contribute significantly to preventing an escalation.

The Actions of the Medical Team

The German Medical Association (*Bundesärztekammer*) prescribes in its guidelines for medical treatment of the terminally ill that the information given to a dying person about his or her condition and treatment options must be truthful. This information and the way it is delivered "must however take account of the dying person's situation and present fears" (*Bundesärztekammer* 2004, 1).

The doctor in charge may withhold information about the hopeless situation of his or her patient if she is convinced that this would clearly and unequivocally cause damage to the patient. He or she should withhold an unfavorable diagnosis (1) if the patient himself explicitly asks the doctor to do so, (2) if the doctor is convinced that such information would lead to a suicide attempt, and (3) if this information would cause serious psychological disturbance. Family members may be informed about such a diagnosis only with the permission of the patient (*Bundesärztekammer* 2004, 1).

These principles are firmly based on the respect for the patient's personal rights, particularly the right of self-determination. Medical treatment therefore requires a patient to be informed before having to consent to any intervention (*Bundesärztekammer* 2007). The patient needs to be given information not only about the therapy to be carried out but also about the critical reasons for the specific therapeutic measures chosen. In our example, the reasons for stopping conventional cancer therapy and shifting to palliative care should be explained to the patient, requiring him or her to be informed of the infaust prognosis.

The position of the family members in the decision-making process, scarcely attended to by the medical team, can also be traced back to the patient-centered attitude described here. This attitude is based on an anthropocentric individualistic concept of the human being. The procedure adopted by the medical team also implies a cultural invariance claim as if in no culture the family had normative significance for decision-making unless explicitly desired by the patient. It should be noted that this attitude led to the escalation of the conflict.

Medical guidelines and legal regulations allow medical practice to be performed more simply and, in the course of time, lead to a certain routine. This routine is based on well-considered ethical arguments; it is however easily interrupted as soon as culturally conditioned ethical problems arise. The way the medical team acted may be viewed as a conventional attitude based on the ethical norms and legal regulations described above. It remains to be considered, though, whether there could be further pragmatic reasons for this attitude.

One reason for the behavior of the medical team could be wanting to stay on the right side of the law. Following the parents' wishes without the consent of the patient could have legal consequences. Legal sanctions now increasingly play a major role in the decisions and actions of doctors, especially those with less professional experience. Critical discussions and concerns debated among academics and the public produce headlines such as "the making of medicine into law" or "the dictatorship of legal constraints" (Ulsenheimer 2008).

A further reason can be a lack of time for a detailed conversation with family members or with the patient (Hancock et al. 2007). Time pressure has long been a phenomenon in everyday medical practice and may present a barrier to an ethically appropriate delivery of medical care. One example is the decrease in time devoted to informing patients or discussing treatment options in detail. Despite this situation, it is necessary to find an appropriate context for longer conversations not only with the patient but also with family members. "Time pressure must play no role," says the training brochure for further education that is published by the German Medical Association (*Bundesärztekammer* 1998, 114).

An additional problem can arise from a lack of *intercultural competence*. Intercultural competence means the ability to discern and analyze the basic elements of an intercultural conflict and to integrate them into the medical and ethical decision-making process (Ilkilic 2008). In the absence of this competence, the reality of cultural components in a conflict might initially be overlooked. In this case, the integration of culture-specific values and connected wishes into the decision-making process is prevented.

It is also difficult to clarify the normative significance of culture-specific attitudes and preferences for practice. One cannot, of course, expect such a difficult achievement from a medical team; nevertheless, there should be some sensitivity to the cultural phenomena in everyday life. In complex cases where the team faces a challenge for which it feels unprepared, outside experts can be called upon, and the clinical ethics committee or clinical ethics consultants can be involved (Paul 2008; Gordon 2010).

Establishing the Will of the Patient

Finding out the patient's actual will to be informed of an unfavorable diagnosis and prognosis and the parents' attitude(s) is of central importance. In an intercultural setting of this kind, it is difficult for the doctor to "take account of [the patient's] present fears" (*Bundesärztekammer* 2004, 1). It is conceivable that a conversation with family members might be able to clarify the patient's attitude to being informed about an unfavorable diagnosis and prognosis. It is more likely that an appropriate approach could be found on this basis. This attempt requires however a certain degree of caution.

There is no reason to expect from the outset that the family members will communicate this information perfectly. Given a conflict of interests, the patient's real attitude may be concealed or misrepresented. Here, a relationship of trust between the family members and the medical teams is necessary. In certain circumstances this information could be checked against statements made by acquaintances or friends of the patient. However, this may be impossible because of the lack of time or personnel.

Finding out the will of the patient directly by means of a conversation between the patient and his doctor may be difficult because of the linguistic and cultural barriers. The presence of an interpreter creates another barrier to a direct conversation. Sensitive nuances and subtle formulations can be lost in translation. Similarly, the doctor will be unable to interpret certain gestures and expressions of the patient's body language because, first, she might not know the meaning of the patient's movements in his cultural context and, second, the content transmitted by emphasis is easily lost in the interpreter's rendition. Thus, access to the patient's will is filtered through multiple layers of mediation. These difficulties can be minimized by use of interpreters specifically trained for such situations.

In any case, gaining an adequate understanding of the patient's preferences requires an optimized strategy. The difficulty in choosing such a strategy consists, among other things, in the alien appearance of the patient's culture. For this reason, a preliminary conversation can be helpful to allow access to the patient's personality. In a conversation of this kind, one can discuss the patient's current knowledge of his or her condition and possibly also ask about any expectations regarding treatment options or the course of the medical condition. The significance and value of his family can also be addressed in this conversation. One can even ask directly whether a direct involvement of family members in the decision-making process would be in accordance with his wishes.

The information and impressions gained in the initial conversation can be helpful for determining the strategy for the second talk. They can also help to eliminate strategies found to be inappropriate. Sensitivity and caution should accompany the doctor's actions in these conversations. "The question about the truth about the seriousness of the illness is therefore ultimately a question about the appropriate truth" (*Bundesärztekammer* 1998, 114).

Family and Truth-Telling

Withholding an unfavorable diagnosis or prognosis on the request of family members is not a rare occurrence in some countries in the world. Such a practice is often encountered outside the Western world, in particular in Asian and South American countries, but also in the Near East and Muslim countries (Berger 1998; Mobeireek et al. 2008). The medical ethicist Yali Chong, from the Peking University Health Care Center, emphasizes the importance of the family in decisions about informing the patient of his condition. He even speaks of the model of family–patient–doctor in the Chinese–Confucian culture (Cong 2004).

Here, the seriousness of the illness also determines the influence of the family on the procedure to be adopted. "If the illness is very easy to cure, the family member will directly disclose all the information to the patient, or allow the patient to do so. Otherwise, the family member offers only partial information or lies to the patient" (Cong 2004, 152). Jotkowitz and his colleagues argue similarly on this topic and speak of a similar reserve with respect to informing a patient fully about a bad diagnosis and prognosis in the Jewish tradition (Jotkowitz et al. 2006).

In Turkey, family members' desire to be involved in determining medical treatment is also strong if the illness is incurable and terminal (Ozdogan et al. 2006; Aksoy 2005). It is common for family members to express to the doctor their wish that the patient not be informed of a bad diagnosis, often before the diagnosis has even been made. It is also not rare for the doctor, in the case of an unfavorable diagnosis, to discuss the further procedure with family members first. The attitude of the parents in the case described above can be viewed as a typical instance of such cases.

It would certainly be wrong to see this attitude as a merely cultural attitude without any moral foundations. Two forms of argumentation can be constructed from the perspective of the Turkish–Islamic culture that is rarely made explicit in practice. The first one assumes that informing patients about an incurable disease or imminent death would upset them and thus cause a psychological burden. This action is to be viewed as unequivocally harmful and hence to be avoided.

Here, the classical medical–ethical principle of avoiding harm comes to the fore. This form of argumentation is not foreign to western European medical ethics and also not insignificant in common practice. The important difference consists in the normative interpretation of the individual assessment of this practice. In the Turkish–Islamic culture, this principle of doing no harm is initially independent of an individual attitude. Family members are involved in the decision-making process on this basis. The central importance accorded to the family in social life generally makes this involvement easier. Even from an individualist perspective, this action is not *eo ipso* to be seen as detrimental to the patient's well-being. Whether this action is harmful can be decided only on the basis of the patient's own attitude to this practice.

The attitude of the family members in the above-mentioned case can also be justified by Islamic belief. In Islamic thought, the time of death is set by God and remains hidden from human beings (Quran Sura 56: 60). Humans can speculate about it with the means at their disposal, but they cannot predict this moment with absolute certainty. A predictive statement about end of life is viewed critically from this religious perspective. "One is ultimately not God" is the reaction to such statements. It is worth noting that such reactions more frequently follow negative prognoses. Such an assertion is also seen as an open attack on the theological concept of hope.

To take away the hope of healing would contradict the implicit attributes of God in Islamic belief since this attitude would deny God's omnipotence. This theological foundation would also make the family's attitude in the situation described above plausible, from the perspective of their religious beliefs, even if it was not made explicit at the time.

PART 3: UNIVERSALISTIC AND PARTICULARISTIC APPROACHES TO TRUTH-TELLING

When it comes to medical–ethical conflicts in an intercultural setting, such as those discussed and analyzed above, the conceptualization of the cultural phenomena, their ethical evaluation and integration into the decision-making process take on central importance. As the example has shown, cultural phenomena are often given little attention in the procedure followed by the medical team.

At this point, it is important to ask whether the approach adopted in this conflict is the only ethically legitimate course of action or whether a different procedure might provide a better way of dealing with the conflict. In other words, is an anthropocentric, individualistic ethical approach, based on human dignity, personal rights, and the right to self-determination, able to take account of cultural phenomena and to integrate them into the decision-making process? The latter question is directly connected with the ethical assessment of culturally specific values. This and similar questions have already been addressed by medical ethicists in discussions about the universality of the principle of respect for patient autonomy. In what follows, two basic positions on the topic of truth-telling will be examined.

American bioethicist Ruth Macklin argues that established fundamental ethical principles can adequately address cultural phenomena in medical care and integrate them into the decision-making process in an appropriate way. She distinguishes between the principles of "respect for the person" and "respect for autonomy" and subordinates the latter principle to the former (Macklin 1998). Autonomy, a self-evident consequence of the principle of respect for the person, does not in her opinion exclude withholding an unfavorable diagnosis and taking family members' choices into account during the decision-making process.

Provided the patient agrees, family members can contribute to the health care team's deliberations. In the same way, the patient's wish not to be informed about an unfavorable diagnosis can be honored by the physician (Macklin 1998, 7). Note that this approach claims universal validity and is thought capable of resolving conflicts in an intercultural physician–patient relationship.

Chinese medical ethicist Ruiping Fan denies the universally binding character of "Western bioethical principles" and questions their "abstract content," which would offer a basis for the moral evaluation of medical practices in all cultures (Fan 1997). He argues his position, taking the principle of autonomy as an example and discussing two forms of determination that can be derived from it, namely, self-determination and determination by the family.

In his opinion, the Western principle of autonomy leads to self-determination where the starting point is individual free will and the subjective determinability of moral goods. Determination by the family can be derived, on the other hand, from the East Asian principle of autonomy. This form of determination claims an objective understanding of moral goods and emphasizes the value of harmonious dependency within the family. These two concepts of autonomy cannot, according to Fan, be equated with each other, as they imply different moral actions.

Fan illustrates these theoretical discussions with instances of truth-telling in the case of an unfavorable diagnosis and prognosis. From the Chinese or Confucian perspective, withholding a diagnosis and prognosis can be ethically justified. First, the family members should be informed and, subsequently, the further procedure should be decided upon in consultation with the family. If the family decides to withhold information from the patient, the doctor should respect this decision (Fan and Li 2004). According to Fan and Li's particularistic approach, this procedure rests on the following conditions:

1. The physician finds evidence of manifest mutual concern of the family members for the patient.
2. The family's wishes are not egregiously in discord with the physician's professional judgment regarding the medical best interests of the patient.

If either or both of the two necessary conditions are not met, the physician should communicate directly with the patient (Fan and Li 2004, 189).

CRITICAL DISCUSSION OF UNIVERSALISTIC AND PARTICULARISTIC APPROACHES

A major concern of the universalistic approaches argued by Macklin and others is the prevention of harm, which can reach the degree of a violation of human rights. For this reason, every medical action must first be examined to assess whether it represents a violation of human rights. In a second step, the intervention should be evaluated from the patient's perspective. Only then can it be ethically legitimated in medical practice.

This approach presupposes a hierarchy among ethical principles, according to which patient autonomy is most important (Macklin 1998). To argue for the universal application of this approach assumes the validity of this hierarchy among ethical principles. Yet, as long as such a hierarchy in the form just described is not accepted in a given culture, this approach cannot be applied ("unbridgeable moral gap between Western individualism and non-Western communalism"; Baker 1998, 212).

A further deficiency of the universalistic approach is its inability to ethically assess culturally dependent moral phenomena like family autonomy. It is not able to ascribe a normative value to such phenomena. This approach is always dependent from the individualistic under-standing of the human being. Therefore, this ascription of ethical value thus has a *hypothetical* character and not an *a priori* one.

If one applies the entire approach to our case study, the attitude of the medical team can be ethically legitimated on its basis. The medical team deliberately ignored the wishes of the family and instead turned to the patient himself. The reason given was the patient's autonomy. As long as the patient does not assent, no normative value can be ascribed to the wishes of the family. It is obvious that this ignorance of the cultural phenomena led to the escalation of the conflict.

In addition, this approach presupposes a responsible adult and informed patient with whom one can communicate perfectly without linguistic or cultural barriers. A further diffi-culty comes in when the patient is not able to express himself, as is the case for example with an incompetent or comatose patient, infant, or fetus.

Despite these difficulties, this approach possesses an important strength for a multicultural society, the constituent groups of which are by no means homogeneous. It is ethically unjus-tifiable to decide about the treatment given to a patient merely on the basis of his (perceived) membership in a religious or ethnic group. An indiscriminate application of the knowledge gained about the patient's culture or the extrapolation from previous individual experiences can turn out to be mistaken in a current case. For this reason, it is always important to uncover the individual patient's attitude to a specific practice.

The normatively relativist or particularistic approach promises a better account of cultural phenomena in making ethical judgments than universalistic ones. Particularists can derive moral maxims for actions from culturally specific phenomena. Because the moral judgments within a culture are affected by other cultural phenomena, they receive as such a normative value—without being examined according to fundamental ethical principles. Thus, with-holding an unfavorable diagnosis, for example, is morally right if this practice is morally accepted within a certain culture. This position is clearly supported, especially by cultural anthropology.

Unfortunately, this approach implies a *culturalistic fallacy.* I understand under the cultur-alistic fallacy that the ethical justification of a moral practice or attitude is only through its existence in a certain group. According to this attitude, a reflection upon or criticism of a culture's moral practice is impossible.

A comprehensive application of this approach is not only problematic because of the cultur-alistic fallacy but also because of its prerequisite moral homogeneity within a given ethnic group. In the age of globalization, a profound change in values is taking place, even in societies considered closed to the outside world, so that disparate values emerge within each culture. If the members of a certain culture live in another country, the influence of the dominant values in the host country would be strong and thus support the heterogeneity of values within this ethnic group.

If one applies this approach to our case study, the relatives' wish attains normative value and can under certain circumstances be acted on. If the patient's expectations agree with those of the family, this approach is better able to take account of the cultural phenomena. If the patient does not agree with the family's wishes, however, the patient could then be restrained in his decisions, even disenfranchised. An insoluble problem is also presented by the juridical justification of the medical team's actions. Withholding medical information without the patient's assent can have legal, as well as moral, repercussions for the doctor.

CONCLUSION

The disclosure of an unfavorable diagnosis and infaust prognosis to a patient, communicating essential (and existential) information to the person most immediately concerned, has historically been a controversial topic. Today, it has lost nothing of its controversial status. On the contrary, we encounter this question in medical practice much more frequently and with a growing complexity. Truth-telling in the intercultural setting of a value pluralistic society requires a better founded and more comprehensive discussion of the problem than has hitherto taken place.

From the comprehensive discussion and analysis presented above, the following conclusions on a practical and theoretical level can be developed:

- An ethically appropriate way of handling the disclosure of an unfavorable diagnosis and infaust prognosis in an intercultural setting requires first of all culturally sensitive and successful communication, especially in case of a conflict of preferences and interests, in order for the conflict parties to reach a mutual understanding of their values and of the specific reasons for their attitude. Translation by relatives or hospital staff has often proven counterproductive and ethically problematic; hence, communication should be mediated by professional interpreters trained for medical practice.
- An ethically legitimate resolution of such conflicts often requires intercultural competence, to be understood as the ability to recognize and analyze the goods at stake in an intercultural conflict and to integrate them into medical–ethical decision-making. The availability of such competence cannot, however, be taken as a given. It should be imparted during medical studies and supported in professional life by means of further training. Intercultural competence must also be recognized as an important competence for members of ethics committees in a value pluralistic society.
- The decisions and actions of doctors must be taken within the limits of the law and conforming to the regulations of professional institutions. These regulations should be laid down in such a way as to leave sufficient space for taking account of cultural phenomena. Equally, in a culturally determined medical–ethical conflict, it should be investigated whether a procedure diverging from the conventional practice is possible. For reasons presented above, it often happens that options that are in principle available for medical decision-making are not pursued. With a culturally sensitive attitude and intercultural competence, additional options can be better integrated into medical decision-making.
- The ethical problems that arise in applying the universalistic and particularistic approaches were discussed in detail above. A rigid application of any of these approaches appears to be problematic in many respects. Instead, an integrative procedure should be followed. This procedure entails taking account of the ethical goods at issue in the conflict from the perspective of the conflict parties. This does not mean prioritizing either patient autonomy or family autonomy but, rather, contextualizing these forms of autonomy sensitively in concrete terms.

Only then can both the wholesale application of patient autonomy often found in conventional practice and the overruling of the individual patient's wishes based on his presumed belonging to a certain culture be prevented. This process of argumentation and reflection, however, presents a challenge for the medical team, which should therefore in complex situations have access to expertise from a competence center or to ethical consultancy by a clinical ethics committee or clinical ethics consultant.

ACKNOWLEDGMENT

The author would like to thank Dr. Rainer Brömer for his important comments and critical perusal of this manuscript.

REFERENCES

Aksoy, S. 2005. "End-of-Life Decision-Making in Turkey." In *End-of-Life Decision-Making: A Cross-National Study*, edited by R. H. Blank and J. C. Merrick, 183–195. Cambridge, MA: MIT Press.

Baker, R. 1998. "A Theory of International Bioethics: Multiculturalism, Postmodernism, and the Bankruptcy of Fundamentalism." *Kennedy Institute of Ethics Journal* 8, no. 3: 201–31.

Berger, J. T. 1998. "Culture and Ethnicity in Clinical Care." *Archives of Internal Medicine* 158, no. 19: 2085–90.

Brody, H. 1997. "The Physician-Patient Relationship." In *Medical Ethics*, second edition, edited by R. W. Veatch, 75–101. Boston: Jones and Bartlett Publishers.

Brown, K. H. 1995. "Information Disclosure." In *Encyclopedia of Bioethics*, edited by W. Reich, 1221–24. New York: The Free Press.

Bundesärztekammer. 1998. *Gesundheit im Alter. Texte und Materialien der Bundesärztekammer zur Fortbildung und Weiterbildung*. Köln.

———. 2004. Grundsätze der Bundesärztekammer zur ärztlichen Sterbebegleitung. *Deutsches Ärzteblatt* 19: 1–2.

———. 2007. *Berufsordnung für die deutschen Ärztinnen und Ärzte*.

Chadwick, R. 1997. "Das Recht auf Wissen und das Recht auf Nichtwissen aus philosophischer Sicht." In *Perspektiven der Humangenetik*, edited by F. W. Silvia Petermann and Michael Quante, 195–207. Paderborn: Ferdinand Schöningh.

Cong, Y. 2004. "Doctor-Family-Patient Relationship: The Chinese Paradigm of Informed Consent." *Journal of Medicine and Philosophy* 29, no. 2: 149–78.

Faden, R. R., and T. L. Beauchamp. 1986. *A History and Theory of Informed Consent*. New York: Oxford University Press.

Fan, R. 1997. "Self-Determination vs. Family-Determination: Two Incommensurable Principles of Autonomy: A Report from East Asia." *Bioethics* 11, no. 3–4: 309–22.

Fan, R., and B. Li. 2004. "Truth Telling in Medicine: The Confucian View." *Journal of Medicine and Philosophy* 29, no. 2: 179–93.

Hancock, K. et al. 2007. "Truth-Telling in Discussing Prognosis in Advanced Life-Limiting Illnesses: A Systematic Review." *Palliative Medicine* 21, no. 6: 507–17.

Ilkilic, I. 2002. "Der muslimische Patient. Medizinethische Aspekte des muslimischen Krankheitsverständnisses in einer wertpluralen Gesellschaft." Diss., Münster London: Lit.

———. 2007. "Medizinethische Aspekte im Umgang mit muslimischen Patienten." *Deutsche Medizinische Wochenschrift* 132, no. 30: 1587–90.

———. 2008. "Kulturelle Aspekte bei ethischen Entscheidungen am Lebensende und interkulturelle Kompetenz." *Bundesgesundheitsblatt Gesundheitsforschung Gesundheitsschutz* 51, no. 8: 857–64.

Jameton, A. 1995. "Information Disclosure: Ethical Issues." In *Encyclopedia of Bioethics*, edited by W. Reich, 1225–332. New York: The Free Press.

Jotkowitz, A. et al. 2006. "Truth-Telling in a Culturally Diverse World." *Cancer Investigation* 24, no. 8: 786–89.

Kagawa-Singer, M., and L. J. Blackhall. 2001. "Negotiating Cross-Cultural Issues at the End of Life: 'You Got to Go Where He Lives.'" *JAMA* 286, no. 23: 2993–3001.

Krakauer, E. L. et al. 2002. "Barriers to Optimum End-of-Life Care for Minority Patients." *Journal of the American Geriatric Society* 50, no. 1: 182–90.

Macklin, R. 1998. "Ethical Relativism in a Multicultural Society." *Kennedy Institute of Ethics Journal* 8, no. 1: 1–22.

———. 1999. *Against Relativism: Cultural Diversity and the Search for Ethical Universals in Medicine.* New York: Oxford University Press.

Mobeireek, A. F. et al. 2008. "Information Disclosure and Decision-Making: The Middle East versus the Far East and the West." *Journal of Medical Ethics* 34, no. 4: 225–29.

Novack, D. H. et al. 1979. "Changes in Physicians' Attitudes toward Telling the Cancer Patient." *JAMA* 241, no. 9: 897–900.

Oken, D. 1961. "What to Tell Cancer Patients: A Study of Medical Attitudes." *JAMA* 175: 1120–8.

Ozdogan, M. et al. 2006. "Factors Related to Truth-Telling Practice of Physicians Treating Patients with Cancer in Turkey." *Journal of Palliative Medicine* 9, no. 5: 1114–19.

Paul, N. W. 2008. "Klinische Ethikberatung: Therapieziele, Patientenwille und Entscheidungsprobleme in der modernen Medizin. In *Grenzsituationen in der Intensivmedizin*, edited by T. Junginger, 208–17. Berlin: Springer.

Pilchmaier, H. 1999. "Wahrheit und Wahrhaftigkeit am Krankenbett." *Deutsches Ärzteblatt* 96, no. 9: 536–37.

Salomon, F. 2003. "Wahrheit vermitteln am Krankenbett." *Deutsche Medizinische Wochenschrift* 128, no. 23: 1307–10.

Steinhart, B. 2002. "Patient Autonomy: Evolution of the Doctor-Patient Relationship." *Haemophilia* 8, no. 3: 441–6.

Sullivan, R. J. et al. 2001. "Truth-Telling and Patient Diagnoses." *Journal of Medical Ethics* 27, no. 3: 192–7.

Surbone, A. 2006. "Telling the Truth to Patients with Cancer: What Is the Truth?" *Lancet Oncology* 7, no. 11: 944–50.

Tuckett, A. G. 2004. "Truth-Telling in Clinical Practice and the Arguments for and Against: A Review of the Literature." *Nursing Ethics* 11, no. (5): 500–13.

Ulsenheimer, K. 2008. *Arztstrafrecht in der Praxis.* Heidelberg: C. F. Müller.

Valente, S. M. 2004. "End of Life and Ethnicity." *Journal for Nurses in Staff Development* 20, no. 6: 285–93.

Van de Loo, J. 2000. "Aufklärung / Aufklärungspflicht." In *Lexikon der Bioethik*, edited by W. Korff, 284–7. Gütersloh: Gütersloher Verlagshaus.

Volker, D. L. 2005. "Control and End-of-Life Care: Does Ethnicity Matter?" *American Journal of Hospital Palliative Care* 22, no. 6: 442–6.

Walter, U. 2000. "Aufklärung / Aufklärungspflicht: Rechtlich." In *Lexikon der Bioethik*, edited by W. Korff, 287–8. Gütersloh: Gütersloher Verlagshaus.

NOTE

1. This paper was developed out of the project Medical Ethical Decisions at the End of Life in Intercultural Settings, supported by Johannes Gutenberg University Mainz (Förderlinie der Stufe I).

5

Bioethics as Environmental Ethics

Ontogeny Recapitulates Environment

Peter Tagore Tan

ABSTRACT

This chapter is a critical reflection on the relationship between bioethics and environmental ethics. Presently, they are understood as separate subdisciplines of ethics, each covering different subjects that overlap when environmental issues affect human health and well-being. This relationship creates a bioethical model that tends to argue for an overspecialization of bioethics and an anthropocentric concept of human health, both of which are passively reactive to environmental problems and can paradoxically frustrate the end of human well-being itself. Following the lead of Van Renssaeler Potter, the founder of bioethics, and especially Aldo Leopold, the founding figure of the ecological movement whose concept of a land ethic directed Potter's writings, a better relationship can be found by understanding bioethics as a specific type of environmental ethics instead. This relationship can be expressed with a concept from recapitulation theory—ontogeny recapitulates environment. The second part of this article will explore what this means for bioethics. Bioethics deepens our understanding of ethics and must therefore be an agent of conservation and land complexity, characteristics that are crucial to understanding the bioethical component in the three major types of environmental challenges, those of anthropogenic climate change, pollution, and land depletion. The article concludes by considering what bioethics must be once it is developed as a specific type of environmental ethics.

> That man is, in fact, only a member of a biotic team is shown by an ecological interpretation of history. Many historical events, hitherto explained solely in terms of human enterprise, were actually biotic interactions between people and land. The characteristics of the land determined the facts quite as potently as the characteristics of the men who lived on it.
>
> —Aldo Leopold (*A Sand County Almanac*, 205)

WHAT IS BIOETHICS? WHAT HAS IT BECOME?

Born from the habit to differentiate and separate, philosophy has satisfied itself by distinguishing ethics from other philosophical investigations and to further subcategorize ethics into its more specialized parts. Two of these subdivisions are the focus of this article—environmental ethics and bioethics. As current public awareness of anthropogenic climate change joins previous eras' awareness of environmental pollution and depletion of wild spaces in our collective knowledge of ecological concerns, the close relationship between these two subdisciplines of ethics has become impossible to ignore. What relationship exists, however, is understood to be between two separate but equal domains, each of them applying ethical problem solving to different subjects.

The traditional way to approach bioethics and the environment would be to adopt this model and to list well-known and recent environmental disasters that have led to health problems and then to analyze the issues using classical ethical theories, now in their bioethical guise because they relate to human health. But there are good reasons to question this model and to choose another.

The title of this article is meant to challenge this structure of understanding the subdisciplines of ethics. It is pointedly not about bioethics *and* environmental ethics but bioethics *as* environmental ethics, and it means to position environmental ethics as the more generic study and bioethics as a more specific instantiation of it. Bioethics, I will argue, is actually a highly refined type of environmental ethics, but as it is practiced now it is so far removed from any of all but the grossest connection to environmental concerns that it seems a discipline apart. There are roughly three major types of cases of such environmental concerns—anthropogenic climate change, pollution, and resource depletion. Only when the effects of one or more of them threaten our health do we think to connect environmental ethics with bioethics. In other words, when philosophy thinks in terms of bioethics *and* environmental ethics, it is in the sense of a bioethical reaction to environmental collapse that finally registers as having negative consequences for human health, but, when it thinks of bioethics *as* an environmental ethic, there is such reaction of course, but there is also an active engagement and negotiation with the general health of our environs, the health of which is also the source for the health of humans.

This approach of nesting bioethics within environmental ethics is far from new, and it is actually the point of the original analysis by Van Rensselaer Potter in *Bioethics: Bridge to the Future*. Potter is credited with coining the term *bioethics*, and connecting medicine (Potter was a research oncologist by vocation) to ethical action in the *bios*, the life characterized by one's way of living, was so self-evident to him that he later expressed surprise and concern that what he meant by bioethics could be so misconstrued by those who would claim to champion it.

Potter was part of the generation that witnessed the hubristic terror brought on by the atomic age and came to realize that the rapid growth in scientific knowledge was accompanied with a similarly rapid decrease in the wisdom to properly apply it. The environmental movement by that time had fully absorbed Rachel Carson's *Silent Spring*, Lynn Townsend White Jr.'s "The Historical Roots of Our Ecological Crisis," and Garrett Hardin's "Tragedy of the Commons." Potter himself dedicated his first book to the conservationist Aldo Leopold whose *A Sand County Almanac* challenged the antagonistic human versus nature relationship and even included Leopold in the title of his second book, *Bioethics: Building on the Leopold Legacy*. Leopold's ecological concepts will figure heavily later in this article.

Potter thus had in mind to, in Cristina Richie's words, "[locate] bioethics in the *bios*—the life in the world—and drew a connection between medicine and conservation" (Richie 2014). According to James Dwyer, Potter "hoped this field would include broad issues about population health, acceptable survival, and the natural environment" (Dwyer 2009). Bioethics today, of course, has no such breadth and reach. More often than not, following Daniel Callahan in 1973, the 1974 *Belmont Report*, and Tom Beauchamp and James Childress in 1979, it means bio*medical* ethics instead, which is to say moral issues involving medical professionals and patients and subjects, research protocols in medical investigations, clinical trials, and access to medical services, to name a few. Gone is any mention of our environs, the home in which we humans reside, the condition for the possibility of human health, a home that we nevertheless despoil to the detriment of our well-being.

There are I believe two main reasons to argue for bioethics as an environmental ethics. The first is that bioethics understood and developed otherwise has become too specialized; the second is a natural outcome of this, that the anthropocentrism of bioethics focuses too closely on the medical health of humans such that it paradoxically jeopardizes the very health of humans.

Bioethicists as Specialists

The specialization critique is derived from John H. Evans's sociological analysis of the growth of bioethics and Carl Elliott's survey of how bioethics allowed itself to be co-opted by medical corporate money. Both Evans and especially Elliott level unorthodox criticisms that, while overreaching at times, ought to at least give bioethics a needed check on whether its own historical narrative is indeed as ethical as the advice it dispenses.

Evans gives a descriptive account of the rise of bioethics as a profession and identifies its success on the fact that bioethicists were able to furnish medical institutions and the governmental bureaucracies that are supposed to oversee them with the proper formal language that could serve as universal and ready-to-use principles. This was done in order to, in Evans's words, "enhance calculability, or in the more common language, to simplify bioethical decision making" (Evans 2000, 88).

These principles have been codified in Beauchamp and Childress's widely used *Principles of Bioethics*. Albert Jonsen refers to them as the "common coin of moral discourse" (Jonsen 1998, 103), and, while such common ethical coinage sought to universalize ethical applicability, it also served to restrict the numbers of those who had the expertise and specialized knowledge to apply the level of ethical formalism necessary for proper ethical judgment. "As bioethics has matured," writes Elliott, "its practitioners have aspired to a kind of professional expertise. Bioethicists have gained recognition largely by carving out roles as trusted advisors" (Elliott 2018, 146–47).

Carl Elliott catalogs the problems that arise when the expert few who have the specialized skill to pass ethical judgment on biomedical issues run headfirst into the corporations whose products oftentimes create these biomedical issues. In most cases, the bioethicist is absorbed into the corporation, perhaps as a way to buy their silence, but most definitely as a way to legitimize medical practice. The bioethicist's role as an industry critic vanishes. As Elliott puts it, "[When] bioethicists seek to become trusted advisors, rather than gadflies or watchdogs, it will not be surprising if they slowly come to resemble the people they are trusted to advise" (Elliott 2000, 147). When this happens, it becomes "unclear . . . whether hired ethicists actually have the power to stop unethical actions. Do they modify company policy in a meaningful way, or are they hired to make selling easier?" (Elliott 2000, 137). Whether it is pharmaceutical companies funding centers for bioethical research, or giving substantial award money to individual bioethicists, or using bioethicists to give controversial practices a clean bill of ethical health, or once independent bioethicists starting profit-driven independent review boards whose services can be bought to clear clinical trial protocols, the specialization of bioethics as a field unto its own self all too easily created a trap of its own making.

There is another type of specialization that is important to this article and tangentially referred to in Evans. This is not a bioethics issue as much as it is that of the modern Western approach to ethics. It is the assumption that the proper way to determine ethical action in a social setting is to reduce society to its component parts in order to pay specific attention to the atomic element of social interaction.

This is the practical meaning of *specialis*, the Latin term for "particular" and "individual": if we can somehow understand what is ethically correct on the individual level, we will have found the atomic unit for basic ethical judgment for society at large, thus mirroring perfectly in ethical argumentation what Abraham Bosse's illustration depicts in his famous frontispiece gracing Thomas Hobbes's *Leviathan*. While virtue theory—whether Confucian, Aristotelian, or care based—offers a strong counterpoint to this reductionism, deontological, consequentialist, rights-based ethics and the principlism that Beauchamp and Childress forward as a way to unite these modern forms of morality all perform this *reductio ad singula*.

As we shall see below with a pre-Aristotelian analysis of *ethos*, ethics is neither primarily nor originally about abstract concepts of autonomy or permissibility or wrongness or rights—it is about how we create a proper sense of being where we find ourselves to be. This sense of social creation is what bioethics as environmental ethics is meant to retrieve and why it finds the modern development of bioethics highly constrained and refined in its stress on individual decision-making.[1] Taken together, the specialization of bioethics has created deracinated concepts of moral propriety that are removed from its communal basis and is resistant to real-world checks as to whether its special status confers on it at least as many practical problems as it does advantages on the academic stage.

Bioethical Anthropocentrism

Unlike that of the specialization of bioethics, the anthropocentric critique is not as readily apparent and needs to be qualified. It is not that bioethics is anthropocentric because it is centered on humans. That claim is a given—since we're talking about human health, of course it will be centered on humans. The charge is rather that it cannot fathom any other kind of health other than human health, which brings with it a related inability to note and assess long-term actions whose consequences span more than a human generation.

The problem of bioethical anthropocentrism is thus that it simply assumes that practices developed to increase human health will at the same time increase the overall state of health in general, as if taking care of human health will simultaneously take care of the health of the environment in which humans live. The conflation of the human world to include the world at large is perhaps understandable. Culturally the Western approach to ethics in general is based on both a metaphysics that holds human essence to be separate from that of mere natural stuff and a theology that teaches humanity is the crown of creation.

When bioethicists talk about health—even WHO's more inclusive definition as a "state of physical, mental and emotional well-being, not merely the absence of disease or infirmity" (WHO 2019)—it is human health apart from anything else that matters, not the environmental conditions that work in concert with human interests to sustain that health. Mirroring ecologist Arne Næss's distinction between shallow and deep ecology, this might be considered a "shallow" bioethics concerned with human well-being only (Næss 1983).

This is of course a highly anthropocentric point of view but is not the only definition of health. Aldo Leopold gives another from an ecological perspective: "health is the capacity of the land for self-renewal" (Leopold 1949, 221). "Self-renewal," and its near-synonym, self-healing, refers to the health of the land and all that is part of it, humans included, and we can call this, again after Næss, a "deep" bioethics. This relationship will be analyzed below and is in fact the meaning of the title of this article, but the important point to note for now is that it is entirely possible to be healthy according to WHO's shallow measure of health and yet be unhealthy according to Leopold's deep measure of self-renewal. Sometimes, this is done on purpose. Prescription drugs are in fact specifically designed for just this sort of attainment of shallow health; they allow humans to increase their immediate health, but their side effects often make humans vulnerable to other diseases that hinder self-healing.

But many human activities do not have this trade-off in mind and are done with the assumption that the short-term attainment of a shallow health simply leads to a long-term attainment of a deep health. Practices in food-chain production involve technologies meant to increase human flourishing through better nutrition, but the herbicides, fertilizers, growth hormones, and pesticides used are active agents in increasing human suffering instead (Union of Concerned Scientists 2019). Products meant to address safety and health, anything from antibiotics to flame retardants to tamper-proof packaging, have introduced entire suites of chemicals in the ecosystem and therefore humans that disrupt healthy human function (Holden 2019).

Humans in fact do many things in the name of healthier living that have a set of consequences more damaging on other health fronts not measured, not yet measured, or much less measurable at the present time. Some challenges to human flourishing take decades or generations to unfold. Only now in the first half of the twenty-first century, when technologies, practices, and habits accrued over decades and even centuries specifically established to maximize the well-being of the developed world led not just to a Rachel Carson–like silent spring, but the entire collapse of ecosystems that harm humanity—it is only now that bioethics is finally reacting to anthropogenic health calamities that were environmentally a long time of our own making.

BIOETHICS AS ENVIRONMENTAL ETHICS

Leopold's Land Ethics

If the specialization and anthropocentrism of bioethics results in conflating human well-being for the well-being of the place humans live, clearly we need a different way to understand this relationship. Fortunately, we have such an alternative in Van Rensselaer Potter's founding text on bioethics. Unfortunately, Potter's project to bridge the "traditional boundaries [of biology] to include the most essential elements of the social sciences and the humanities" (Potter 1971, viii) is difficult to precisely define given its transdisciplinary nature. Part of this is due to his slightly rambling zeal: many parts of the book are wandering and lack cohesion, and between the seventeen years that separated his two books, even his usage of what bioethics was supposed to mean shifted in a way that was not acknowledged by Potter himself. And yet for all this, his central claim that bioethics needed to engage with the world more fully still resonates.

One way to better understand Potter's project and thus to better understand the proper relationship between bioethics and the environment is to refer to Potter's intellectual mentor, Aldo Leopold, whose environmentalism anticipates Potter's critique of bioethical anthropocentrism more than two decades prior. The seven pages near the end of *A Sand County Almanac*, subtitled "The Land Pyramid," serves as a succinct and much needed guide to grasping the importance of the environment in understanding human health. A key passage indicates that what we take for granted as the land on which we live is actually what sustains biotic—not just human—existence in general.

> Land, then, is not merely soil; it is a fountain of energy flowing through the circuit of soils, plants, and animals. Food chains are the living channels that conduct energy upward; death and decay return it to the soil. The circuit is not closed; some energy is dissipated in decay, some is added by absorption from the air, and some is stored in soils, peats, and long-lived forests. But it is a sustained circuit, like a slowly augmented revolving fund of life (Leopold 1949, 216).

Combining the language of poetic metaphor and environmental science, Leopold means to shake us free of our anthropocentric blinders. Humans for him are part of the land and placed on the same ontological level as all other life forms, precariously balanced in food chains, in the process of growth and death. Leopold forces us to situate life in the much larger milieu of the land, or what we are calling the environment. To experience the world and manage to selectively notice and analyze only the human element is self-aggrandizing and self-defeating. Acting without the environment in mind is to create pathways—channels of energy, to use Leopold's words—that operate against human self-interests by forgetting our cooperative existence with the land. From an environmental perspective, Leopold recontextualizes human activity and decenters human importance. The question is not whether humans can or cannot create a sustained circuit. Because humans are part of the land, whatever humans do *will* result in a sustained circuit. The question is rather whether humans can create a circuit in a way that is amenable to human flourishing or whether humans will create a circuit that will frustrate human well-being instead.

Leopold's ecological vision necessitates such a rewiring of our basic concepts regarding human essence, dignity, and autonomy; it means revisiting the Platonic dualism and Aristotelian hylomorphism that inform the philosophical habit of pitting humans against nature. I suspect that this is why it is difficult for the field of bioethics to recognize the worth of Potter's writings. Theirs is a bioethics borne from this comfortable philosophical position, and it is being asked to understand a bioethics that does not share its anthropocentric assumptions.

When the former cannot fit the latter into the specific categories of its own understanding, it labels it imprecise and confused and leaves it at that. Potter languishes as a footnote in bioethics textbooks (if at all) because the metaphysical commitment needed to fully process the Leopoldian vision of land is too involved and seemingly distracts the reader from getting to the "real" issues of bioethics. Nothing could be further from the truth. Leopold's concept of land gives us a much more nuanced and deeper understanding of the relationship between bioethics and environmental ethics. Instead of answering this question of relationship by referring to bioethics *and* environmental ethics, the structure of his land pyramid implies a nested relationship where bioethics is a specific form of environmental ethics.

Recapitulation

This is of course the meaning of the subtitle of this article: bioethics ought to be understood *as* part of environmental ethics because we cannot undo the relationship between human behavior and the land. How this relationship operates is the meaning of the subtitle, and it freely borrows from Ernst Haeckel's well-known aphorism ("Ontogeny recapitulates phylogeny") regarding the evolutionary development of organisms. Haeckel's biogenetic theory has been discredited on the individual embryonic level: embryos do not morphologically repeat their evolutionary ancestors. But recapitulation theory in general allows us to appreciate the dynamic relationship humans have with their environment. Bioethics is a part of environmental ethics because human biology and human behavior are constituted by and of the environment.

Modernity has reified human individualism to the extent that it has forgotten the importance of land relationships in the creation of the individual. Bioethics as environmental ethics seeks to remind us of this interconnectivity when it states that *ontogeny* (the origins and development of each human organism) *recapitulates* (repeats the basic features of) *environment* (literally, "that which encircles us," our inhabitation). We humans are a microcosm of the place we inhabit such that the health of the place in which we live determines the health of human beings.

Just how we humans are determined by where we live is usually attributed to the geographic features of our habitation. Every place humans inhabit, whether it is mountainous terrain, land surrounded by large expanses of water, swaths of desert, or tropical jungles, demands the development of habits that allow the proper negotiation of the geographic constraints of their world. Those habits that have proven successful turn into prized characteristics, and, of those characteristics, a few have been so important to negotiated survival that they become the social virtues that have come to define particular peoples from particular places. This is the anthropological or historical account of how human existence is related to the environmental condition of the world.

But, in the context of this article, there is another sense of how humans are determined by our place of habitation, and this happens when our own despoilment of that place changes our health for the worse. We are where we live, but where we live turns out to be dependent on what we do to it. "Our major concern is no longer with the disease organisms that once were omnipresent," writes Rachel Carson. "Today we are concerned with a different kind of hazard that lurks in our world—a hazard that we ourselves have introduced into our world as our modern way of life has evolved" (Carson 1962, 187).

Carson could not know in 1962 just how correct she was. Our "modern way of life" has altered our environment enough that it alters our existential prospects. When populations increase such that human activity routinely exceeds the carrying capacity of the land, human ontogeny recapitulates the environment as much as the environment recapitulates human ontogeny in a feedback loop that exhausts the health of both the land and humans.

This is apparent in the problem of anthropogenic climate change. When bioethics is anthropocentrically focused on immediate human well-being, it fails to notice that the very human way in which we negotiate and conduct our doings with the world to attain this end implicates us in activities that are destructive to human well-being and the land. The US Global Change Research Program (2019) cites several ways anthropogenic climate change affects human health: extreme heat results in increasing occurrences of heatstroke and heat-related deaths; overall global warming results in increased cardiovascular and respiratory illnesses, along with decreasing precipitation and intense weather activity; rising sea levels threaten coastal populations with drowning and injury and inadequate access to medical facilities; changes in temperature extremes and weather patterns increase the population of disease vectors; increasing temperatures also increase waterborne diseases and food-related pathogens;

more destructive weather increases the level of exposure to trauma through disasters and increases the likelihood of mental health consequences.

Human activity is of course responsible for much more than anthropogenic climate change. There is the type of pollution from pesticides and herbicides and nuclear waste that Carson writes about, but to that list must be added additional sources of pollution that she could not have known about at her time. Noise pollution has, for example, been linked to hypertension, heart disease, and decreased developmental performance in children (Passchier-Vermeer and Passchier 2000). Light pollution similarly disrupts circadian rhythms that increase the risk of certain cancers (Redhwan and Anil 2016) and diabetes and obesity (Fonken et al. 2010) while also altering the behavior of pollinators important for agriculture and the food industry (MacGregor et al. 2015). Microplastics are so prevalent in even tap water and air that they are found in animal tissue and human waste, which means there is a strong chance that we have microplastics embedded in our own tissue as well (Lancet Planetary Health 2017).

What the health effects of microplastics are on humans are thus far unknown, but plastics are known to contain endocrine disruptors that directly affect reproductive and developmental growth (Meeker et al. 2009). And CO_2 is not just a potent greenhouse gas; excessive amounts acidify ocean water, disrupting the very bottom of the food chain and putting the entire food web at risk of collapse (National Oceanic and Atmospheric Administration 2019). Pollution, especially in amounts beyond which the land can safely absorb, is the unfortunate marker of human success. As much as tektites announce the Cretaceous-Paleogene boundary in the geological rock column, microplastics could well be the geological marker for the Anthropocene. Ontogeny recapitulates the environment that we have made.

A Different Ethics in the Making

Where does this all leave ethics, and bioethics in particular? Here is Leopold's answer to the first question: "Ethics are possibly a kind of community instinct in-the-making" (Leopold 1949, 203). This is a difficult quasi-definition for the anthropocentric tradition to analyze. *Instincts* are understood to be dispositions innately fixed by genetics and thus proper to lower organisms. *Habit* is what we humans ethically develop, and habits are dispositions learned via culture and institutions (if one is virtuously inclined) or our innate rationality (if one is a philosophical modern). And yet ethics is here developed as an instinct. Can it be that appealing to something like the categorical imperative is an instinct that better secures social interaction? And if ethics are an instinct common to all organisms, is it possible that other nonhuman organisms practice an ethics of their own? And what of the fact that ethics are "in-the-making"? What of the virtues or the prima facie duties of human rights? Are they not universally accepted and justified according to universal principles of reason that have withstood the test of time?

These are all the correct questions to ask of this new nonanthropocentric ethics. But there are two points to make in its general defense. The first is that what anthropocentrism means by universal is far from actually being universal. Ethics as developed is a *particular* ethics that refers only to humans and fails to even acknowledge the biotic and nonbiotic relationships that ground human beings. The community referred to by Leopold requires us to have a far more expansive grasp of what we mean by ethical universality. It certainly cannot refer to a universal Ideal essence leftover from Plato, nor modernity's identification of only rational humans as ethical agents. Ethics as community instinct in-the-making means that ethics is universal when as many biotic and nonbiotic systems in the land pyramid are properly accounted for to achieve general ecological well-being. A nonanthropocentric ethical stance is far more universal in scope than any ethical system that relies only on human essence, agency, rationality, or purposivity. What humans take to be human accomplishments are really not just human accomplishments. As Leopold states in the opening quote of this article, they are communal accomplishments requiring biotic relationships within the larger domain of nonbiotic material and phenomena.

Second, the fact that ethics is in-the-making does not mean it is relativistic and absent an unchanging prescriptive rule. There is one such prescriptivism—in all cases we ought to preserve the health of the land. How that preservation of health becomes realized is entirely open to pragmatic application, and any other analysis regarding duties, intuitions, rights, consequences, emotions, and virtues is at the service of this end.

Bioethical Ethos, Conservation, and Biotic Complexity

What must be true of bioethics if indeed ontogeny does reciprocate the environment? There are I believe three interconnected issues. The first is that the *ethics* in bioethics becomes deeper and more profoundly connected to human experience. If we set the recapitulation statement to human scale, it refers to the developmental sequence of human beings as they negotiate where they are in the world—in their home, their habituated gathering place, their *ethos*. This is a different and older understanding of what is meant by *ethos*.

According to theologian Paul Lehmann, το ηθος originally refers to an animal stall or dwelling. The verb ειωθα means being accustomed to and is more in line with the formation of habits that Aristotle had in mind. To Lehmann, "the relationship between stability and custom was a kind of elemental datum of experience. It was really the primary office of custom to do in the human area what the stall did for animals: to provide security and stability" (Lehmann 1963, 24). Nancie Erhard writes that Homer used the word to refer not just to human-made stables but also to those "accustomed places of animals [much as] Herodotus . . . applied it to the habitual places of lions, and Oppianus to those of fish" (Erhard 2007, 12). In its original instantiation, *ethos* really meant those safe havens, those comfortable grottoes and dens that animals would habitually return to to rest, feed, heal, and retire. "Ethos thus has a fragrance of wildness at the same time that it conveys accustomed and proper place. It is much more akin to our word 'habitat'" (Erhard 2017, 12). The ethics in Homer situates humans in these well-worn habitations of our choosing.

Given Homer's seminal influence in Greek thought, one way to read Aristotelian ethics is to understand it as a project that answers what Homer left unstated: How do and how should (for Aristotle is both descriptive and prescriptive in scope) people who inhabit their living spaces—call them homes, towns, cities, etc.—behave to ensure the well-being of their inhabitation? Ethics thus contains what Jenell Johnson calls "[a] multifaceted, polysemic sense of ethos—comprising character, credibility, individual habit, cultural convention, and wild habitat" (Johnson 2016). The interplay of all these levels of meaning is present in the ethics developed here. Philosophy is well aware of Aristotle's use of *ethos*, which states that humans are what humans habitually do, but it is not as aware of Homer's, which states that what humans habitually do is determined by the place that they, literally speaking, in-habit.[2]

The type of ethics developed here is not just about discerning what is permissible and what is not: it is really about the existentially fraught reasons why and how permissibility is determined. What is good is that which gives the greatest chance of survivability in that our measure of *ethos* is in large part determined by how well we are able to guarantee the health of the land that maximizes our survival. We have somehow turned the ethical question away from "what will ensure the survivability of as many species in a balanced account of the land?" toward the instrumentalism behind "what can I get away with?" In perhaps the most famous quote of *A Sand County Almanac*, Leopold ties this existential need for biotic cooperation with the derivation of ethical judgment: "A thing is right when it tends to preserve the integrity, stability, and beauty of the biotic community. It is wrong when it tends otherwise" (Leopold, 1949, 224–25).

Without this existential claim, what else is there to spur moral compunction? Economic punishment? Loss of social status? Neither necessitates a fundamental change in ethical values and may in fact perpetrate a different form of the same type of enlightened self-interest. Many biomedical judgments and calls to action are of this sort. A land-based bioethics finds an ethical solution to necessarily involve the larger question of how best to inhabit and create a place of living that maximizes the integrity, stability, and beauty of the land in order to bring about biotic health and well-being.

Clearly, humans are as healthy as the environment in which they live. This may seem as an obvious truism, but the prevailing philosophy practiced in the West denies such an ethical parity between humans and the world and to begin instead by assuming a human versus nature dichotomy. But absent that assumption, conservation now can be reinterpreted to mean more than the protection, preservation, and management of natural resources through prohibitions, rules, and laws, as if to say that conservation is needed to preserve "nature" from human encroachment. There is of course no such thing: what is made by humans is, as a matter of fact, made in and by nature. Leopold understands human encroachment as but a natural process of land systems. The natural tendency of successful organisms is to increase their biological foot-print, and the natural processes that keep that footprint in check lead to the collapse of those organisms by unintended pathways that are nevertheless of their own making.

Population dynamics reminds us that the last phase of a closed biotic system occurs when populations decrease exponentially because of a lack of nutrients and an increase in waste products. When the successful organisms in question are human and the closed system the earth, such a collapse is precisely what bioethics must address and prevent. Bioethics should be about conserving the ability for the environs to self-heal such that human ontogenesis can repair itself as part of that environmental self-healing process. This deep sense of conserva-tion means that bioethics cannot just be the academic study of what duties medical sciences have in addressing ensuing health problems, or what rights patients have in gaining access to treatments caused by environmental pollutants, or deriving a principlist determination of the moral culpability of companies that have contributed most to environmental despoilment. It is all that, but also so much more. Bioethics must be about the active role humans have in the ability of their place of inhabitation to heal itself. It is about the health of the biosphere that funds the health of humans and other organisms.

As a particular type of environmental ethic, bioethics is actually arguing for biotic complexity as a way to ensure human health, understanding that what is necessary for life are ultimately nonbiotic land systems consisting of geography, atmospherics, and water. "The velocity and upward flow of energy depend on the complex structure of the plant and animal community[.] This interdependence between the complex structure of the land and its smooth functioning as an energy unit is one of its basic attributes," writes Leopold (1949, 216). Focusing only on human health and well-being has the effect of altering Leopold's land pyramid. Complex pathways are straightened, intermingled symbioses pruned, and multiple currents of energy dammed off to prevent the formation of unwanted tributaries.

The energy circuit is paved and cleaned of biotic and nonbiotic debris in our attempt to redirect the energy circuit to suit human needs. Heavily manipulated, the ecology of the place adjusts and changes, but at a price; "the land recovers, but at some reduced level of complexity, and with a reduced carrying capacity for people, plants, and animals" (Leopold 1949, 219). Human intervention thus has the tendency toward complication when we simplify the biotic land pyramid, and complication is not complexity. Biotic complexity ensures evolutionary growth; complication ensues when the complexity of the land is stunted by humans who reduce ecological relationships to a handful of biotic simples.

CONCLUSION

Such an interpretation of bioethics requires a substantive reworking of the bioethical landscape. Now linked to environmental issues, concepts such as land-carrying capacity and land health must now be factored in the bioethical framework, even as human health and well-being have to be factored into what were previously purely environmental concerns. These issues are not easily worked out.

Because humans are part of the land, a question of biotic balance must be addressed. Humans present an existential risk to some organisms, but it is equally true that some organisms present a similar risk to human beings. How should we determine the biotic balance in the land pyramid? And what do we do about one of the primary drivers of ecological collapse, human overpopulation? Bioethics would now need to take the lead on this issue, keeping in mind Garrett Hardin's curt abstract: "The population problem has no technical solution; it requires a fundamental extension in morality" (Hardin 1968). What exactly constitutes such an "extension of morality"?

This article has sketched out the basic contours of a bioethics as an environmental ethics. Left behind has been any talk about what this would mean for environmental ethics. But one advantage of this recasting of bioethics is that it can mediate the debate in contemporary environmental ethics regarding the anthropocentric content of environmentalism. Deep ecologists like Næss and biocentric environmentalists like J. Baird Callicott and Laura Westra make the point that a true environmental ethics must be based on the intrinsic value of nature; "weak" anthropocentrists like Bryan Norton claim that, when it comes down to determining the policies meant to expand environmental protection, there is no practical difference between those who hold nature as having intrinsic value, and those who hold that it has instrumental value.[3]

Because bioethics has been identified as an anthropocentric study within environmental ethics, it can slot in as the point of convergence between the weak and the nonanthropocentric accounts. The difference is of course that bioethics does not concern itself with just environmental policy—it is always environmental policy for the sake of human well-being, an assumption behind Norton's convergence hypothesis, but developed explicitly here.

As with any concept or discipline that is being reframed from its traditional meaning, there are many questions that need to be answered and many difficult issues to resolve. But bioethics as an environmental ethics offers a new approach that avoids the pitfalls of hyperspecialization and an unchecked anthropocentrism. It does this by contextualizing bioethics in something larger and more important than itself, and this allows it to address the complex interplay between ecosystems and human ontogenesis, here understood both as anthropological development and individual development.

The resulting bioethics thus has a different feel than bioethics in its current iteration. Its ethical basis is older than Aristotle's, the ethical roles that humans play are more profound than in Confucian humanism, and it is far more suspicious than modernity can be of human rationality becoming instrumental. It looks at consequences, but not as consequentialists do with their eyes set on anthropocentric utility; it is virtuous, but with an excellence measured by the telos of the land; it has a sense of duty, but openly embraces heteronomy because human autonomy means violating its own categorical imperative: never treat the land solely as a means to an end.

REFERENCES

Baker, Robert. 2002. "On Being a Bioethicist" (review). *American Journal of Bioethics* 2, no. 2, (Spring): 65–69.

Carson, Rachel. 1962. *Silent Spring*. New York: Houghton Mifflin Harcourt Publishing.

Dwyer, James. 2009. "How to Connect Bioethics and Environmental Ethics: Health, Sustainability, and Justice." *Bioethics* 23, no. 9: 497–502.

Elliott, Carl. 2010. "The Ethicists." In *Beyond Bioethics*, edited by Osagie K. Obasogie and Marcy Darnovsky, 132–49. Berkeley: University of California Press.

Erhard, Nancie. 2007. *Moral Habitat: Ethos and Agency for the State of the Earth*. Albany: SUNY Press.

Evans, John. 2000. "A Sociological Account of the Growth of Principlism." In *Beyond Bioethics*, edited by Osagie K. Obasogie and Marcy Darnovsky, 85–93. Oakland: University of California Press.

Fonken, Laura K., Joanna L. Workman, James C. Walton, Zachary M. Weil, John S. Morris, Abraham Haim, and Randy J. Nelson. 2010. "Light at Night Increases Body Mass by Shifting the Time of Food Intake." *Proceedings of the National Academy of Sciences of the United States* 107, no. 43: 18664–669.

Hardin, Garrett. 1968. "The Tragedy of the Commons." *Science* 162, no. 3859: 1243–48.

Holden, Emily. 2019. "Is Modern Life Poisoning Me? I Took the Tests to Find Out." *The Guardian*. Accessed 5/23/2019. https://www.theguardian.com/us-news/2019/may/22/is-modern-life-poisoning-me-i-took-the-tests-to-find-out.

Johnson, Jenell. 2016. "Bioethics as a Way of Life: The Radical Bioethics of Van Rensselaer Potter." *Literature and Medicine* 34, no. 1 (Spring): 7–24.

Jonsen, Albert. 1998. *The Birth of Bioethics*. New York: Oxford University Press.

Lancet Planetary Health. 2017. "Microplastics and Human Health—An Urgent Problem." *The Lancet*. Accessed 5/23/2019. https://www.thelancet.com/journals/lanplh/article/PIIS2542-5196(17)30121-3/fulltext.

Lehman, Paul L. 1963. *Ethics in a Christian Context*. New York: Harper and Row Publishers.

Leopold, Aldo. 1949. *A Sand County Almanac*. New York: Oxford University Press.

MacGregor, Callum J., Michael J. O. Popcock, Richard Fox, and Darren M. Evans. 2015. "Pollination by Nocturnal Lepidoptera, and the Effects of Light Pollution: A Review. *Ecological Entomology* 40, no. 30: 187–98.

Malpas, Jeff. 2017. *Heidegger and the Thinking of Place: Explorations in the Topology of Being*. Cambridge, MA: MIT Press.

Meeker, J. D., S. Sathyanarayana, and H. S. Swan. 2009. "Phthalates and Other Additives in Plastics: Human Exposure and Associated Health Outcomes." *Philosophical Transactions B of the Royal Society* 364, no. 1526: 2097–113.

Minteer, Ben A., and Robert E. Manning. 2000. "Convergence in Environmental Values: An Empirical and Conceptual Defense." *Philosophy and Geography* 3: 47–60.

Næss, Arne. 1983. "The Shallow and the Deep, Long-Range Ecology Movement." *Inquiry* 16: 95–100.

National Oceanic and Atmospheric Administration. 2019. "Ocean Acidification." Accessed 5/19/2019. https://www.noaa.gov/education/resource-collections/ocean-coasts-education-resources/ocean-acidification.

Passchier-Vermeer, W., and W. F. Passchier. 2000. "Noise Exposure and Public Health." *Environmental Health Perspectives* 108 (Supplement 1): 123–31.

Potter, Van Rensselaer. 1971. *Bioethics: Bridge to the Future*. New York: Prentice Hall Publishing.

Redhwan, A. Al-Naggar, and Shirin Anil. 2016. "Artificial Light at Night and Cancer: A Global Study." *Asian Pacific Journal of Cancer Prevention* 17, no. 10: 4661–64.

Richie, Cristina. 2014. "A Brief History of Environmental Bioethics." *AMA Journal of Ethics* 16, no. 9: 749–52.

Union of Concerned Scientists. 2019. "Hidden Costs of Industrial Agriculture." Accessed 4/28/2019. https://www.ucsusa.org/food_and_agriculture/our-failing-food-system/industrial-agriculture/hidden -costs-of-industrial.html#.

US Global Change Research Program. 2019. "The Impacts of Climate Change on Human Health in the United States: A Scientific Assessment: Summary." Accessed 5/24/2019. https://www.theguardian .com/us-news/2019/may/22/is-modern-life-poisoning-me-i-took-the-tests-to-find-out.

World Health Organization. 2019. "Constitution." Accessed 4/29/2019. https://www.who.int/about/ who-we-are/constitution.

NOTES

1. The claim is not that modern theories do not consider social action in their ethical judgments. Consequentialism, of course, does exactly that. It is that, even in consequentialism, the ability to make an ethical decision can be performed by any given individual who follows a version of the utilitarian calculus.

2. This deep philosophical reflection of place, of *topos*, is also developed extensively by Heidegger. *Dasein*, his primordial existential entity, does after all mean "being there," where *there* is the world into which it finds itself thrown. The central relationship between existence and place, or what Jeff Malpas calls "the topology of being" (Malpas 2017), is similarly developed, albeit with a German accent instead.

3. This topic has been fairly and ably covered by Ben A. Minteer and Robert E. Manning's (2000) excellent article, "Convergence in Environmental Values: An Empirical and Conceptual Defense."

6

Lost in Translation

Can We have a Global Bioethics without a Global Moral Language?

Søren Holm[1]

ABSTRACT

This chapter will analyze the question of whether a global bioethics can be established if we do not have a prior common moral language. The first part will analyze two contenders for a global moral language: (1) human rights and (2) a set of core principles (looking closely at Macklin's work). It will argue that neither constitute a shared moral language and will identify the reasons they don't. The second part will then discuss whether a hybrid approach involving core human rights interpreted in the light of core moral principles can form the basis for a global bioethics. It will again be argued that such an approach is problematic. The third part will then consider whether we are not better off by accepting that there are irresolvable moral differences at both theoretical and practical levels and accepting that the real moral task is to mediate between these differences in concrete situations.

INTRODUCTION

It is a trite platitude that we live in a connected global world where the consequences of our actions may spread far and wide and where perhaps, more importantly, we are aware that the consequences of our actions may spread far and wide. How are we to deal with the global moral problems that occur in such a world? One suggestion is that because the problems are global they should be analyzed and resolved within an agreed global moral framework. It is this suggestion that will be analyzed critically in this chapter. I will outline the epistemic and social conditions necessary for convergence on a common position and apply this analysis in relation to convergence on a common set of core or fundamental moral principles. I will also consider the use of human rights as the common minimal framework.

   In the analysis I will use the principle of "respect for persons" as the main example of a potentially universal moral principle and the important 1998 book *Against Relativism: Cultural Diversity and the Search for Ethical Universals in Medicine*, by Ruth Macklin, as the main source of examples. I have chosen to use Macklin's book in this way because I take it to be one of the strongest, best, and clearest defenses of an unabashed universalist position in bioethics.

I furthermore agree with Macklin's universalism at the theoretical level but disagree with her concerning the conditions under which theoretical universalism can be converted into concrete ethical judgments. This makes her book and analysis an appropriate touchstone for the more skeptical view I develop here.

The analysis will mainly relate to the possibility of a global ethics, but many of the arguments are also relevant to the possibility of a common ethics within a single multicultural society. But, before proceeding any further, it is important briefly to make the case for why a common, global ethics might be considered desirable. The world in which we live is not "the best of all worlds." The rights of millions of people are breached without justification, unjustifiable resource inequalities are perpetuated and widened, and the strong are often allowed to prey on the weak with impunity.

There are thus many ways in which the world could be made a better place, ethically speaking. Although each of us can do much on our own to make the world a better place, there are also many things that can be changed only if individuals or states work together. The necessary cooperation will plausibly be easier if it is possible to reach agreement on what features of the world we ought to change and why we ought to change them. And this agreement might be believed to require a common set of ethical principles. If we, for instance, want to identify unjustifiable resource inequalities that ought to be rectified, this seems to presuppose agreement on some account of what justice requires. We may be able to proceed some of the way in the absence of a common global ethics, but getting all the way seems to require one. And it would therefore be a major achievement if we could agree on one.

CONDITIONS FOR CONVERGENCE

Under what general conditions can we reasonably expect convergence on a common moral framework, in a situation where moral agents (1) start from radically different positions, (2) are able to communicate with each other and engage in moral discourse, and (3) are willing to engage in moral discourse in good faith?[2]

Let us first note that the answer to this question is independent of whether we assume a foundationalist or a coherentist account of moral justification. On either of these accounts, the process by which convergence is achieved in discourse between real moral agents is going to be a coherence-seeking process involving all the elements of wide reflective equilibrium as inputs (i.e., beliefs and facts about the world, considered moral judgments, and moral theories) (Daniels 2008). We will never be in a situation where we try to agree on our common moral principles without any prior moral commitments. Agreeing on foundationalism or coherentism will be an outcome of the process, not an initial assumption, and it might not even be a necessary outcome.

As a starting point in a convergence-seeking process, the participants will need to try to reach agreement on the ground rules for the process. Here, there are major stumbling blocks. The one that is commonly discussed is whether considered moral judgments that are based on (religious) comprehensive worldviews are admissible in the process (Audi and Wolterstorff 1997; Rawls 1996). Robert Audi, for instance proposes two principles of secular reason and motivation as side constraints on interventions in public political debates.

The Principle of Secular Rationale

"One has a prima facie obligation not to advocate or support any law or public policy that restricts human conduct, unless one has, and is willing to offer, adequate secular reasons for this advocacy or support" (Audi and Wolterstorff 1997, 25).

The Principle of Secular Motivation

"One has a (prima facie) obligation to abstain from advocacy or support of a law or public policy that restricts human conduct, unless one is sufficiently *motivated* by (normatively) adequate secular reason" (Audi and Wolterstorff 1997, 28).

Admitting moral judgments based on religious worldviews will make it more difficult to reach consensus, but not admitting them is also problematic. There are no participants in the process who do not hold a comprehensive worldview that influences their concrete judgments. Only some of these comprehensive worldviews are religious,[3] but a specific nonreligious worldview can be as idiosyncratic, held as strongly, and influence concrete judgments as much as a religious one (e.g., a Marxist–Leninist worldview) (Luther 1986).

If nonshared components of comprehensive worldviews are excluded *ab initio*, it is likely to have one of two effects. It will either mean that those who are strongly committed to their comprehensive worldview will be less interested in engaging with the process, or it will mean that they cannot engage in good faith. They will not be able to state their views in what they see as the strongest possible way but will be forced to find ways of stating them that are less satisfactory from their point of view.

Here, we seem to be between a rock and a hard place, philosophically speaking. Either we complicate our coherence-building process by letting participants state their initial ethical views clearly and with their own justification, or we run the risk of making it impossible for some participants to engage in the process in good faith. If we choose to exclude nonshared components of comprehensive worldviews, we further have the problem that it becomes unclear how the persons who hold these views should view the outcome of the process.

Let us imagine that wide reflective equilibrium has been obtained around a set of global ethical principles. It then seems possible to claim that participants in the process should accept these principles because they are a way of making their own moral views more coherent and thereby, presumably, more justifiable. But, if the input is not "their own moral views," it is difficult to see why they should have any commitment to accepting the outcome.

A slightly different issue that is often confused with the religion issue is the issue of nonnegotiable commitments. If any party in the process has nonnegotiable commitments, it may block the achievement of coherence, and it may therefore be a necessary component of good faith that everything is up for grabs. But nonnegotiable commitments can be held for a variety of reasons, not only religious ones.

The other stumbling block is that real-life coherence seeking does not take place behind a veil of ignorance. All participants are aware of who they are and of what consequences a given set of common ethical principles will have for them and their descendants. In an ideal world where everyone is motivated by ethical concerns, only this would not matter, but it will matter for real-world consensus building.

We can therefore not expect agreement on common, global ethical principles to be reached quickly or without contention. What we can expect is a slow process moving forward in a piecemeal fashion, and maybe not even always moving forward. We may be able to reach agreement that a specific ethical construct is a fundamental ethical principle and part of a common global ethics, whereas other constructs still have only the status of plausible candidates or still have vague scope and content.

What we cannot expect, even if we are committed theoretical universalists, is that agreement on the universal principles is reached quickly or easily.

HOW PRECISE A CONSENSUS CAN WE REACH?

Let us, despite the problems alluded to above, assume that we have reached a consensus that "respect for persons" is a fundamental and universal ethical principle[4] that should guide our global ethics. Are we then in a position to make concrete ethical judgments?

Let us first consider a case where "respect for persons" is the only moral consideration that is engaged. No other principles are in play, and it is clear that everyone involved falls within the scope of the principle[5] (i.e., that they are persons). In such a case, we would still need to specify the content of the principle in order to form a judgment. It is a well-known and often repeated criticism of Beauchamp and Childress's principlist approach that, whereas we might be able to agree on the importance of the four principles when they are fairly content-less labels, it is much more difficult to agree on their precise content (e.g., how much beneficence is required). And the same question must be raised here: What does "respect for persons" actually mean? A brief survey of the literature makes it clear that this is a highly controversial question. John Harris argues that respect for persons has two distinct aspects:

> Respect for persons requires us to acknowledge the dignity and value of other persons and to treat them as ends in themselves and not merely instrumentally as means to ends or objectives chosen by others. Respect for persons has two distinct dimensions:
>
> 1. Respect for autonomy.
> 2. Concern for welfare.
>
> When I suggest that these elements are crucial to any conception of respect for persons I mean simply that no one could claim to respect persons if their attitude to others failed to take account of, and indeed exhibit, these elements." (Harris 2003, 10)

But respect for autonomy and concern for welfare seem to be two very different things. Macklin explicates respect for persons primarily as respect for personal autonomy that avoids many interpretative problems, being primarily a negative condition and therefore a potential candidate for a strict and complete duty.

If, however, Harris is right and respect for persons also encompasses concern for welfare, we are left with the further problem of how to explicate welfare.[6] Is the welfare of a person a purely subjective matter to be decided only from the first-person perspective, or is it (at least partly) an objective matter? To agree on this will be important in order to come to concrete judgment in cases where a person wants to perform actions that will negatively affect some objective assessment of their welfare or interest. But are we likely to reach consensus on the explication? Or likely to reach consensus on what should be incorporated in a list of objective goods conducive to welfare?

This might, initially, seem not to matter if we take the more restrictive Macklin line equating respect for persons with respect for autonomy and relegating welfare considerations to some other fundamental ethical principle. But thinking that this move will solve the problem is partly an illusion because welfare ceases to matter only if we take respect for autonomy to be absolute in the sense that paternalistic action is never justifiable. If we accept that there are instances where paternalism in respect of a competent person is justified, the question of our account of welfare again raises its head. And, given that no philosophical agreement has yet been reached on this issue, we would surely expect too much of our consensus process if we believed it would give us a firm answer.

A more complicated problem occurs when we have more than one fundamental moral principle in play and where they are in potential conflict.[7] This is a very old problem, and most moral systems have ways of dealing with it (e.g., the processes of specification and balancing in Beauchamp and Childress's work) (2009).

But, in the global context, what sometimes happens is that someone brings a moral consideration to the table that is new in the sense that it is outside of the moral system of the other participants in the discourse. This would still happen even if we had an agreed set of global moral principles because, unlike in ideal philosophy, not everyone will have been at the discourse where these principles were agreed.

Let me illustrate this problem with an extended example from Macklin's book. In a chapter on death and birth, she discusses organ transplantation in the Philippines and the role of traditional Filipino morality in shaping the practice:

> The dead person whose organs are removed is not in a position to make a proper "donation" in an act that stems from the right sort of moral motivation. The relevant concept in the traditional Filipino value system is known as *kusang loob*. For an act to have moral worth it must be done out of *kusang loob*, an idea similar to free will but not exactly the same. If a person needs to be told what to do, or is coerced into performing an action, the act does not come out of *kusang loob*. To have moral worth, an action must also be done without anticipation of reward or personal gain and not purely out of a sense of duty.
>
> The implications for the morality of organ donation are rather straightforward. If a person is not in a position to act from the proper moral motivation, that is, out of *kusang loob*, it is better for the action not to have been done at all. Presumably, then, only if a person had signed an organ donation card, done so in an uncoerced manner and not purely out of a sense of duty, would the donation qualify as being done out of *kusang loob*. [. . .]
>
> What follows from this picture for ethical relativism? Should we conclude that the medical practice of organ transplantation is ethically wrong in the Philippines because of the value attached to the concept of *kusang loob* but ethically right elsewhere as long as the proper safeguards are followed? [. . .]
>
> The Filipino concept of *kusang loob* is a feature of a moral system in that culture that does not appear to have an exact counterpart in our own society, at least not with respect to organ donation. *Kusang loob* falls under the category of moral motivation, an aspect of ethical behavior that may legitimately differ from one society to another and is therefore an example of one of the things that turns out to be relative. The application of this concept to organ donation yields the result that organ donation itself is neither morally right nor morally wrong, but its rightness or wrongness depends (among other things) on the moral motivation of the individual whose organs are harvested for transplantation. This marks a cultural and ethical difference from organ donation in other cultures where a donation need not stem from a particular moral motivation. This difference is not at the level of fundamental ethical principles, so it does not confirm the proposition that ethical principles vary from one culture to the next with no deeper underlying principles. (Macklin 1998, 143–44)

I agree with Macklin that nothing in this account of the implications of traditional Filipino values for organ transplantation confirms "the proposition that ethical principles vary from one culture to the next with no deeper underlying principles," but I disagree with the way she justifies this conclusion.

Believing that moral motivation is important in deciding whether an act is morally right or wrong is not a peculiar Filipino concern. The non-Filipino philosopher Immanuel Kant famously argued that motivation in the form of a good will was the only thing that decided rightness and wrongness:

> Nothing can possibly be conceived in the world, or even out of it, which can be called good, without qualification, except a good will. [. . .]
>
> A good will is good not because of what it performs or effects, not by its aptness for the attainment of some proposed end, but simply by virtue of the volition; that is, it is good in itself, and considered by itself is to be esteemed much higher than all that can be brought about by it in favor of any inclination, nay even of the sum total of all inclinations. (Kant 1985)

And the characteristics that make an action problematic in the Filipino case have some overlaps with what makes an action heteronomous and therefore without value in Kantian philosophy. Similar concerns related to motivation or intention can also be found in many other ethical systems. It is therefore impossible to drive a wedge between fundamental ethical principles and concerns with motivation in the way Macklin does. That the right motivation matters in the moral assessment of actions may eventually be one of the fundamental ethical principles that emerge from a consensus process.

There is nothing inherent in the concept of a "fundamental ethical principle" that precludes this. A fundamental ethical principle does not have to be about rights or duties. But if we can't just discount *kusang loob* as a particular Filipino ethical value that can never count as a fundamental ethical principle, how are we to deal with it? If we are really committed to universalism and to moral discourse in good faith, it seems that we will minimally have to consider whether we need to augment our set of fundamental ethical principles with a principle about right, ethical motivation. This will not be necessary if we can plausibly claim that our current set of fundamental ethical principles already contains all the principles that can count as fundamental ethical principles. But it is difficult to see how such a claim can be sustained, at least at the present stage of the discourse where we are still moving forward toward a global, common ethics.

So the introduction of *kusang loob* into the debate as a possible important ethical consideration will, at least temporarily, destabilize our set of fundamental ethical principles. It is only after we have seriously considered whether *kusang loob* or some suitable modification can make our set of principles even more coherent that we can make a concrete judgment concerning Filipino as well as non-Filipino organ donation.

This is not a problem if *kusang loob* is an isolated instance of a prima facie valid ethical consideration found in a specific culture, but there are of course likely to be many such examples and therefore many circumstances where concrete judgment might elude us because our set of global common ethics cannot be claimed to be complete.

HUMAN RIGHTS AS THE COMMON FRAMEWORK

But is the analysis above not far too complicated and hairsplitting? Could we not simply sidestep the philosophical issues and seek convergence in the area of international human rights law?

The link between public health, medicine, ethics, and human rights was first analyzed in detail by Jonathan Mann, and a turn toward human rights has been prominent in recent developments in "global ethics" (Mann 1997). Most have argued that ethics and human rights are complementary, but at least some commentators foresee a development where human rights law will eventually subsume bioethics and make bioethics more or less redundant (Faunce 2005).

Roberto Andorno furthermore argues that human rights are best understood as a result of a consensus-seeking process that allows consensus on principles without requiring consensus on justifications. The agreed set of human rights may not be the result of wide reflective equilibrium, but they are nevertheless agreed:

> The global success of the human rights movement in contemporary society is probably due to the fact that a practical agreement about the rights that should be respected is perfectly compatible with theoretical disagreement on their ultimate foundation (14). The Universal Declaration of Human Rights of 1948 is the best example of this phenomenon, because it was drafted by representatives of particularly diverse, even opposed, ideologies. Upon this strong legislative foundation has been built an extensive network of human rights mechanisms designed to develop international standards, monitor their implementation and investigate violations of human rights. (Andorno 2002, 960)

The advantages of moving to a human rights arena are according to proponents of such a move many: (1) states voluntarily agree to be bound by human rights and such rights therefore have undisputed normative force, (2) that human rights jurisprudence provides an interpretative system for determining the scope and meaning of human rights, and (3) that specific institutions (e.g., the European Court of Human Rights [ECHR] can provide authoritative interpretations with legal force). If we, therefore, as an example want to know the scope and meaning of the right to private and family life enunciated in Article 8 of the European Convention of Human Rights, we can look at ECHR jurisprudence. Article 8 states that:

1. Everyone has the right to respect for his private and family life, his home and his correspondence.
2. There shall be no interference by a public authority with the exercise of this right except such as is in accordance with the law and is necessary in a democratic society in the interests of national security, public safety or the economic well-being of the country, for the prevention of disorder or crime, for the protection of health or morals, or for the protection of the rights and freedoms of others.

In relation to sexual matters we would then find that the Article 8 rights in general protect against discrimination because of sexual orientation or activity but also that not all kinds of sexual activity are protected. In the judgment in *Laskey, Jaggard and Brown v. the United Kingdom* (judgment of 19 February 1997), the ECHR, for instance, found that the organized, consensual sadomasochistic activities carried out by a group of men were not protected by Article 8.

The human rights framework thus specifies the rights of individuals and provides mechanisms for authoritative interpretation. These rights are furthermore universal in scope and consensually agreed, at least within the relevant set of jurisdictions (member states of the Council of Europe in the case of the ECHR). It thus seems that human rights give the universalists everything that they could reasonably want and that they circumvent all of the problems about agreement on precise content discussed above because of the existence of authoritative interpretations.

One possible criticism of this positive picture is that there are problems with our current enumerations of human rights and that we should add some and perhaps also remove some from our lists of binding human rights. I think this a valid criticism (Holm 2009), but not one that I will be pursuing here.

The criticism that I want to pursue here is based on the fact that the precise content of specific human rights is an area of huge contestation. The lawyers for Laskey, Jaggard, and Brown argued that their activities were protected by Article 8, and many commentators have agreed with them, but the ECHR disagreed. It is a standard legal fiction that courts interpret laws; they do not make them. Or, to put it differently, when a court makes a decision on a point of law, it simply states what the legal position is; it does not change the legal position. According to this fiction, the lawyers for Laskey et al. simply made a legal mistake.[8] Article 8 did not protect these kinds of sexual activities and it had never done so.

But, given recent changes in sexual mores, it is quite likely that the *Laskey* judgment will one day be overturned. This will be of no help to Laskey et al., who have long since served their prison sentences. But it will mean that Article 8 suddenly protects activity that the court had previously denied it protected. Or, to put it differently, if *Laskey* is overturned, it will illustrate that the content of human rights is much more fluid and malleable than we might initially believe. It will also illustrate that the initial, voluntary consent of states is almost completely irrelevant to the normative force of their current human rights commitment. The rights that the original signatories signed up to in 1950 when the European Convention on Human Rights and Fundamental Freedoms was signed was a set of rights with very different content than the rights in 2010.

Human rights do give us legal enforceability in some regions of the world, but they do not substitute for a common global ethics. They are a parallel normative system with as many interpretative problems and as much vagueness of content.

THE DISMAL CONCLUSION?

In this paper, I have argued for the conclusion that the likelihood that we will be able to agree on a global moral framework that is sufficiently specific to lead to concrete judgment concerning global moral problems is very small indeed. The justification for this conclusion is not that moral relativism is true. I believe that there are compelling arguments showing moral relativism to be unsustainable as a theoretical position and there are good arguments for accepting moral universalism, but that is a matter for another paper.

Alas, the falsity of moral relativism does not guarantee actual convergence on one commonly accepted moral framework. In the paper, I have presented arguments showing that there are very large epistemic and social obstacles standing in the way of actual moral convergence and that we should not expect overall convergence to happen. And, even if we could achieve convergence on principles like "respect for persons," it is unlikely that we could converge on the precise interpretation of that principle.

This may sound like a dismal conclusion, but one way of seeing it in a more positive light is by realizing that it is essentially the position we have been in since the inception of philosophical ethics among the pre-Socratics. Agreement has rarely been achieved in the theoretical realm, but that has not precluded genuine moral progress and agreement on concrete judgments. We may still not agree on exactly why chattel slavery is wrong, but is it not a sufficient cause for joy that most of us now have an unshakeable belief that it is wrong, that laws are in force banning it, and that these laws are almost universally enforced?

In one sense, it would be strange indeed if we, at this precise moment in time, achieved what has eluded all our philosophical forerunners, that is, an agreed set of universal, content-full ethical principles.

REFERENCES

Andorno, R. 2002. "Biomedicine and International Human Rights Law: In Search of a Global Consensus." *Bulletin of the World Health Organization* 80: 959–63.

Audi, R., and N. Wolterstorff. 1997. *Religion in the Public Square*. Lanham, MD: Rowman & Littlefield.

Beauchamp, T., and J. Childress. 2009. *Principles of Biomedical Ethics*, sixth ed. New York: Oxford University Press.

Daniels, N. 2008. "Reflective Equilibrium." In *The Stanford Encyclopedia of Philosophy*, Fall 2008 ed., edited by Edward N. Zalta. Published April 28, 2003. http://plato.stanford.edu/archives/fall2008/entries/reflective-equilibrium/.

Faunce, T. A. 2005. "Will International Human Rights Subsume Medical Ethics? Intersections in the UNESCO Universal Bioethics Declaration." *Journal of Medical Ethics* 31: 173–78.

Harris, J. 2003. "Consent and End of Life Decisions." *Journal of Medical Ethics* 29: 10–15.

Holm, S. 2009. "Global Concerns and Local Arguments: How a Localized Bioethics May Perpetuate Injustice." In *The Philosophy of Public Health*, edited by A. Dawson, 63–72. Farnham: Ashgate.

Kant, I. 1985. *Fundamental Principles of the Metaphysics of Morals*. Translated by Thomas Kingsmill Abbott. http://en.wikisource.org/wiki/Groundwork_of_the_Metaphysics_of_Morals.

Luther, E. 1986. *Ethik in der Medizin*. Halle: Martin Luther Universität.

Macklin, R. 1998. *Against Relativism: Cultural Diversity and the Search for Ethical Universals in Medicine*. New York: Oxford University Press.

Mann, J. M. 1997. "Medicine and Public Health, Ethics and Human Rights." *The Hastings Center Report* 27, no. 3: 6–13.

Rawls, J. 1996. *Political Liberalism (With a New Introduction and the "Reply to Habermas")*. New York: Columbia University Press.

NOTES

1. Professor Søren Holm, Centre for Social Ethics and Policy, School of Law, University of Manchester & Centre for Medical Ethics, University of Oslo.

2. The good-faith requirement is necessary, but, unfortunately, often absent from real-life moral discourse where participants often expect other people to change their views without themselves being willing to change.

3. We will here sidestep the issue of trying to define *religion* or *religious*.

4. Without necessarily assuming foundationalism.

5. In reality, we know that reaching agreement on the scope of the person concept at the beginning and end of life is highly contentious.

6. This is, of course, a quite general problem in ethics.

7. I here assume that there is more than one fundamental moral principle, although that is, of course, disputed.

8. As did Laskey et al. themselves if they thought that their actions were protected.

Part I Discussion Topics

Wanda Teays

1. If we think about international and cross-cultural issues in medicine, health care, public health, and biomedical research, we need to consider what is important for a global bioethics.
   - How can we bring in a range of voices and concerns to address injustice in health care?
   - What kinds of changes should occur in the training of doctors, nurses, and other caregivers to be more inclusive of different ethnicities and socioeconomic groups?

2. In chapter 1, Bernard Gert sets out the following moral rules that he thinks are universal: (1) Do not kill, (2) do not deceive, (3) do not cause pain, (4) keep your promises, (5) do not disable, (6) do not cheat, (7) do not deprive of freedom, (8) obey the law, (9) do not deprive of pleasure, and (10) do your duty.
   - What do you think of his list? Would you make any additions or changes?

3. Gert argues that "Duties in [the] everyday sense are not derived from our common morality, but in each society duties develop from social roles and from the history and practice of the professions in that society." This statement ties "duty" to social roles (which affect individuals) and professional roles (for medical personnel, researchers, etc.).
   - Are there any other things that shape our sense of duty?

4. In chapter 2, on universal morality, Tom Beauchamp notes: "True cultural relativists . . . subscribe to the thesis that no moral principles of any sort, general or particular, are valid independent of the cultural contexts in which they have arisen and shaped to their present form." Consider this: when there are language barriers, we turn to translators to ensure channels of communication are in place.
   - Should there be something like culture translators to enable better communication in the health care setting? Share your thoughts and offer three to four recommendations as to how this might be achieved.

5. Tom Beauchamp points out that "It is often difficult to determine which group, society, or institution constitutes the culture that should be followed." For example, in pre-Taliban Afghanistan, women were often well educated and worked in professions, but, under the Taliban-imposed culture, they were not allowed to work or seek an education beyond the age of eight. He then asks, "Should we say that women should be governed by either of these conflicting sets of norms?"

   • What do you think?

6. How much truth should doctors and nurses share with patients? To what degree should values and traditions shape truth-telling?

7. The notion of the duty to inform usually focuses on diagnosis. The California case of *Arato v. Avedon* (1993) raised the issue of whether a doctor has to inform the patient of a dire prognosis. Mark A. Rothstein pushes the issue further, arguing that access to information is not as burdensome as it once was. He, thus, asserts that doctors have a duty to notify patients of new medical information. Share your thoughts as to whether we should change doctors' duties to inform, in light of Rothstein's observations:

   > Physicians generally have had no ethical or legal duty to notify patients about new medical information discovered after a visit, notwithstanding the health care benefits to patients that might flow from receiving the information. The rule was based on the relatively high burdens that notification would impose on physicians compared with the likelihood of benefits to patients. This established view, however, no longer may be appropriate in light of new physician-patient relationships and the reduced burden of patient notification using new types of health information technology (HIT).
   >
   >   [As a result, there is a] duty to inform patients and former patients about relevant, medical development subsequent to their episode of care. It concludes by recommending the recognition in ethics and law of a limited, ongoing duty to notify patients of significant information relevant to their health. (Mark A. Rothstein, "Physicians' Duty to Inform Patients of New Medical Discoveries: The Effect of Health Information Technology," *The Journal of Law, Medicine & Ethics* 39, no. 4 (2011)

8. Is there a way to mediate disputes around bioethical issues and, thus, go beyond the traditional debate (or adversarial) model? Not all moral problems have a clear "winner." Offer two or three ideas for constructing or applying a mediation model.

9. How can global bioethics address concerns of ordinary people around the world and not just privilege the views of doctors and researchers?

10. Assuming there is merit to Peter Tagore Tan's view that bioethics *is* environmental ethics, how might this change our response to environmental disasters like Chernobyl and Fukushima (nuclear accidents) and Bhopal (gas catastrophe)?

11. Søren Holm asks whether global bioethics requires a global *moral* language. What do you think? Would that help address cultural or other obstacles we might face?

12. When looking at theoretical perspectives of global health, we also need to consider how we define our terms. Look, for example, at the controversy over the eighteen-year-old Montreal swimmer Victoria Arlen, a Paralympic gold medalist in the 100-meter freestyle. Arlen spent almost two years in a coma and is now confined to a wheelchair. On August 10, 2013, she was disqualified from the Paralympic Swimming World Championships in Montreal due to "insufficient evidence to suggest there was a permanent impairment," according to Craig Spence, the Paralympic committee spokesperson (See Rachel Lau, "Swimmer and Olympic Gold-Medalist Disqualified for Not Being 'Disabled' Enough," *Global News*, August 14, 2013).

   • Share your thoughts on whether Arlen should have been disqualified.
   • Offer a working definition of disability for swimmers in the Paralympics.

Part II

HUMAN RIGHTS

1

Bioethics and Human Rights

A Historical Perspective[1]

Robert Baker

> The sacred rights of Mankind are not to be rummaged for among old parchments or musty records. They are written, as with a sunbeam, in the whole volume of human nature by the hand of Divinity itself, and can never be erased or obscured.
>
> —Alexander Hamilton, 1787[2]

> Philosophers like myself . . . see our task as a matter of making our own culture—the human rights culture—more self-conscious and more powerful.
>
> —Richard Rorty, 1993[3]

Bioethics and human rights were conceived in the aftermath of the Holocaust, when moral outrage reenergized the outmoded concepts of "medical ethics" and "natural rights," renaming them "bioethics," and "human rights" to give them new purpose. Originally, principles of bioethics were a means for protecting human rights, but through a historical accident, bioethical principles came to be considered as fundamental. In this paper I reflect on the parallel development and accidental divorce of bioethics and human rights to urge their reconciliation.

THE 1948 UN DECLARATION:
FROM THE RIGHTS OF MAN TO HUMAN RIGHTS

The immediate precursor to "human rights" are the *droits de l'homme*, the "natural, inalienable, and sacred rights of man" to "liberty, security, property, and resistance to oppression" declared by the French Republic in 1789.[4] The rights, in turn, derive from the God-given inalienable rights to life, liberty, and the pursuit of happiness in the 1776 American Declaration of Independence. Yet, despite this heritage, the rights of man were moribund in the first part of the twentieth century.

All . . . attempts to arrive at a bill of human rights were sponsored by marginal figures—a few international jurists without political experience or professional philanthropists supported by the uncertain sentiments of professional idealists. The groups they formed, the declarations they issued, showed an uncanny similarity in language and composition to that of societies for the prevention of cruelty to animals. No . . . political figure of any importance could possibly take them seriously; and none of the liberal or radical parties in Europe thought it necessary to incorporate into their program a new declaration of human rights.[5]

Individual human rights began to receive attention only after the failure of the system of ethnically based *group* rights negotiated at the end of World War I. One of Woodrow Wilson's war aims had been to "make the world safe for democracy by render [ing] it a secure habitation for the fundamental right of man to be governed by rulers accountable to him."[6] Ethnic groups were to rule themselves.

In the treaties drawn up after World War I, the multinational Austro-Hungarian and Turkish empires, and various Middle Eastern colonies were dissolved and reconstructed as ethnically and religiously cohesive nation-states. This process of nation creation inevitably stranded some ethnic and religious minorities in the new nation-states—Muslims in Europe, Christians in the Middle East, and Jews everywhere. These minorities, however, were recognized and protected in the treaties that created the new nation states.

The nature of "human rights" was left unspecified until the 1948 Universal Declaration of Human Rights. Specification was prompted by the 1947 Nuremberg trials, at which doctors, lawyers, scientists, and soldiers were indicted for "crimes against humanity." The trials taught the world what it meant to strip a human of rights. Shortly after the Nuremberg trials commenced, Eleanor Roosevelt convened a committee to draft a declaration of human rights. Thus Jews in Nazi Germany became surrogates for all humans without rights, and the details revealed daily at Nuremberg gave content to the rights recognized by Articles 4 through 20 of the Declaration.

Articles 4, 5, and 9 prohibited the "slavery or servitude," "arbitrary detention or exile," and "torture, or cruel, inhuman, or degrading treatment or punishment" concurrently on display at Nuremberg. Articles 6, 8, 10, and 11 ensure that never again would Nazi-style laws strip individuals of citizenship: "everyone has a recognition everywhere as a person before the law."

Article 12 prohibits future Crystal Nights, yellow Stars of David, and other stigmatizing actions by protecting individuals' privacy, family, and home against attacks on honor and reputation. Mindful of the Nazi Racial Purity laws and the laws stripping Jews of their nationality and their property, Article 16 declares that everyone has a right to marry freely and to found a family "without any limitations due to race, nationality, or religion."

Article 15 states that everyone has a right to a nationality and Article 17 affirms that everyone has a right to own property. Finally, Article 13 guaranteed that, unlike the Jews of the 1930s and 1940s, victims of human rights abuse would have the right to flee from persecution. Article 14 grants a right of asylum. The Declaration proclaims nine additional rights—rights of participation, rights to social security, rights to education, and so forth—but the first 20 declarations of human rights were designed to prevent anyone from ever undergoing the treatment accorded to the Jews by the Nazis.[7]

The Universal Declaration of Human Rights was shaped, not only by the failure of minority rights and by outrage at the discovery of the Holocaust, but by the need, underlined by the events unfolding at Nuremberg, to make transcultural, transnational, and transtemporal moral and legal judgments. Unlike their precursors, the *droits de l'homme* and the God-given natural rights of Jefferson and Hamilton, human rights *had* to be globally acceptable.

They had to be neutral between all religious and secular worldviews. Individuals might still subscribe to Hamilton's view that rights are "written, as with a sunbeam, in the whole volume of human nature by the hand of Divinity itself," but, in laying claim to universality, the U.N. Declaration abandoned all claims to religious authority.

To protect an individual's right to practice religion, the emerging human rights culture had to be neutral about religion. As philosopher Charles Taylor has observed, "the concept of human rights could travel better if separated from some of its underlying justifications."[8]

THE NUREMBERG CODE AND THE PRINCIPLIST PRECEDENT IN AMERICAN BIOETHICS

The Preamble to the Universal Declaration of Human Rights reminds the world that it originates as a reaction to "barbarous acts which have outraged the conscience of mankind." The same has been said of the Nuremberg Code: it is "impossible to analyze the origins of the Nuremberg Code apart from the historical setting of atrocities and murders committed in Nazi Germany."[9] Like the Declaration, the Code is a post-Holocaust document.

Why did the tribunal need to *invent* a code of ethics to condemn the Nazi researchers? To quote the defense for the Nazi doctors, at that time there was "an almost complete lack of written legal norms"[10] on human-subjects research. There were two notable exceptions: 1931 German Health Ministry regulations and 1946 American Medical Association (AMA) research principles.

The Ministry regulations prohibited research on German *patients* without their informed consent. The AMA principles prohibited research on *persons* without their consent—it thus anticipated the bioethical turn by using the language of principles to expand the traditional protections of medical ethics from "patients" to "persons."[11]

Read literally, however, neither the regulation nor the principle was applicable to the German researchers. Physicians and scientists working at the camps dealt with *inmates*, not with *patients* covered by the German health insurance,[12] and, as *Germans*, they were not answerable to *American* ethics principles. The researchers' conduct thus seemed to elude the scope of extant medical ethical principles, legal standards, and applicable regulations.

To deal with these problems, the prosecution turned to two American physicians: Colonel Leo Alexander, a psychiatrist who had treated concentration camp survivors, and Professor Andrew Ivy, former scientific director of the Naval Medical Research Institute at Bethesda— and the official observer for the AMA. Both argued that unconsented human experimentation was impermissible, appealing to Hippocratic tradition.[13]

Ivy, however, also appealed to the "*laws of humanity* and the *ethical principles* of the medical profession."[14] The expression "laws of humanity" was the language of the Nuremberg indictment; "ethical principles" was the language of the AMA, which had parsed ethics as "principles" since its 1903 "Principles of Medical Ethics."[15] Ivy went further than the AMA, however, by grounding his principles in human rights: "The involved Nazi physicians and scientists ignored . . . ethical principles and rules . . . which are necessary to insure the *human rights* of the individual" (emphasis added).[16] Ivy's conception of ethical principles as mechanisms for protecting human rights circumvents the defense arguments about the time and place at which specific rules were formulated.

Human rights are inviolable irrespective of any principle, rule, or law stating their inviolability. Thus, even if no ethical principle or law accepted in Germany in the 1930s and 1940s was violated, "physicians and scientists whose conduct is contrary to the laws of humanity and human rights . . . should be prosecuted as criminals."[17] For, to reiterate, unlike laws and principles, human rights are inviolable regardless of whether a rule, principle, or law was formulated prohibiting a specific act of violation.

The Nuremberg judges incorporated aspects of both Alexander's and Ivy's testimonies into their judgment condemning the Nazi doctors. They accepted Ivy's principlist discourse but ignored his elegant suggestion that transcultural ethics could be grounded in human rights. Instead, they fabricated a fiction or, if one prefers, a myth.

They claimed that, "*All agree*, that certain *basic principles* must be observed in order to satisfy moral, ethical, and legal concepts." Consequently, they argued, because the Nazi experiments were contrary to "the principles of the law of nations as they result from the usages established among civilized peoples, from the laws of humanity, and from the dictates of public conscience,"[18] the Nazi doctors were guilty of crimes against humanity.

Because the Tribunal grounded its case on the myth of converging civilized opinion, the Nuremberg Code should be regarded conceptually, as well as chronologically, as an artifact of the pre–human rights era. This historical accident is significant because the research ethics decalogue promulgated at Nuremberg was appropriated by the American bioethics movement of the 1970s as a foundational document. Its *universally agreed basic principles* thus set a precedent for the language and justifications offered in American bioethics—and rights discourse was ignored.

THE REBIRTH OF HUMAN RIGHTS AND BIOETHICS IN THE 1970s

It was an accident of history that human rights and the principles of bioethics were reborn in the 1970s in government documents (The Final Declaration of Helsinki, the Belmont Report) in which they were presumed to serve symbolic functions—which is to say, no real function at all.

The Final Declaration of Helsinki was intended to legitimate the Soviet Empire . . . yet, as political theorist Michael Ignatieff notes, the human rights movements legitimated by the Declaration of Helsinki would eventually bring "the Soviet system crashing down."[19] For, unlike its precursor, "minority rights," "human rights" discourse served to unify. Appeals to "minority rights" tended to imply rights for *my* minority, not for yours; by contrast, no one's human rights came at the expense of anyone else's.

By 1966, evidence of the abuse of human subjects was apparent enough to prompt the National Institutes of Health (NIH) to mandate a system of peer review to protect research subjects.[20] In that same year an article published in the *New England Journal of Medicine* by Henry Beecher himself found that 22 research papers published in such leading journals as *JAMA* and the *New England Journal of Medicine* between 1948 and 1965 were morally questionable.[21]

In the absence of substantive guidelines, however, peer review alone did not prevent research abuses. In 1973 Senator Edward Kennedy investigated a study by the U.S. Public Health Service on untreated syphilis in African-American males, which was conducted without their informed consent. The public was outraged, and federal response was swift.

Tuskegee [margin annotation]

On July 12, 1974, President Nixon signed the National Research Act (NRA), forming a National Commission for the Protection of Human Subjects of Biomedical and Behavioral Research to develop substantive rules for protecting the human subjects of federally funded research. In the next four years the National Commission published several reports recommending regulations to protect research subjects. Internationally, there was a parallel move, starting with Helsinki II (Tokyo, 1975).

The most influential report issued by the National Commission concerned *principles*. In 1978, it issued the three-volume *Belmont Report*,[22] in which it asserted that three basic ethical principles should regulate research on human subjects—the principles of respect for persons, beneficence, and justice. Following the Nuremberg precedent, the Commissioners justified these principles in terms of convergence: the principles were deemed binding because "all agreed" that they ought to be binding.[23]

Convergence was a liberating concept. Tom Beauchamp and James Childress were perhaps the first to appreciate this point. In *Principles of Biomedical Ethics* (first published in 1979),[24] they construct bioethics[25] in terms of four "basic" principles—autonomy, beneficence, nonmaleficence, and justice—one more than the three used in the *Belmont Report*. These principles, in turn, are justified by a presumed *convergence* of reflective ethical thought.

By placing convergence at the level of principles, Beauchamp and Childress liberated bioethics from the ethical theories that happened to be in vogue, philosophically. By so doing, it not only unified the ethical analysis of researcher and clinician conduct, it also deprofessionalized medical ethical discourse. Thus, just as human rights discourse could become a public discourse only if freed from conceptions of divine and human nature, so too, bioethics discourse could serve as a public discourse only if freed from conceptions of the medical profession, its nature, and mission.

The new discourses open the domain of diplomats and doctors to ordinary people, who have no professional pretensions whatsoever. Bioethics and human rights are thus kindred democratizing and deprofessionalizing public discourses that transform the ethics of elites into everyday ethics.

BIOETHICS AND HUMAN RIGHTS: SOME PARALLELS

The parallels between bioethics and human rights as concepts, discourses, movements, and fields are striking. Both were conceived out of horror of the Holocaust, both draw strength from the resolve that "never again" would any vulnerable population be treated as the Nazis had treated the Jews, both support respect for persons, both stake claims to universality, both were born in governmental documents that explicitly justify transnational, transtemporal, transcultural moral judgments, both became unfashionable in the era of Cold War realism, both are international, and thus (perhaps not surprisingly) both refer to Helsinki declarations, both were resurrected in the mid-1970s, both are supported by an unusual alliance of governmental and nongovernmental organizations, both became widely disseminated by disassociating themselves from earlier metaphysical and philosophical moorings, and both use a public discourse to democratize the domain of professional elites, although, ironically, both are supported by professional groups who consider themselves expert in the domain of the discourses. Yet, despite these similarities—and even though one of the progenitors of the Nuremberg Code, Andrew Ivy, envisioned principles as mechanisms for protecting human rights—American bioethics has been ill at ease with the idea of human rights.

It is time to reconsider. Pandemics leap from continent to continent, companies peddle their cures around the world, biomedical experiments sponsored in the developed world are conducted in the developing world, and, in all corners of the globe, the new biology foments culture shock. Bioethical issues do not stop for border crossings. Thus we need global bioethics. But the principlism that has served American bioethics so well is too parochial to play on an international stage, and so to meet the challenges of global bioethics, we need to turn to the more cosmopolitan concept of human rights.

Once bioethics enters the international stage, the ideal of converging principles becomes unsustainable. Different cultures embrace different principles and differ in their interpretations of common principles. If principlism is to function internationally, it must be reconceptualized to shed its parochialism.

RECONCILING BIOETHICS WITH HUMAN RIGHTS

It is time to reconsider Ivy's proposal that we construe the principles of international bioethics as mechanisms for protecting human rights. Rights discourse is already the accepted language of international ethics. As members of the United Nations, virtually all the nations on Earth have pledged themselves to accept as "a common standard," that "all human beings are born free and equal in dignity and rights." As philosopher Richard Rorty has observed, ours is already a human-rights culture.

A global bioethics that envisions principles as mechanisms for protecting human rights will thus inherit an internationally accepted ethical discourse.[26] Rights discourse is the best means available for achieving the shared goal of both bioethics and human rights theory: the moral demand that never again will anyone be treated in the manner that Nazis treated Jews.

An international bioethics based on respect for human rights will also be free from the feckless dispute over whose principles are preferable. Principles are preferable insofar as they effectively protect human rights. Because effectiveness is partially a function of cultural experience, different societies may properly employ different principles—respect for persons, respect for families, solidarity—insofar as they effectively protect human rights in the culture in question. The proposed reconciliation of human rights and bioethics thus recognizes cultural variation in principles and does not challenge American principlism within its home cultural sphere.

Grounding international bioethics discourse in human rights will not be a panacea. Human rights discourse may be the lingua franca of the international community, but the scope and limits of human rights should properly be subject to intense debate, as should the principles and rules that we create to protect these rights. The depth of the dilemmas that we must address will not dissipate merely because we use a common mode of moral discourse to address them. The transcultural scope of human rights discourse can, however, dissipate problems of moral parochialism.

Each culture has a deeply rooted predilection to treat its own conception of morality, its own moral concepts and principles, as primary. Human rights discourse was designed to be as cosmopolitan and international as the United Nations itself; it permits us to transcend our parochialism and thus to focus on the substance of the profound moral challenges that we face.

ACKNOWLEDGMENTS

I should like to thank Joseph d'Oronzio for inviting me to compare the historical development of bioethics and human rights, thereby providing me with an excuse to engage in an exceptionally illuminating exercise. This paper draws on my earlier work on human rights, which has been enriched by discussions at the International Association of Bioethics (Tokyo), the Hastings Center, New York University, the Mount Sinai Medical Center (especially with Rosamond Rhodes and Stephen Baumrin), and by critiques by Tom Beauchamp and Ruth Macklin.

NOTES

1. *Cambridge Quarterly of Healthcare Ethics* (2001), 10, 241–52. Printed in the USA. Reprinted with permission.

2. A. Hamilton in *Nonsense upon Stilts: Bentham, Burke and Marx on the Rights of Man*, edited by Jeremy Waldron (London: Methuen, 1987), 18.

3. R. Rorty, "Human Rights, Rationality, and Sentimentality," in *On Human Rights: The Oxford Amnesty Lectures*, edited by S. Shute and S. Hurley (New York: Basic Books, 1993), 117.

4. French Assembly, "Declaration of the Rights of Man and the Citizen, 1789," in *Nonsense upon Stilts: Bentham, Burke and Marx on the Rights of Man*, edited by Jeremy Waldron (London: Methuen, 1987), 26.

5. H. Arendt, *The Origins of Totalitarianism* (New York: Meridian Books, 1958), 292.

6. E. Schwelb, *Human Rights and the International Community: The Roots and Growth of the Universal Declaration of Human Rights, 1948–1963* (Chicago: Quadrangle Books, 1964), 24.

7. J. Morsink, *The Universal Declaration of Human Rights: Origins, Drafting, and Intent* (Philadelphia: University of Pennsylvania Press, 1999).

8. C. Taylor, "Conditions of an Unforced Consensus on Human Rights," in *The East Asian Challenge for Human Rights*, edited by J. R. Bauer and D. A. Bell (London and New York: Cambridge University Press, 1999), 126.

9. M. Grodin, "The Historical Origins of the Nuremberg Code," in *The Nazi Doctors and the Nuremberg Code*, edited by G. A. Annas and M. Grodin (London and New York: Oxford University Press, 1992), 135–36.

10. J. Katz, *Experimentation with Human Beings* (New York: Russell Sage Foundation, 1972), 300.

11. The AMA adopted this principle but only in 1946, that is, only at Ivy's insistence and only after the Nazi researchers were indicted.

12. Although this point was not raised at the trial, Gypsies, Jews, and homosexuals had been stripped of German citizenship and were considered *Untermenschen*, subhumans, and thus were not protected by regulations covering *Menschen*, humans. For the 1931 regulations in English and German, see H. M. Sass, "Reichrundschreiben 1931: Pre-Nuremberg German Regulations Concerning New Therapy and Human Experimentation," *The Journal of Medicine and Philosophy* 8 (1983): 104–9.

13. L. Alexander, "Ethics of Human Experimentation," *Psychiatric Journal of the University of Ottawa*, 1 (1976): 40–6. See also Grodin, "The Historical Origins of the Nuremberg Code."

14. M. Grodin, ed., *The Nazi Doctors and the Nuremberg Code* (London and New York: Oxford University Press, 1992), 134–35.

15. A. C. Ivy, "Report on War Crimes of a Medical Nature Committed in Germany and Elsewhere on German Nationals and the Nationals of Occupied Countries by the Nazi Regime during World War II," Document JC 9218, American Medical Association Archives, 1946: 9.

16. American Medical Association, "Principles of Medical Ethics (1903)," in *The American Medical Ethics Revolution*, edited by R. Baker, A. Caplan, E. Emanuel, and S. Latham (Baltimore: Johns Hopkins Press, 1999).

17. Ivy, "Report on War Crimes of a Medical Nature," 11.

18. Ibid., 13–14.

19. Katz, *Experimentation with Human Beings*, 305.

20. M. Ignatieff, "Human Rights: The Midlife Crisis," *The New York Review of Books* 46 (1999): 59.

21. W. J. Curran, "Governmental Regulation of the Use of Human Subjects in Medical Research: The Approach of Two Federal Agencies," *Daedalus* 92 (1969): 576–78.

22. H. Beecher, "Ethics and Clinical Research, *New England Journal of Medicine* 274 (1966): 1354–60; National Commission for the Protection of Human Subjects of Biomedical and Behavioral Research, *The Belmont Report* (Washington, DC, 1978).

23. For a detailed critique of the convergence justification and replies, see R. Baker, "Multiculturalism, Postmodernism, and the Bankruptcy of Fundamentalism," *Kennedy Institute of Ethics Journal* 8 (1998): 210–31; R. Baker, "A Theory of International Bioethics," *Kennedy Institute of Ethics Journal* 8 (1998): 233–74; R. Baker, "Negotiating International Bioethics: A Response to Tom Beauchamp and Ruth Macklin," *Kennedy Institute of Ethics Journal* 8 (1998): 423–55; T. L. Beauchamp, "The Mettle of Moral Fundamentalism: A Reply to Robert Baker," *Kennedy Institute of Ethics Journal* 8 (1998): 423–55; R. Macklin, "A Defense of Fundamental Principles and Human Rights: A Reply to Robert Baker," *Kennedy Institute of Ethics Journal* 8 (1998): 403–22.

24. T. L. Beauchamp and J. F. Childress, *Principles of Biomedical Ethics* (London and New York: Oxford University Press, 1979, 1983, 1989, 1994).

25. Ironically, Beauchamp and Childress tend to avoid the term *bioethics*. The term was coined in the early 1970s perhaps by Sargent Shriver, or by André Hellegers, or by Van Rensselaer Potter. It achieved canonical status when the Library of Congress entered it as a subject heading, citing as its authority an article, "Bioethics as a Discipline," published by Daniel Callahan in the first volume of the *Hastings Center Report*. Callahan can thus also be credited with coining the term. See A. R. Jonsen, *The Birth of Bioethics* (London and New York: Oxford University Press, 1998), 26–27; and W. T. Reich, "The Word 'Bioethics': The Struggle for Its Earliest Meanings," *Kennedy Institute of Ethics Journal* 4 (1994): 319–36; 5 (1995): 19–34.

26. Transnational medical ethics has already done this: thus, the Preamble to the Convention for the Protection of Human Rights and Dignity of the Human Being with Regard to the Application of Biology and Medicine: Convention on Human Rights and Biomedicine, adopted by Council of Europe in 1997, the term "rights" or "human rights" appears eight times—no mention is made of "principles." "Convention for Protection of Human Rights and Dignity of the Human Being with Regard to the Application of Biology and Biomedicine: Convention on Human Rights and Biomedicine," *Kennedy Institute of Ethics Journal* 7 (1996): 277–90.

2

Boundaries of Torture[1]

Wanda Teays

ABSTRACT

In this chapter I look at the boundaries of torture and the ethical issues they bring to light. I employ Nel Noddings' notion of three components of evil as a framework of analysis. Each one is applied to torture—recognizing prohibitions set out by the UN Convention Against Torture in 1984. One change over the years has been the increasing use of abusive practices that leave no scars or other physical evidence. Examples are sleep deprivation, isolation, threats to family members, and forced standing. For perpetrators, such tactics offer significant advantages.

We will consider how things can escalate and lead to further abuse. This is referred to as "force drift." In conjunction, I examine two dimensions of pain—physical and mental pain. An instance of the latter is a "mind virus," where victims are made to feel responsible for their maltreatment. To complicate the matter, clustering techniques may be put to use, thereby ratcheting up the suffering. Another concern is the role language has played in allowing inhumane tactics to be authorized. For example, replacing the term "prisoner" with "detainee" stripped away a host of protections and left "detainees" vulnerable to all sorts of mistreatment.

> The therapeutic mission is the profession's primary role and the core of physicians' professional identity. If this mission and identity are to be preserved, there are some things doctors must not do.
>
> —M. Gregg Bloche and Jonathan H. Marks

INTRODUCTION

Nel Noddings characterizes evil as having three components—pain, separation, and helplessness (1989, 95 and 118). This provides us with a useful framework to approach torture. We tend to think of torture in terms of pain, with the infliction of severe pain as an indicator of torturous acts. That being the case, let's first consider forms of torture having a physical component and then turn to other forms, such as mental and/or psychological.

Torture can have both physical and mental aspects in terms of the experience of pain. That both physical and mental suffering are aspects of torture is acknowledged by the UN Convention against Torture and Other Forms of Cruel, Inhuman or Degrading Treatment or Punishment, which was instituted in 1984. We see this in the following definition:

> For the purposes of this Convention, the term "torture" means any act by which severe pain or suffering, whether physical or mental, is intentionally inflicted on a person for such purposes as obtaining from him or a third person information or a confession, punishing him for an act he or a third person has committed or is suspected of having committed, or intimidating or coercing him or a third person, or for any reason based on discrimination of any kind, when such pain or suffering is inflicted by or at the instigation of or with the consent or acquiescence of a public official or other person acting in an official capacity. (Adams, Balfour and Reed 2006, 684)

Note also Article 3 of UN Resolution 37:

> It is a gross contravention of medical ethics, as well as an offense under applicable international instruments, for health personnel, particularly physicians, to engage, actively or passively, in acts which constitute participation in, complicity in, incitement to or attempts to commit torture or other cruel, inhuman or degrading treatment or punishment.

WHERE DO WE FIND TORTURE? AND BY WHOM?

There are many settings in which torture takes place. Most of the examples in this chapter focus on the degradation and abuse of detainees. However, brutality is across a wider spectrum and doctors are in the thick of it. The participation of medical personnel is not merely the result of dual loyalties in which they are torn between their professional duties and those related to combating terrorism. For some, acts born of patriotism take precedence—and the consequences leave a lot to be desired.

For example, Journalist Sophie Arie (2011) reports that, "In Italy, doctors and nurses at the prison where G8 protesters were detained in 2001 have been accused of suturing some detainees without anesthesia, leaving them undressed for long periods of time, and hitting and beating them." It's hard to fathom medical professionals exhibiting such callousness and tossing their fiduciary duties to the wind. Such actions reveal a moral failure.

THE INFLICTION OF PAIN

With this greater picture in mind, let's turn to the infliction of pain in acts of torture. The range of cases illustrates the sorts of pain that torture can cause. On one end of the spectrum is the physical aspect of pain—physical torture—that can spin out of control and escalate. At the other end is the mental aspect of pain—psychological torture—that can cause long-lasting effects, such as PTSD.

First, keep in mind the scope of the problem and the extent to which health professionals are involved. It's not just one country or an assortment of yahoos tossing their ethics to the wind. According to Dan Agin, the British had doctors present at interrogations of IRA members in the 1970s. The French used physicians to assist in the interrogations during the war with Algeria. And so on. Agin points out that, "The list is long, and now history will add Americans of the early 21st century as a people who tortured prisoners. History has put blood on our hands" (2009).

We shouldn't look for monsters in the collection of perpetrators and enablers. The list of physical and mental torture is certainly long, as is the list of those who put them to use. Torture and degrading treatment are not just committed by those with a tenuous hold on morality. Perfectly "normal" citizens and groups of individuals consider torture a viable option.

One reason for the assumption that torture is worthwhile is the view that, if you inflict enough pain, torture works. Evidence does not support this belief. Nevertheless, the popular view is that even the most stalwart individual can be broken and, therefore, torture should be a viable option. That reality means we need to cast a wide net in assessing culpability.

We see, for instance, the excesses of "civilized" countries like Britain. Speaking of British torture techniques, David Ignatius (2005) asserts that:

> The British put hoods on their IRA prisoners, just as U.S. interrogators have done in Iraq. The British approved other, harsher methods: depriving IRA prisoners of sleep, making them lean against a wall for long periods, using "white noise" that would confuse them.
>
> The clincher for British interrogators was mock execution. The preferred method in the mid-1970s was to take hooded IRA prisoners up in helicopters over the lakes near Belfast and threaten to throw them out if they didn't talk. Sometimes, they actually were thrown out. The prisoners didn't know that the helicopter was only a few yards above the water.

THE "FIVE TECHNIQUES"

In 1972, following an investigation into the treatment of prisoners in Northern Ireland, then-Prime Minister Edward Heath banned the use of hooding, white noise, sleep deprivation, food deprivation and painful stress positions—known as the "five techniques" (British Broadcasting Corporation 2011). His action made it clear that a line had been crossed and it was time to put an end to these practices.

The "five techniques" found a modified version in acceptable tactics on the part of the U.S. For example, the Department of Defense considered the following interrogation techniques to be humane and legally permissible: "isolation for more than 5 months, sleep deprivation lasting 48 to 54 days during which interrogation took place 18 to 20 hours per day, degradation, sexual humiliation, military dogs to instill fear, and exposure to extremes of heat and cold and loud noise for long periods and combinations of these techniques" (Justo 2006, 1462). Unfortunately, the criteria for judging this "humane" by the Department of Defense was not made public.

THE DOMAIN OF PAIN: TORTURE ON THE PHYSICAL PLANE

The range of torture involving physical pain includes "walling," where the victim's head is slammed into a wall, beatings, sexual assault, being hung by the wrists from the ceiling, short shackling, hypothermia, and bodily injury. In addition to "physical roughing up; sensory, food, and sleep deprivation," detainees were also subjected to a water pit in which they had to stand on tiptoe to keep from drowning (Savage 2004).

There has also been the use of waterboarding (simulated drowning) on high-profile suspects. In many cases (e.g., at Guantanamo Bay), hunger-striking detainees were force-fed and/or subjected to "rectal hydration," both of which cause physical pain and mental distress—and typically involve the participation of health professionals.

Human Rights Watch (2000) cites a recent case of torture from Chechnya in 2000:

> From the time they entered the Chernokozovo facility, when Russian guards would force them to run a gauntlet of guards who would beat them mercilessly, through their stay in cramped and sordid conditions, to the time they were released, detainees had no relief from torment. Fearing identification and possible future retribution, Russian soldiers in Chechnya frequently wore camouflage uniforms with no division patches or pins that would identify them.
>
> Human Rights Watch calls for a full investigation by the Russian authorities of what happened at Chernokozovo in January and February 2000, for those responsible for human rights violations committed there to be brought to justice, and for compensation to be granted to victims or their relatives.

Furthermore, the fact the guards abusing the detainees in Chechnya sought to obscure—hide—their identity from their victims makes it clear that they knew what they were doing and that it was wrong.

THE USE OF MENTAL AND PSYCHOLOGICAL ABUSE

Physical torment is a central concern. So, too, is mental and psychological suffering. Examples of torture involving mental pain are environmental manipulation such as 24 hour lighting or darkness, piercingly loud music, solitary confinement or being confined to a box, and threats to family members. In addition, the exploitation of phobias (e.g., fear of vermin) contributes to the victim's level of distress. That reality did not prevent doctors from enabling such a practice.

Medical historian Giovanni Maio (2001) observes that methods of torture have changed by expanding the types of mental abuse that are used:

> Traditional methods mainly used physical pain, whereas modern torture also involves psychiatric-pharmacological and psychological techniques. Brainwashing is the oldest form of psychological torture; other methods include further deprivation (e.g., sleep deprivation), apparent execution, isolation, dark cells, personal threats, and forced observation of others being tortured.
>
> These techniques are used often because they leave no visible evidence of torture; torture today must be impossible to prove, which would not be possible without medical skills.

The Senate Committee Report on Torture (2014) discusses the use of sleep deprivation that, as Maio states, is now "used often." This is because it does not leave marks and certainly would be experienced as disorienting and extraordinarily stressful. As noted by the Senate Intelligence Committee on Torture (2014):

> Sleep deprivation involved keeping detainees awake for up to 180 hours, usually standing or in stress positions, at times with their hands shackled above their heads. At least five detainees experienced disturbing hallucinations during prolonged sleep deprivation and, in at least two of those cases, the CIA nonetheless continued the sleep deprivation. . . . CIA medical personnel treated at least one detainee for swelling in order to allow the continued use of standing sleep deprivation.

In addition, the Inspector General's report describes several forms of abuse not previously reported that, from a medical and legal perspective, constitute torture (Physicians for Human Rights 2009). These include: (1) mock executions and threatening detainees by brandishing handguns and power drills; (2) threatening harm to family members, including sexual assault of females and murder of the detainee's children; and (3) physical abuse, including applying pressure to the side of a detainee's neck resulting in near loss of consciousness (Physicians for Human Rights 2009).

JUSTIFYING TORTURE WITH HYPOTHETICALS

We may wonder why such harsh practices are seen as justifiable. The commonly cited argument for employing torture is nuclear terrorism; namely, that there is the equivalent of a "ticking bomb" set to go off in some large metropolitan area such as Paris or New York City and time is not on our side.

Members of the pro-torture faction, including such luminaries as Supreme Court Justice Antonin Scalia and US president Trump, think this justifies lifting the restraints against torture. That the hypothetical scenario is merely speculative is not given much weight. Journalist/editor Matt Ford (2014) explained in *The Atlantic* that,

> The Senate torture report shows how detached this hypothetical scenario is from reality. In the real world, CIA personnel tortured hundreds of detainees, including ones who committed no crimes. CIA officers and contractors waterboarded detainees, in some cases hundreds of times. CIA medical personnel flooded their orifices with nutrients via plastic tubes for "behavior control." CIA officials denied detainees access to sanitary facilities and forced them to use diapers for humiliation.
>
> They forced detainees to stand on broken ankles. They subjected one to sleep deprivation for 56 hours until he could barely speak and was "visibly shaken by his hallucinations depicting dogs mauling and killing his sons and family." They threatened to murder detainees' children and sexually assault their mothers. They used the taped cries of an "intellectually challenged" detainee to coerce family members. They even shackled one detainee named Gul Rahman, naked, to a concrete floor in a "stress position," where he died of hypothermia. (Ford 2014)

No time bomb ticked as this happened, as Ford points out.

THE SLIPPERY SLOPE OF "FORCE DRIFT"

Consider the physical aspects of pain. When looking at torture, Wisnewski and Emerick (2009) observe that the use of force can easily escalate, making it difficult to control. This is the point where "force drift" comes into play and an interrogator can "slide" into coercion. Attributing the term to psychologist Michael Gelles, they explain how it evolves:

> [The] tendency to slide into coercion was documented by Dr. Michael Gelles, the chief psychologist at the Naval criminal investigation service. Dr. Gelles warned his superiors of what he called a 'force drift': a natural inclination "to uncontrolled abuse when interrogators encounter resistance."
>
> He further warned that, "once the initial barrier against the use of force had been breached, 'force drift' would almost certainly begin. . . . And if left unchecked, force levels including torture, could be reached" (2009, 110).

PUTTING "FORCE DRIFT" TO WORK

One factor contributing to the loss of control in "force drift" is the objectification and dehumanization of the other. Acts of coercion and brutality are more likely to occur when there is a power differential between those involved. And when the victim has a lesser moral status, as with so-called unlawful or unprivileged combatants, it's even harder to stop the slide into abuse. Visions of mob violence come to mind, in that normal inhibitions get swept aside.

Humanities professor Colin Dayan points out the consequences; namely, "Once stigmatized categories are created, whether they are labeled 'security threat groups' or 'illegal enemy combatants,' torture can be administered readily by those in power" (2007, 57).

Here's where categorizing others as "enemies" opens the door on abuse and mistreatment. The dehumanization of our enemies can swiftly lead to disrespect and degradation. In short, the "enemy" merits few protections. With that, notions of non-maleficence and beneficence are made inoperable.

MENTAL PAIN AND TORTURE

Another dimension of pain involves the mental or psychological aspects. Long after the physical scars have faded and the pain has been relegated to past memories (or nightmares), there may still be long-term effects. Such effects become more apparent as time goes on.

For example, in 2016, the *New York Times* investigated the mental pain of torture of suspects who were rounded up after the 9/11 attacks. They found that psychological and emotional scars haunted the men because of the interrogations at secret C.I.A. "Black Sites" and at Guantanamo Bay. On October 21, 2016, the editorial board asserted that,

> A disturbingly high number of these men were innocent, or were low-level fighters who posed so little threat that they were eventually released without charge. Yet despite assurances from lawyers in the Department of Justice that "enhanced interrogation techniques" should have no negative long-term effects, *The Times* found that many of the men still suffer from paranoia, psychosis, depression and post-traumatic stress disorder related to their abuse. They have flashbacks, nightmares and debilitating panic attacks. Some cannot work, go outside, or speak to their families about what they went through.

The U.S. Senate Report shows us how bizarre this can be, in detailing the interrogation of Ridha al-Najjar (2014, 60). He was held at the CIA "Black Site" Cobalt outside of Kabul, Afghanistan, where the mental aspects of his torture were exploited.

The conditions were horrific: in the regular cells, James Wilkinson (2017) reports, they were shackled to a metal ring in the wall, and given a bucket to use as a toilet. In the sleep deprivation cells they were shackled by their hands to the ceiling, and made to defecate in diapers. When diapers were not available, they stood bare from the waist down, or defecated into makeshift diapers created using duct tape. The cells were unheated, and subjected to blaring music.

The U.S. Senate Report on Torture (2014) details al-Najjar's treatment and reveals how vicious were the conditions used to break him—which they succeeded in doing.

> The CIA discussed its interrogation strategy of al-Najjar during June and July [2002]. . . . One cable, dated 16 July 2002, was sent to the CIA Station in Country [redacted], "suggesting possible interrogation techniques to use against Ridha al-Najjar, including: utilizing 'Najjar's fear for the

well-being of his family to our benefit'. . . using 'vague threats' to create a 'mind virus'; that would cause al-Najjar to believe that his situation would continue to get worse . . . manipulating Ridha al-Najjar's environment using a hood, restraints, and music; and employing sleep deprivation through the use of round-the-clock interrogations."

By 26 July 2002, CIA officers were proposing "breaking Najjar" through the use of "isolation, sound disorientation techniques, sense of time deprivation, limited light, cold temperatures, sleep deprivation" (2014, 60).

The report goes on to say that the CIA's interrogation plan for al-Najjar included for the use of "loud music, worse food, sleep deprivation and hooding." In addition,

al-Najjar was tortured throughout August and September 2002, and by 21 September one CIA cable was clear that he was now "clearly a broken man" and "on the verge of complete breakdown" as a result of isolation. Indeed, al-Najjar was now "willing to do whatever the CIA officer asked" (The Rendition Project).

A second example of the mental aspects of physical torture is the case of Mohamed Ben Soud, who was detained by the CIA in Afghanistan. According to a *New York Times* report by Sheri Fink and James Risen (2017), he was subjected to being locked in small boxes, slammed against a wall and doused with buckets of ice water while naked and shackled. The consequences of this abuse are significant, as the following indicates:

He said he still suffered from nightmares, fear, mood swings and other psychological injuries as a result of his captivity. "It comes to me during my sleep and as if I'm still imprisoned in that horrible place and still shackled," he said in his deposition, through a translator. "I get the feeling of worry about my future and about the fear that this could happen again." (Fink and Risen 2017)

Self-inflicted fear and other kinds of distress, as shown with both al-Najjar and Ben Soud, can be mentally debilitating and cause significant harm. We see this with the use of psychological manipulation via the "mind virus."

EMPLOYING A "MIND VIRUS"

Mike Doherty (2015) had the opportunity to interview an ex-CIA interrogator. He spoke of the way mental suffering was put to use when questioning (and trying to break) a suspect. To achieve that goal he employed a "mind virus." He explains:

We capitalize on certain psychological techniques that aren't related to personal threat. Let's say for example you walk in the office tomorrow, and one of your co-workers comes running up to you and says, "The boss wants to see you right away." . . . Do you immediately think, "Today's a great day. I'm going to get promoted"? Probably that's not our thought process. The message you have received has planted what behaviorists would term a "mind virus." We don't know whether or not that would create fear or uncertainty—we don't know where that virus is going in your mind. . . . It's fear that's self-inflicted. (2015)

He acknowledges that this procedure is not always productive. "Mind viruses can be misused," he says, "so if you're in custody and I walk in, and all of a sudden I pull out a Glock 9mm and set it on top of the desk, that's the mind virus, right? But that's not the way to do it. That's the wrong message. We believe that's counterproductive" (Doherty 2015).

In the case of mental aspects of pain from torture, victims may feel responsible for their suffering—their "mind virus"—as if they have some control over its effects. This can get exploited. We see this in the CIA manual recommending that the subject be manipulated into blaming themselves for their suffering.

For example, when a detainee is told, "You leave me no other choice but to . . ." the victim may interpret "You leave me" as something they're in control of (Wisnewski and Emerick 2009, 111). This is quite different from being told "Comply or else," where no options are presented to them. Blaming yourself for being harmed by another can cause long-lasting posttraumatic stress. This makes it a powerful tool and quite useful in establishing control of the victim.

MAKING VICTIMS FEEL RESPONSIBLE FOR THEIR PAIN

Historian Alfred McCoy discusses how people can be manipulated into feeling responsible for their mistreatment. He says,

> Once the subject is disoriented, interrogators can then move on to the stage of self-inflicted pain through techniques such as enforced standing with arms extended. . . . In this latter phase, victims are made to feel responsible for their own suffering, thus inducing them to alleviate their agony by capitulating to the power of their interrogators. (Wisnewski and Emerick 2009, 114–15)

Offering options to detainees so they feel responsible for their own pain and stress can take absurd turns. Consider the choices offered in force-feeding. Colin Dayan observes that:

> Talking to a group of reporters about the chair to which detainees were strapped during the insertion of the feeding tubes, General John Craddock, the head of the United States Southern Command, said, "it's not like 'The Chair.' It's pretty comfortable; it's not abusive. He explained how his soldiers gave detainees a choice of colors for feeding tubes–yellow, clear, and beige—adding, "They like the yellow." (2007, 74–75)

Being able to choose the color of your straw for force-feeding is like getting to pick the belt you are going to be beaten with. In any case, by bringing the victim into the decision-making, the blame for the abuse gets spread wider. One result is this strengthens the mental component of torture.

CLUSTERING: COMBINING METHODS OF ABUSE

The Senate Report on Torture also confirms the theory of a "slippery slope" in interrogation settings, namely, that torture by its very nature escalates in the severity and frequency of its use beyond the approved techniques.

This raises two key points. First, while the techniques are evaluated individually, these techniques were designed to be used in combination, thus enhancing pain and disorientation. This is a game-changer in terms of the effects on the victim of clustered techniques.

Second, to comprehend the severity of the effects of these techniques, it is essential to consider the context of their use. In terms of both long and short-term psychological effects, there is no meaningful equivalence between waterboarding when used in SERE (Survival

Evasion Resistance Escape) training of soldiers who volunteered and consented to the procedure and who trusted the interrogator to protect their safety, and waterboarding a high-value detainee in a setting where the victim fears for his life (PHR 2009, 1). The two situations have little in common in terms of the psychological component.

HOW DOES LANGUAGE FIGURE IN?

Luis Justo (2006) asserts that we need to discuss the "philosophy of torture" (if such a concept exists). This calls for an examination of the various terms of the debate, including ones that obscure or trivialize the pain of torture.

The use of euphemisms such as "enhanced interrogation" to describe torture should be discredited, Justo recommends, since it contributes to public mystification (2006, 1463). With that mystification comes a reluctance to see how much brutality has become tolerable. Furthermore, such "public mystification" entails using or creating terms that have no ready reference to previous uses of language. If a phrase like "enhanced interrogation" can replace "torture," then concerns are less likely to be raised and there's less chance for condemnation—or public outrage.

TWISTING LANGUAGE

As we have seen, the term "prisoners" has generally been replaced by "detainees" to allow fewer protections in the war on terror. "Detainees" are not considered protected by the Geneva Conventions or international ethical codes and treaties. Consequently, "detainees" lack the moral status accorded "prisoners," setting the stage for actions and policies that makes them vulnerable to mistreatment.

The low moral status of detainees relative to that of prisoners was sealed by a linguistic fiat, drawing a sharp distinction between the two groups. This is borne out by the rejection of the Geneva Conventions' guideline requiring the prompt registration of prisoners. That has not been perceived as binding in the case of detainees. Basically, those who are not prisoners do not merit the same treatment; thus their vulnerability.

Once this distinction is in place, attention then could turn to what is allowable treatment. What was prohibited in interrogating "prisoners" was not seen as applicable to "detainees." Even citizenship cannot save a terrorist suspect from being swept up into the class of "detainees" and having but a tenuous moral status. Look, for instance, at the treatment of John Walker Lindh and Jose Padilla, both American citizens. The abuse they experienced indicates how easily human rights can be thrust aside.

We see this also with innocent individuals like Khaled el-Masri. On December 31, 2003, el-Masri was on a tourist bus headed for a vacation at the Macedonian capital, Skopje. At the border stop he was held back and hauled off the bus.

> He said that after being kidnapped by the Macedonian authorities at the border, he was turned over to officials he believed were from the United States. He said they flew him to a prison in Afghanistan, where he said he was shackled, beaten repeatedly, photographed nude, injected with drugs and questioned by interrogators about what they insisted were his ties to Al Qaeda. (Van Natta Jr. and Mekhennet 2005)

All too often the haste to apprehend potential terrorists overrides any presumption of innocence until they are charged with a crime, much less proven guilty. El-Masri has not been able to seek legal remedies, because the U.S. government successfully invoked a "state secrets" privilege (Goldberg 2009).

AND THEN IT'S ALL COUCHED IN SECRECY

Unfortunately there has been a great deal of secrecy about policies that have been instituted and actions that have been taken. One of the most disturbing aspects of secrecy is that detainees lack access to the evidence against them. Clearly, it is hard to defend yourself when the charges and evidence have been withheld.

Access to a lawyer is difficult if not impossible, adding to the obstacles facing detainees. And with the fate of an indefinite detention, once a detainee can feel like *always* a detainee, given there may be no end in sight for those stuck there in this situation.

THE IMPACT OF MANIPULATING LANGUAGE

The policies and regulations that inform medical personnel rest, to a great degree, on definitions, categories, connotations and concepts. The connotations of words can play a significant role in shaping policies. Look, for example at "rampage" v. "massacre" v. "act of terrorism", "extremist" v. "terrorist" and "rebel" v. "soldier." The use of language and reshaping of terms carries weight. Our thoughts and policies are guided by the words we use. As a result, employing terms like "detainees" instead of "prisoners" makes all the difference.

Here's where language comes into play: our soldiers are "lawful combatants," whereas "insurgents" are "unlawful combatants" and not bound by the same standards. To add fuel to the fire, the use of such terms as "illegal combatants," "foreign combatants," and "unprivileged enemy combatants" functions as a signal to distinguish the good guys from the bad guys, the enemies. This lays a foundation for the lesser rights accorded "detainees" and makes it easier to slide into abuse.

And so divisions are established. There are five categories that a terrorist suspect can fall into: (1) "Insurgents"—those yet to be captured; (2) "Prisoners"—those charged with a crime and awaiting trial; (3) "Detainees"—those held at a detention center and have neither been charged nor convicted of a crime; (4) Detainees undergoing "rendition," the transport to a country known to allow torture (they are then considered "rendered"); (5) "Ghost detainees" or "Ghost soldiers"—those held without charge at secret detention centers—CIA "Black Sites"—far from the accessibility of the Red Cross or legal counsel. They are said to have undergone "extraordinary rendition."

Detainee attorney Joseph Margulies notes that: "The horror story of the post-9/11 world is that any foreign national anywhere in the world can be plucked from the streets of anywhere, whisked off to another country, never be heard from again and be utterly beyond the reach of the law" (as noted in Teays 2008). That is bad enough. Even worse is the public indifference to the mistreatment—including torture and indefinite detention—of thousands of innocent people caught up in this war on terror.

The dismal status of detainees explains why executive director of the Center on Law and Security at the New York University School of Law, Karen J. Greenberg refers to them as "this nebulous class of persons." The result, she says, is a "new category of person" that has "extricated the United States from the international obligations that have governed the treatment of prisoners in armed conflict since the middle of the nineteenth century." The resulting shift was used to redefine torture; thus allowing coercive interrogation techniques such as waterboarding (2006, xi, as noted in Teays 2011, 72).

THE LANGUAGE GAMES

All the language games need to be examined. Look, for instance, at the *Hamdi vs. Rumsfeld* decision allowing the president to detain an enemy combatant. "How do you make that determination?" wonders Fourth Circuit Judge Diana Motz. "When I call someone an ostrich, I look in the dictionary for a definition. But what did the president look to in determining whether he [Yasser Hamdi] was an enemy combatant?" (as noted by Dahlia Lithwick 2007). Defining such terms is long overdue, as is their free-wheeling application.

Judge Motz isn't the only one questioning the use and misuse of language in order to put desired policies in place. Social anthropologist Tobias Kelly also discusses the language of torture and the difficulties in nailing down the concept. Those difficulties are exacerbated by the lack of transparency regarding policies and actions. "The recognition of torture presents unique challenges," Kelly argues.

> Torture's particular stigma, as one of the most universally recognized violations of human rights, raises the stakes for those states accused of torture. Very few, if any, states willingly admit that they participate in torture. Furthermore, despite its apparent moral absolutism, torture remains a notoriously slippery category to define because its meaning constantly shifts under pressure. . . . Any attempt to recognize torture must therefore overcome serious political, legal, and epistemological hurdles. (2009, 778)

Given all the hurdles around torture, one of the epistemological tasks is to pay heed to the power of labeling, particularly when it is used to dehumanize people, as we find with prisoners and detainees. That power should not be underestimated.

STRATEGIES FOR JUSTIFYING "FORCEFUL"/"ENHANCED" INTERROGATION

It is instructive to get a sense of techniques of abuse that were sanctified at the highest levels. See, for example, the "torture memos" of the Bush administration, the first of which was drafted by John Yoo and supported by White House counsel Alberto Gonzales. Andrew Cohen of *The Atlantic* reports that the memo was sent to "all the key players of the Bush administration" (2012). Evidently, their assumption that the infliction of physical or mental pain has its merits prevented them from declaring such practices off-limits.

In order to justify the use of forceful interrogation techniques, the U.S. Defense Department adopted two strategies to get around the prohibition on torture, notes Werner G. K. Stritzke (2009). The first asserts that the president's authority to manage military operations is uninhibited by international law and that the use of torture in an interrogation is an act of national self-defense and thus may not be violating the prohibition (2009, 31). This effectively disavows the role and power of international law.

The second strategy advocates for a narrow interpretation of what counts as torture. For example, a Defense Department memo argued that the administration of drugs to detainees violates the prohibition on torture *only if* intended to produce "an extreme effect." Similarly, then U.S. Assistant Attorney-General Jay Bybee insisted that, "Torture must be equivalent in intensity to the pain accompanying serious physical injury, such as organ failure, impairment of bodily function, or even death" (Stritzke 2009, 31).

WHAT ARE THE CONSEQUENCES OF SUCH STRATEGIES?

In setting down such restrictions, Bybee effectively narrowed the domain of what counts as torture so only the most egregious acts would qualify. Given the stakes are high with regard to human rights, it should not be surprising that Bybee would be averse to having the term "degrading treatment" applied to an action sanctioned on the part of the government.

Bybee recommended an interpretation of torture emphasizing the *intention* of the interrogator. An individual could only be said to commit torture if they *intended* to do so. "Thus any interrogator who tortured but later claimed that his intention was to gain information rather than inflict pain was not guilty of torture" (Wisnewski and Emerick, 114–15). That means someone could only be thought guilty of torture if they *sought* to harm or maim the other. Therefore, "Threatening death and inflicting pain would be actionable only when the interrogator intended to harm" (Dayan 2007, 68–69). This puts intentions—not actions—at center stage.

Think about this interpretation. Redefining the term shrinks its range of applicability, or so it is claimed. Wisnewski and Emerick note the consequences:

> This new interpretation of torture removes so much moral substance from the term . . . [so only] the category of "dehumanizing, torture" would remain. . . . As a result, the Geneva Conventions were interpreted less and less broadly, and thus their power to guide interrogations was weakened. (2009, 114–15)

Adopting such an approach would have significant repercussions. It would shift culpability from the perpetrators' actions to their mental state. So long as someone wasn't *contemplating* harm they should not be held responsible for their actions. Only if you are determined to—planning to—inflict pain or suffering should you be thought committing torture. Actions should not be labeled "torture" otherwise.

Such a policy would inject a *mens rea* criterion into assessing an act we might otherwise consider torture. The question is how much emphasis should be placed on the state of mind of the perpetrator—or interrogator.

SHAPING PUBLIC CONSCIOUSNESS

Richard Jackson (2007) asserts that officials create morality-defining narratives to shape the public's acceptance of torture. This is accomplished by replacing existing social reality that prohibits torture with a torture-sustaining reality, one resting on new morality-defining narratives. He contends that torture would then be enabled and practiced routinely.

If that were the case, not only would torturers have to be trained, but also the greater society would have to be prepared and, "in a sense, trained to accept that such things go on" (Jackson 2007, 359). A series of power narratives and representations would then be endlessly reproduced until they become accepted as legitimate forms of knowledge and practice (359). Torture then becomes part of our cultural mindset and is then normalized. At that point a moral transformation will have taken place.

Given the power of narratives, we should not overlook the role of language and the media in making torture more palatable. This merits attention, since we are a society in which stories—narratives—have great appeal. We love stories of heroes vanquishing villains, battles quickly won, and enemies defeated. The dehumanization and objectification of "villains" makes their capture and torture less disturbing than if we did not employ such polar extremes in our descriptions. To make those stories accomplish the goal, the use of terms like "unlawful enemy combatants" and "cowards" come into play.

Similarly, the practice of putting hoods on prisoners or blackened goggles, masks, and earmuffs during transit, makes the enemy "faceless," dehumanized (Jackson 2007, 362). It is much easier to inflict pain on the hooded, faceless Other than to look them in the eye and see their expression (and suffering) as they are being brutalized.

Jackson also discusses the power of images and considers the photographs of detainees (as, for instance, from Abu Ghraib) in huge piles of naked bodies as the ultimate indication of degradation. For a moment in time, he says, the "terrorists" ceased to be individuals and their humanity dissolved (2007, 363–64). And so they are at the mercy of their captors.

THE USE OF LANGUAGE: MEDICAL PERSONNEL

Narratives, images, and revised or invented terminology don't just shape the way we think of detainees. The effects have a greater sweep, extending to health professionals as well. Instead of "doctors" or "medical caregivers" we have the militarized term "medically-trained interrogators," as Philosopher Fritz Allhoff calls them. In his view, "The interrogator's primary task is to facilitate the acquisition of information, not to heal" (2008, 101).

Allhoff is not the only one reshaping concepts. Some perceive doctors in interrogations as *combatants* to whom the Hippocratic Oath does not apply (Stephens 2005). This fundamentally changes what would count as doctors' fiduciary duties and dismantle the patient-doctor relationship.

CONCLUSION

We see how this gets played out: bioethicists M. Gregg Bloche and Jonathan H. Marks (2005) assert that evidence reveals that medical personnel shared confidential documents with potential interrogators. In addition, physicians helped design interrogation strategies, including sleep deprivation and other coercive methods tailored to detainees' medical conditions. Medical personnel also coached interrogators on questioning techniques, Fritz Allhoff points out (2006, 393).

A medical degree is not a sacramental vow, contends David Tornberg, Deputy Assistant Secretary of Defense for Health Affairs. "It is a certification of skill." As he sees it, a medical degree becomes a practical diploma carrying no more ethical weight than a plumber's (Koch, 2006, 250).

Not all agree with Tornberg's downgrading of the medical degree to strip it of its moral significance and ignore the professional codes intended as guidance. See, for example, the UN Committee Against Torture (United Nations 2009). However, many recognize the conflicts that can arise when health professionals are put in a key role with patients. This is acknowledged in the Baha Mousa Public Inquiry Report (2011) regarding the brutal death of an Iraqi civilian held by the British Army:

> The report recognizes the problem of "dual loyalty" in which doctors, particularly in conflict situations, are often torn between their patient and their employer. It also identifies legal and military systems that force doctors into situations where they may risk their jobs or put their own lives in danger by refusing to participate or report torture that they have witnessed. (2011)

Journalist Sophie Arie also notes the concern that British doctors working at immigrant detention centers fail to examine properly or report injuries asylum seekers have received before arriving in the UK.

> This can lead not only to their not receiving treatment they need but also to a lack of evidence supporting the case for asylum for those who have been tortured or abused elsewhere. Military doctors have also failed to report signs of abuse in detainees. (Arie, 2011)

The United States faces the same issues regarding the complicity of doctors in abusing detainees, hiding it or failing to report it. The 2004 CIA Inspector General's report confirms that health professionals were involved at every stage in the development, implementation and legitimization of the torture program.

Legal Officer Stephanie Erin Brewer and social psychologist Jean Maria Arrigo (2009) point out that, "Some commanders may simply order medical personnel to place their loyalty to their country over their medical care for a detainee, including trading medical treatment for information during interrogations" (2009, 11).

This is a problem in need of a solution. Health professionals need to meet this head-on and become advocates for change—change rooted in human rights.

REFERENCES

Adams, Guy B., Danny L. Balfour, and George E. Reed. 2006, September-October, "Abu Ghraib, Administrative Evil, and Moral Inversion: The Value of 'Putting Cruelty First,'" *Public Administration Review*, Vol. 66, No. 5, pp. 680-693. Retrieved January 2018.

Agin, Dan. 2009, April 22. "How It Is: Psychiatrists, Physicians, and Torture," *Huffington Post*, https://www.cchrint.org/2009/09/08/the-huffington-post-how-it-is-psychiatrists-physicians-and-torture/. Retrieved 2 January 2018.

Allhoff, Fritz. 2006. "Physician Involvement in Hostile Interrogations," *Cambridge Quarterly of Healthcare Ethics*, Vol. 15, 392–402, http://files.allhoff.org/research/Physician_Involvement_in_Hostile_Interrogations.pdf. Retrieved 1 May 2018.

———. 2008. *Physicians at War: The Dual-Loyalties Challenge*. Springer.

Arie, Sophie. 2011, September 9. "Doctors Need Better Training to Recognise and Report Torture," *British Medical Journal*, http://www.bmj.com/content/343/bmj.d5766. Retrieved 10 June 2018.

Baha Mousa. 2011. *The Report of the Baha Mousa Inquiry*, June 2018.

British Broadcasting Corporation. 2011, September 8. "Baha Mousa Inquiry: 'Serious Discipline Breach' by Army," bbc.com, http://www.bbc.com/news/uk-14825889. Retrieved 10 June 2018.

Bloche, M. Gregg and Jonathan H. Marks. 2005, January 6. "When Doctors Go to War," *New England Journal of Medicine*, 352(1): 3-6. https://www.nejm.org/doi/full/10.1056/NEJM200504073521423. Retrieved 10 June 2018.

Brewer, Stephanie Erin and Jean Maria Arrigo. 2009. "Preliminary Observations Why Health Professionals Fail to Stop Torture in Overseas Counterterrorism Operations," in Ryan Goodman and Mindy Jane Roseman, Eds., *Interrogations, Forced Feedings, and the Role of Health Professionals*. Cambridge, MA: Human Rights Program, Harvard Law School.

Cohen, Andrew. 2012, February 6. "The Torture Memos, 10 Years Later," *The Atlantic*, https://www.theatlantic.com/national/archive/2012/02/the-torture-memos-10-years-later/252439/. Retrieved 30 March 2019.

Dayan, Colin. 2007. *The Story of Cruel and Unusual*. Cambridge, MA: The MIT Press.

Doherty, Mike. 2015, April 23. "A Former CIA Officer Explains How to Apply Interrogation Techniques to Everyday Life," *Vice*, https://www.vice.com/en_us/article/4wbygn/three-former-cia-officers-want-to-help-you-apply-interrogation-techniques-to-everyday-life-113. Retrieved 10 June 2018.

Editorial Board, The New York Times. 2016, October 21. "Torture and Its Psychological Aftermath," *The New York Times*, https://www.nytimes.com/2016/10/21/opinion/torture-and-its-psychological-aftermath.html21 October 2016. Retrieved 10 June 2018.

Fink, Sheri and James Risen. 2017, June 20. "Psychologists Open a Window on Brutal CIA Interrogations." *The New York Times*, https://www.nytimes.com/interactive/2017/06/20/us/cia-torture.html. Retrieved 10 June 2018.

Ford, Matt. 2014, December 13. "Antonin Scalia's Case for Torture," *The Atlantic*, https://www.theatlantic.com/politics/archive/2014/12/antonin-scalias-case-for-torture/383730/. Retrieved 10 June 2018.

Goldberg, Nicholas. 2009, February 15. "'State Secrets' on Trial," *The Los Angeles Times*, https://www.latimes.com/la-oe-secrets15-2009feb15-story.html. Retrieved 10 June 2018.

Greenberg, Karen J. 2006. *The Torture Debate in America*. Cambridge, MA: Cambridge University Press.

Human Rights Watch. 2000, October, "Welcome to Hell: Arbitrary Detention, Torture, and Extortion in Chechnya—The Chernokozovo Detention Center," *Human Rights Watch Report*, https://www.hrw.org/reports/2000/russia_chechnya4/detention-center.htm. Retrieved 10 June 2018.

Ignatius, David. 2005, December 16. "Stepping Back from Torture," *The Washington Post*, http://www.washingtonpost.com/wp-dyn/content/article/2005/12/15/AR2005121501438_Comments.html. Retrieved 10 June 2018.

Jackson, Richard. 2007, July. "Language, Policy and the Construction of a Torture Culture in the War on Terrorism," *Review of International Studies*, Vol. 33, Issue 3, pp. 353-371, https://www.cambridge.org/core/journals/review-of-international-studies/article/language-policy-and-the-construction-of-a-torture-culture-in-the-war-on-terrorism/5006D871A4E5550BE5EBA0F10CCEDACF. Retrieved 10 June 2018.

Justo, Luis. 2006, June 24, "Doctors, Interrogation, and Torture," *British Medical Journal*, Vol. 332, No. 7556, pp. 1462–1463, http://www.jstor.org/stable/25689660. Retrieved 10 June 2018.

Koch, Tom. 2006, May. "Weaponizing Medicine," *Journal of Medical Ethics*, Vol. 32, No. 5, pp. 249–252, https://www.jstor.org/stable/27719620?seq=1#page_scan_tab_contents. Retrieved 10 June 2018.

Lithwick, Dahlia. 2007, February 1, "The Third Man: The 4th Circuit Does One More Round on Enemy Combatants," *Slate*, http://www.slate.com/articles/news_and_politics/jurisprudence/2007/02/the_third_man.html. Retrieved 10 June 2018.

Maio, Giovanni. 2001, May 19. "History of Medical Involvement in Torture—Then and Now," Department of Medical History, *The Lancet*, Vol. 357, Issue 9268, 1609-1611. https://www.thelancet.com/journals/lancet/issue/vol357no9268/PIIS0140-6736(00)X0242-5. Retrieved 10 June 2018.

Nel Noddings, *Women and Evil*. University of California Press, 1989.

Physicians for Human Rights. 2009, August. "Aiding Torture: Health Professionals' Ethics and Human Rights Violations Revealed in the May 2004 CIA Inspector General's Report."

The Rendition Project, "Ridha al-Najjar," https://www.therenditionproject.org.uk/prisoners/najjar.html. Retrieved 10 June 2018.

Savage, Charlie. 2004, December 27. "CIA Resists Request for Abuse Data," *Boston Globe*, http://www.boston.com/news/globe/. Retrieved 10 June 2018.

Stephens, Joe. 2005, January 6. "Army Doctors Implicated in Abuse," *The Washington Post*, Retrieved 10 June 2018.

Stritzke, Werner G. K., Ed. 2009. *Terrorism and Torture: An Interdisciplinary Perspective*. Cambridge University Press.

Teays, Wanda. 2008, "Torture and Public Health," in Michael Boylan, Ed., *International Public Health Policy and Ethics*. Springer.

———. 2011, "The Ethics of Otherness," in Michael Boylan, Ed., *Morality and Global Justice Reader*. Boulder, CO: Westview Press.

United Nations. 2009. "The UN Committee Against Torture: Human Rights Monitoring and the Legal Recognition of Cruelty, "*Human Rights Quarterly*, https://www.jstor.org/stable/40389967. Retrieved 10 June 2018.

The U.S. Senate Committee. 2014, December 8. *The Senate Committee Report on Torture*. Retrieved 10 June 2018.

Van Natta Jr., Don and Souad Mekhennet. 2005, January 9, "German's Claim of Kidnapping Brings Investigation of U.S. Link," *The New York Times*, http://www.nytimes.com/2005/01/09/world/europe/germans-claim-of-kidnapping-brings-investigation-of-us-link.html. Retrieved 10 June 2018.

Wilkinson, James. 2017, October 10. "CIA Black Site 'Cobalt'," *The Daily Mail (UK)*, http://www.dailymail.co.uk/news/article-4965130/Grim-facts-emerge-CIA-black-site-Cobalt.html#ixzz58S4T8vjo. Retrieved 10 June 2018.

Wisnewski, J. Jeremy and Emerick, R. D. 2009. *The Ethics of Torture*. London: Continuum.

NOTE

1. © Springer Nature Switzerland AG 2019. Wanda Teays, "Doctors and Torture: Medicine at the Crossroads." *International Library of Ethics, Law, and the New Medicine* 80: 57–74. Used with permission.

3

Rights of Persons with Disabilities from a Global Perspective

Akiko Ito

ABSTRACT

In this chapter, I will discuss the implementation phase of the United Nations Convention on the Rights of Persons with Disabilities, to discuss most pertinent issues for policy making to support national implementation of CRPD, with a focus on cultural rights. I will draw from my work at the UN to demonstrate the ways in which the concerns raised are international ones.

INTRODUCTION

In this chapter, I discuss divergent constructions of disability and diverse approaches to equalizing opportunities for persons with disabilities. There has been a shift from the medical model to the socioeconomic/minority rights model, which recognizes principles of bioethics. This shift of disability concept is one of the key driving forces of the development of conceptual frameworks and the establishment of the legal mechanisms related to disability and human rights. The Convention on the Rights of Persons with Disabilities (CRPD) is not only a new human rights tool but also a groundbreaking tool to change society. Emerging issues such as mental health and psychological aspect of disability and bioethics related to disabilities are also examined. It is imperative that we pay more attention to cross-cultural or global dimensions of disability rights. I will conclude with some recommendations regarding the implementation of the CRPD, including mainstreaming disability rights into global priorities.

DISABILITY, CULTURE, AND EMERGING ISSUES

Before 1970, the UN approached disability issues from a social welfare model perspective. In its first ten years of work, the UN focused on promoting the rights of persons with physical disability. Its primary concern was the establishment of international bodies and the

103

development of suitable operational programs to deal with disability issues in cooperation with nongovernmental organizations. In the period from 1955 to 1970, an emphasis on prevention and rehabilitation was established,[1] but little attention was paid to obstacles created by social institutions and society in general.[2]

The social welfare perspective emphasized helping those with disabilities fit into general societal structures. For example, a deaf person might be taught only how to read lips. New approaches stress modifications to the environment to promote the equalization of opportunities for persons with disabilities (e.g., when sign language interpreters are provided at public events). This formulation emphasizes society's responsibility to remove barriers that underpin exclusion of persons with disabilities and denial of basic citizenship rights.[3]

This approach sees persons with disabilities as a minority group. According to Harlan Hahn, discrimination has historically isolated persons with disabilities as a minority group. He states, "people with disabilities are a minority group because they have been the objects of prejudice and discrimination."[4] As discrimination that occurs over time, it reinforces attitudes that, in turn, reinforce discrimination, thus becoming a vicious cycle. He places the focus on public attitudes, rather than physical limitations, as the primary source of difficulties facing persons with disabilities.

The minority-group model specifies that public policy molds all facets of the environment. It further considers government policies to be reflecting societal attitudes and values. As a result, existing features of architectural design, job requirements, and daily life that have a discriminatory impact on disabled citizens cannot be viewed merely as happenstance or coincidence, notes Hahn.[5]

Other scholars contend that a true human rights approach toward the issue of disability differs from approaches focusing on the environment.[6] Where the environmental approach looks at ecological barriers, human rights approaches looks at the rights to which all people, regardless of disability status, are entitled. It analyzes how society marginalizes people with disabilities and how the social environment could be changed.[7]

Given these changes in the ways disability is perceived, the CRPD establishes a major conceptual break from earlier approaches (e.g., in the World Programme of Action, as well as the Standard Rules). It exclusively focuses on ensuring the human rights of persons with disabilities.[8] The CRPD addresses disability prevention and rehabilitation as an aspect of full and comprehensive *human rights protection* for persons with disabilities. Thus, prevention and rehabilitation are directed at ensuring equal access and making all public health programs accessible to persons with disabilities.

Drafters of the CRPD signaled that public health issues, such as protecting the general population from infectious diseases, and implementing public safety policies, such as road safety or industrial accident prevention, are not appropriately addressed within the framework of disability rights.

This tension is particularly pronounced in view of the CRPD. For that reason, its drafters explicitly adopted a comprehensive, rights-based, sociocontextual understanding of disability. The Convention seeks to address the long-standing and as yet unresolved challenge of defining disability within a human rights and social model framework. As a result, it does not specifically define disability.[9]

Instead, the CRPD Preamble took a different approach, stating that, "Disability is an evolving concept and that disability results from the interaction between persons with impairments and attitudinal and environmental barriers that hinders their full and effective participation in society on an equal basis with others."[10]

It further states that, "Persons with disabilities include those who have long-term physical, mental, intellectual or sensory impairments which in interaction with various barriers may hinder their full and effective participation in society on an equal basis with others"[11] (see Article 1).

The Convention thus adopts a broad categorization of persons with disabilities: It moved away from the World Health Organization's more *medical orientation* and embraced a *social model* of disability within which civil, political, economic, social, and cultural rights are enumerated and elaborated. Clearly, this is a major shift, with broad implications. In the next section, I will discuss cultural aspects that should be considered.

CULTURAL AND RELATED EMERGING DIMENSIONS IN DISABILITIES

As discussed above, disability is closely associated with the environment according to the *social model*. It is imperative to pay attention to cultural and anthropological aspects of disability since they play key roles in the environment for persons with disabilities. This includes culture-sensitive implementation of CRPD.

The UN has facilitated regional years and decades on disability mechanisms—as seen in Europe's Year of the Disabled, the Asian and Pacific Decade of Disabled Persons, and the African Decade of Disabled Persons. These mechanisms can be more targeted and more culture-sensitive than those at the international level. They also provide opportunities for intraregional cooperation and technical assistance, which may be more culturally appropriate.

CRPD recognizes the right of persons with disabilities to take part on an equal basis with others in cultural life. This called for appropriate measures to ensure that persons with disabilities have access to (a) cultural materials in accessible formats; (b) TV programs, films, theater, and other cultural activities, in accessible formats; (c) places for cultural performances or services, such as museums, cinemas, libraries, and tourism services; and, as far as possible, (d) monuments and sites of national cultural importance.

CRPD calls for appropriate measures to enable persons with disabilities to have the opportunity to develop and utilize their creative, artistic, and intellectual potential not only for their own benefit but also for the enrichment of society. Further, CRPD calls for all appropriate steps by state parties to ensure that laws protecting intellectual property rights do not constitute an unreasonable or discriminatory barrier to access by persons with disabilities to cultural materials. Persons with disabilities are entitled, on an equal basis with others, to recognition and support of their specific cultural and linguistic identity, including sign languages and deaf culture. This article plays a key role in promoting culture-sensitive mainstreaming of disability into development priorities.

The mental, psychological, and emotional aspect in disability and development is an emerging key issue. It plays a key role in cultural, anthropological, and environmental determinants of disability and in determining quality of life of persons with disabilities and effectiveness of policy implementation. Because persons with mental, psychosocial, or intellectual disabilities are often much marginalized, it is an emerging key priority to pay attention to these aspects of disability.

BIOETHICS IN CRPD

CRPD states that, "State Parties undertake to collect appropriate information, including statistical and research data, to enable them to formulate and implement policies to give effect to the present Convention." The process of collecting and maintaining this information "shall comply with internationally accepted norms to protect human rights and fundamental freedoms and ethical principles in the collection and use of statistics" (see Article 31.1.b). Given the importance of research and the protection of human subjects in the field of bioethics—not to mention the importance placed on codes like Nuremberg and Helsinki—attention needs to be directed to this area of the CPRD.

Similarly, CPRD's position on respect for the family, the right to decide freely and responsibly on the number and spacing of their children and to have access to age-appropriate information and reproductive and family planning education, is recognized, and the means necessary to enable them to exercise these rights are provided; the right to retain their fertility on an equal basis with others is specifically elaborated (see Article 23).

Finally, CPRD's statement on health holds that state parties shall provide persons with disabilities with the same range, quality, and standard of free or affordable health care and programs as provided to other persons, including in the area of sexual and reproductive health and population-based public health programs (see Article 25).

IMPLEMENTATION: CULTURE-SENSITIVE MAINSTREAMING INTO MDGS

Mainstreaming disability in development policies, processes, and mechanisms has been on the UN agenda for more than a quarter of a century. Since the mid-1990s, many development agencies, funds, and programs have taken significant steps to mainstream disability at the policy level.

At the global level, the UN has adopted the World Programme of Action as an international policy framework for disability-inclusive development, and the Standard Rules for the equalization of opportunities, which reaffirmed the principles of inclusive policies, plans, and activities in development cooperation and provided further guidance on disability-inclusive measures.

The World Programme of Action, marking a "slow shift towards a rights-based model" of disability is a hybrid instrument evoking the emergence of a human rights–oriented approach. It clearly articulates some of the core human rights issues of concern for persons with disabilities. At the same time, it reflects some of the more traditional conceptions of disability, with a focus on disability prevention and rehabilitation. That said, it captures the social context of disability in observing that, "It is largely the environment which determines the effect of an impairment or a disability on a person's daily life."[12]

The Standard Rules, while not legally binding, remain a practical framework in defining obstacles and barriers on the equalization of opportunities for person with disabilities. It also helps target areas of action. They should serve as a guide to states that have not yet signed and ratified the CRPD—but should be fully informed by it. In addition, the Standard Rules may be used as an instrument to foster further integration of disability with the UN system against the fuller framework of the CRPD. The latter provides an additional mandate for inclusion within and across the UN system.

As an instrument for promoting both human rights and development, the CPRD provides a comprehensive normative framework for mainstreaming disability in the development agenda with new opportunities. It is also legally binding. The Convention recognizes the importance of international cooperation and its promotion for the realization of the rights of persons with disabilities and their full inclusion into all aspects of life (see Article 32).

In particular, Article 32 stipulates that international cooperation measures should (a) be inclusive of and accessible to persons with disabilities; (b) facilitate and support capacity-building, including through the exchange and sharing of information, experiences, training programs, and best practices; (c) facilitate cooperation in research and access to scientific and technical knowledge; and (d) provide technical and economic assistance, including by facilitating access to and sharing of accessible and assistive technologies and through the transfer of technologies.

As noted by the president of the General Assembly, the CPRD represents "a great opportunity to celebrate the emergence of comprehensive guidelines the world so urgently needs."[13] The World Programme of Action and the Standard Rules were important milestones to developing a legally binding human rights convention that would apply human rights to persons with disabilities.

The Standard Rules contributed to the development of the CRPD in articulating accessibility as a priority area for targeted reforms and in raising awareness as a core component in achieving rights for persons with disabilities. The CRPD takes these and other concepts further. It situates them within a framework that is comprehensive in its coverage of specific substantive rights and provides principles and obligations applicable to the achievement of civil, political, economic, social, and cultural rights.

Following these significant advances, the UN agencies, funds, and programs have started to mainstream disability in their development policies. For example,

- UNFPA and WHO developed a guidance note on sexual and reproductive health of persons with disabilities for their headquarters, regional, and country offices, after UNFPA's integration of disability in its Strategic Plan 2008–2013 as a cross-cutting issue.
- UNAIDS developed a policy brief on HIV and disability with its ten cosponsors.
- UNDP has started developing a guidance note on integrating disability into its development activities.

Development of processes and mechanisms to implement these policies are still under way. In addition, there are still some UN agencies that have not yet fully addressed the policy and implementation issues of mainstreaming disability.

The mainstreaming of disability in development cooperation is also relatively new to most development partners. The Nordic countries and the United States (through USAID) began the process of mainstreaming disability into their development cooperation during the 1990s. Australia, Austria, Canada, European Union, Japan, New Zealand, and the United Kingdom have also started integration of development in their development policies. However, there has not been extensive experience in mainstreaming disability at a program level, and so there has been little opportunity to evaluate best practices or share information on implementation.

Given that persons with disabilities comprise an estimated 10 percent of the world's population, of whom 80 percent live in developing countries, it is an urgent priority to mainstream disability as a cross-cutting issue in the development policies and in processes and mechanisms at the global, regional, subregional, and national levels. To achieve this, it is necessary to pay more attention to emerging aspects of disability, such as culture and mental well-being.

The CRPD approach to disability and human rights is not a simple addition to the international human rights mechanisms. It is groundbreaking in changing the global society with its social model perspective, its attention to accessibility for all, and its inclusion of persons with disabilities in all the processes of decision-making and implementation. Together with gender equalization efforts and efforts to mainstream mental, psychological, and emotional aspects of development, the CRPD will play a key role in forming a new sustainable community and better quality of life for all people.

NOTES

1. United Nations Secretariat, Division for Social Policy and Development, *The United Nations and Disabled Persons: An Historical Overview: First Fifty Years* (New York: United Nations, 1997), 14–15.

2. Ibid., 15.

3. Victor Finkelstein, *Attitudes and Disabled People* (New York: World Rehabilitation Fund, 1980); Michael Oliver, *Social Work with Disabled People* (Basingstoke, UK: Macmillan, 1983); Michael Oliver, *The Politics of Disablement: Social Work with Disabled People* (Basingstoke, UK: Macmillan, 1990).

4. Harlan Hahn, "The Political Implications of Disability Definitions and Data," *Disability Policy Studies* 4, no. 3: 47.

5. Ibid., 46.

6. Marcia H. Rioux, "Disability: The Place of Judgement in a World of Fact," *Journal of Intellectual Disability Research* 41, no. 2 (1997): 102–11.

7. Michael Oliver, "Changing the Social Relations of Research Production," *Disability, Handicap and Society* 7, no. 2 (1992): 101–14.

8. *Id.* at art. 1 ("The purpose of the present Convention is to promote, protect and ensure the full and equal enjoyment of all human rights and fundamental freedoms by all persons with disabilities, and to promote respect for their inherent dignity.").

9. *See* CRPD, *supra* note 1 at Preamble, para. (e) and art. 1.

10. *Id.* at preamble, para. (e).

11. CRPD, *supra* note 1 at art. 1.

12. World Programme, *supra* note 3 at para. 21.

13. Statement by H. E. Sheikha Haya Rashed Al Khalifa, President of the United Nations General Assembly, at the Adoption of the Convention on the Rights of Persons with Disabilities (13 December 2006), http://www.un.org/ga/president/61/statements/statement20061213.shtml.

4

Medical Tourism

Justice, Autonomy, and Power

Virginia L. Warren

ABSTRACT

"Medical tourism" refers to patients traveling across national borders for medical treatment. My primary focus is on patients living in the United States who travel to low-income countries for medical care. The main reasons for medical tourism include—above all—saving money, cutting waiting time, and getting medical treatment unavailable at home. I consider traveling for major surgery, for kidney transplants from poor people who illegally sell a kidney, and for experimental treatment not yet available in the United States. The principal moral concerns I discuss are based on patient autonomy, harms to the patient and to others back home (such as drug-resistant infections), and harms to poor people in the destination country—including injustice due to "brain drain" when international patients come for medical treatment.

Many solutions to these objections to medical tourism have been offered, and more could be devised. However, a fundamental problem works against their being tried or fully enforced: the power of money and its impact on politics. I close by offering an approach to bioethics that directly addresses power in health care. I expand the discussion of autonomy, as usually understood, to include empowering patients, health care professionals, and the general public—both individually and in partnership with others. I then advance the following principle: *The duty to confront power, often in coordination with others, in order to further other important moral principles and values.* It is not free-standing; it concerns how and when one should act to carry out other moral duties. It is the duty that whistle-blowers follow, although I have expanded it—in the age of #MeToo—to accentuate the power of working together. Confronting power may help more people to fulfill their right to basic health care—both in the United States and in destination countries—and help justice be better served.

INTRODUCTION

Medicine has become a global market, with a growing number of patients traveling to other countries for medical treatment. In the biomedical literature, "medical tourist" is the commonly used name for patients who travel across national borders for medical treatment. I. Glenn Cohen (2015, xv) writes: "I will define them as individuals who travel abroad for the primary purpose of getting health care (as opposed to expatriates who receive care while living abroad, or individuals who get sick on vacation)." Peta Cook et al. (2013, 63) rely on a similar definition: "we view medical tourism as the phenomenon of patients travelling to foreign or international locales with the motivation to receive invasive medical treatment, usually because cost or availability confers some financial or personal advantage."

While I also adopt this narrower interpretation of medical tourism, some sources consider broader ones. For example, Halina Kotikova and Eva Schwartzhoffova (2013) write about traveling to health spas and other health care–related businesses. Cook et al. (2013, 63) note that when the medical treatment is less burdensome, "medical tourism" is sometimes used to "include the practice of packaging together holidays with medical treatments. The marketing of medical tourism often concentrates on nearby attractions and/or vacation packages" for the patient and family or other caretakers. In these two examples, the "tourism" label seems a felicitous match.

Discussions of medical tourism refer to the *home* (or source) country in which patients live and the *destination* country and/or specific medical center to which they travel for medical care. Cohen (2015, 1–37) offers a comprehensive overview of medical and legal terms, along with occupations and groups, related to medical tourism. "While medical tourists come predominantly from the developed world, medical-tourist sites are found globally, with many medical tourists flowing to world-class facilities in the developing world" (Cook et al. 2013, 61–62).

My primary focus is on patients living in the United States who travel to low-income countries for medical care. Reasons for medical tourism include—above all—saving money, as well as cutting waiting time, and getting medical treatment unavailable at home. The principal moral concerns I discuss are the patient's autonomy (avoiding coercion and having sufficient correct information to make an informed decision), harms to the patient (due to poor medical quality) and to others back home (such as drug-resistant infections), and possible harms to poor people in the destination country—especially, if they suffer injustice because their right to basic health care is undermined when international patients come for medical treatment. As we will see, some moral issues raised about medical tourism mirror issues raised when patients stay in the United States.

A TOOLBOX OF MORAL PRINCIPLES FOR BIOETHICS

The field of bioethics began its modern development with the Nuremberg Code (1947) on human experimentation, which was endorsed by many nations after World War II in response to the horrors of experiments forced on human subjects by the Nazis. It emphasizes autonomy and begins: "The voluntary consent of the human subject is absolutely essential."

The moral framework of bioethics further developed during the 1960s and 1970s. After a period of wide-ranging exploration of how to approach ethical issues in medicine and biology, a short list of moral principles (which were put forth by, among others, Tom L. Beauchamp and James F. Childress [1979] in the first edition of their basic textbook) gained prominence: autonomy, nonmaleficence, beneficence, and justice. Also considered are the value of life and other rights and utilitarianism. Later, virtue ethics and to some degree feminist ethics have been added.

I will examine three reasons US patients might choose to get medical care in other countries and a possible objection based on treating poor people in destination countries unjustly. I close by offering an approach to bioethics that addresses the impact of economic and political power on health care. I expand the discussion of autonomy, as commonly understood, to include empowering patients, health care professionals, and the general public—both individually and in partnership with others. I then advance the following principle: *The duty to confront power, often in coordination with others, in order to further other important moral principles and values.*

FIRST REASON FOR MEDICAL TOURISM: PATIENTS SAVE MONEY

Without question, saving money is the principal reason many US patients travel to other countries for medical care. Comparing prices in the United States with those in destination countries is eye-opening. Neil Lunt et al. (2011) produced an influential report—with a chart (included by Cohen [2015, 4] and Lunt et al. [2013, 34]) comparing the costs of medical procedures in the US with nine other countries where medical tourism is common—including India, Thailand, Singapore, Malaysia, and Mexico. Rounding off, hip or knee replacement surgery may cost about one-quarter as much as in the United States, heart bypass surgery may cost about one-tenth as much, and heart valve replacement surgery may cost somewhat over one-twentieth as much. Even after adding in travel and temporary living expenses, the savings for patients can be considerable. The evidence of cost saving for medical tourists living in the United States (and in many other high-income countries) for many medical procedures is well established.

Compared with other high-income countries, the United States on average spends considerably more per capita on health care and a larger percent of its GDP, and gets poorer health outcomes; among the higher expenses paid in the United States are physician services, drugs, and administrative costs (Papanicolas et al. 2018). In the United States, the practice of medicine has much less government regulation than in other high-income countries, where governments hold down prices, and, alone among those countries, many in the United States have no health insurance at all. Medical debt is a significant problem in the United States, even for those who are insured (Hamel et al. 2016).

Several moral objections may be raised to US medical tourists seeking less expensive medical care elsewhere, including based on patient autonomy, quality of care, harm to others, and injustice to poor people in the destination country.

Medical tourists from the United States may have their autonomy compromised in several ways. They may feel forced to travel by the burden of high medical costs at home; they may even face bankruptcy. However, patients will find it difficult to get reliable information to make the decision to go to a specific country. Comparing medical costs of a procedure in the United States with those in various destination countries is difficult, in part, because US medical prices—which should be transparent and available—may be as opaque as cement.

According to Cohen's (2015, 76) careful research,

> Quality of care remains one of the—and probably *the* most—frequently cited concern about medical tourism. Although one can find many anecdotal instances of poor care being delivered as part of medical tourism, the kind of data one would need to make a full-fledged assessment is currently largely absent. . . . At the same time, the existing often-touted signals of high quality—JCI [Joint Commission International] accreditation, number of Western-trained physicians [a kind of reverse brain drain going toward destination countries, but Lunt et al. (2011, 35–36) question its significance], partnerships with prestigious facilities in the developed country—seem more about branding and less about rigorous measures of quality.

Hence, medical tourists may be harmed by inferior medical care, and making a truly informed choice based on quality is, once again, quite difficult.

Justice may be a concern. Below, we discuss possible injustices associated with medical tourists. It may be that injustice in the United States—where many are denied the right to basic, affordable health care—could lead to poor people in destination countries receiving even worse health care as a result.

SECOND REASON FOR MEDICAL TOURISM: AVOIDING LONG WAIT TIMES

In some countries, long wait lines for nonemergency medical care can be a significant problem, making faster care one reason patients travel to other countries. For example, patients in European Union countries may travel to other EU countries that have less waiting time for a specific procedure, and Canadians may travel to the United States (Cohen 2015, 6, 9–10). Moreover, saving time for patients may also save money for insurers. For example, Lunt et al. (2011, 31) cite evidence that, if the UK's health service sent patients to India for total hip and knee replacement surgeries, the health service might save over a hundred million pounds a year, in addition to reducing the waiting lists with tens of thousands of UK patients.

While avoiding long wait lines is not a main factor leading US patients to travel to other countries, there is a major exception. In the United States, there is a long wait to receive kidneys for transplantation. There are simply not enough donated kidneys for all who need them. Most are from deceased donors who register to have their organs removed upon their death, and some are from volunteer living donors. Many on dialysis die before receiving a kidney.

Among the moral objections to medical tourism for kidney transplants raised below, the first two concern how the kidneys are obtained: they are bought and sold. It is illegal to pay people to donate organs in the United States, and worldwide only Iran has legalized selling organs (and Iran regulates it); still, black markets for buying organs exist in many places in the world (Cohen 2015, 263).

First, it can be objected that using purchased kidneys is intrinsically wrong because selling an organ debases the seller's human dignity. Nikola Biller-Andorno and Zümrüt Alpinar (2014, 773–74) consider this line of argument unhelpful. They argue that the concept of human dignity is either too vague to be helpful, or—if based on Kantian ethics or the values of specific religions—not widely enough shared to persuade people generally. They find autonomy a more convincing objection. I am sympathetic to the human dignity objection, although I agree that it is philosophically intricate.

Second, it can be objected that kidney sellers are not acting autonomously. To begin with, they are desperate for money, or they would not be selling parts of their body. Further, "The brokers who manage the trade are often affiliated with organized crime and rely on misinformation, pressure, and sometimes threats to recruit sellers" (Cohen 2015, 313). Sellers are regularly lied to about how long and difficult recovery is and then cheated out of much of their promised payment. They often regret their decision (Cohen 2015, 300, 313) because they are worse off physically and financially than before the surgery. Given real-world conditions, this objection is conclusive against medical tourists receiving purchased kidneys.

Third, the quality of medical care for medical tourists may be questioned: are medical outcomes worse in the destination country than if patients had transplant surgery and follow-up care in the United States? While reliable data from destination countries is hard to come by since the procedure is illegal (Cohen 2015, 281), we may surmise that the quality is generally low. However, if patients are quite *un*likely to receive a donated organ in the United States, then their comparison with transplant surgery elsewhere would be to continue their poor quality of life at home without the surgery—which is an easier comparison to beat.

Fourth, the autonomy of kidney transplant tourists may also be examined. Again, because the procedure is illegal—and patients are not discussing medical tourism with their home physicians—it is unlikely that kidney transplant tourists are fully and correctly informed about the quality, conditions, and cost of the medical treatment elsewhere.

So far, I am following the way patient autonomy is usually construed in bioethics: compare the risks and benefits *for the patient* of different alternatives. However, we may wonder whether the kidney recipients were informed, more broadly, about the true situation for kidney *sellers* in that destination country: their likely medical results, whether they would probably be lied to or cheated out of money, and whether afterward they would likely suffer greatly, leaving them awash with regret. I think we know the answer, and not only because the brokers from destination countries lie to medical tourists as well. For the information that patients are usually deemed to require—in order to make an autonomous medical decision—does not include whether others may suffer a harm or injustice as a result, or whether there is a serious environmental impact, or a host of other possible effects. We will return to possible injustice caused to others when discussing brain drain below.

There is general agreement that buying kidneys for transplant in the black market is morally wrong, and I concur. Responses offered by Biller-Andorno and Alpinar (2014, 781) and Cohen (2015, 314) include shutting down organ trafficking in destination countries, through monitoring by international bodies and/or through having better police enforcement of existing laws prohibiting such sales; increasing the supply of donated kidneys in home countries by passing laws that presume consent for organ donation at death; and lessening demand by preventing kidney failure. For many in the United States who currently face kidney failure, focusing on long-term supply and demand for donated kidneys will leave their dreams of a healthier life to fade and die. However, for the foreseeable future, that is all we have.

THIRD REASON FOR MEDICAL TOURISM: EXPERIMENTAL PROCEDURES NOT LEGALLY AVAILABLE IN THE HOME COUNTRY

Currently, patients living outside the United States may become medical tourists for abortions or physician-assisted suicide if they are unavailable where they live. In the case of finding surrogate mothers willing to be pregnant (usually with an embryo from the sperm and/or egg of the adopting parents) and to relinquish that child for adoption—a type of fertility tourism—people may come from other countries to the United States, where surrogacy is legal (Cohen 2015, 372–73).

I focus here on experimental drugs, medical devices, and procedures that are not legally available for patients in the United States because the Federal Drug Administration (FDA) has not yet approved them. Current examples include stem cell therapy (Cohen 2015, 421–78; Hall 2013b, 12–16; Hall 2013a, 204), and transplanting parts of animals into humans, such as cells from the pancreas of pigs to potentially help patients with type 1 diabetes (Cook et al. 2013, 65).

Regarding drugs, the FDA approval process in the United States takes many years. "It has been estimated that, from start to finish, the FDA approval process can take up to ten years for a successful drug. Until a drug is approved, it is illegal to sell the drug to willing patients, unless the drug qualifies for one of FDA's narrow exceptions" (Cohen 2015, 422). Even with recent attempts to fast-track some potentially life-saving drugs, the average approval time of eight years has been reduced to about seven (Healy 2017). Relatively few patients are accepted into clinical trials and, even then, one has a 50 percent chance of being randomly assigned to a placebo (or, in cases where there is already an established treatment, to that existing treatment). Patients in the United States who want access to unapproved drugs or medical devices may seek them elsewhere.

Moral objections to medical tourism for unapproved experimental drugs and procedures include, above all, risk of harms to the patient that are not balanced by the chance of compensating benefits for the patient (weighing nonmaleficence against beneficence). Human stem cell therapy, for example, is of unproven value (Lunt et al. 2013, 42–43). Moreover, harm may be done to others in the United States upon return. Drug-resistant bacteria may be transported back, after infections are caught in destination hospitals (Hall 2013a, 207–9). Cook et al. (2013, 65) warn that experimental surgeries using parts of nonhuman animals are especially risky since viruses completely new to humans could be introduced from other species. Further, financial burdens may be placed on the US health care system if patients return in need of significant follow-up treatment after poorly done procedures. Of these objections, the risk of overall harm to the patient is viewed as the greatest concern by medical tourists, the risk depending on the specific procedure and place. Whether the patient can get reliable information upon which to base a decision also varies.

OBJECTION: INJUSTICE—INCLUDING FROM BRAIN DRAIN—TO THOSE IN THE DESTINATION COUNTRY

An important and frequently discussed objection to medical tourism concerns justice. That poor people in the destination country may be treated unjustly rests on a general claim about human rights: everyone has a right to the basic necessities of life, including food, clothing, shelter, and health care. One specific version of this objection concerns brain drain. In general, brain drain occurs when professionals choose not to work in areas where patients are most in need in order to work elsewhere—usually to be paid more, although getting higher status or better working conditions may also be involved. Poor people in a destination country may have their health unjustly harmed when medical professionals—and medical centers and equipment—are allocated away from serving their health needs to those of incoming medical tourists. The argument is as follows:

1. Poor people in a destination country for medical tourism have a right to basic health care, and in many countries this right is not, in general, being fulfilled.
2. [*causal connection*] If medical tourists come to a destination country for medical treatment and doing so *causes* many poor people there (who may already have inadequate health care) to have health care that is both worsened *and* less than what they have a basic right to, then an injustice is done to those poor people.
3. [*specific case*] Specific evidence must support the claim that medical tourists to *this* destination country for *this* medical treatment cause such an injustice.

4. Therefore, it is unjust for there to be medical tourism to *this* destination country for *this* medical treatment.

   a. [*specific responsibility*] Therefore, it is unjust for medical tourists to choose to go to *this* destination country for *this* medical treatment.
   b. [*specific responsibility*] Therefore, it is unjust for physicians and other medical professionals in *this* destination country to work in medical centers within this country that actively serve—and advertise to attract—medical tourists from other countries, when they could serve poor people in *this* country instead.
   c. [*specific responsibility*] Therefore, it is unjust for physicians and other medical professionals in *this* destination country to leave to work in *other* countries that actively serve patients who can pay more, when they could stay and serve poor people in *this* country instead.

Cohen (2015) carefully underscores that evidence is needed to prove the causal connection (premise 2) between medical tourists traveling for a specific treatment and poor people of a specific country having worse health care as a direct result (premise 3). After painstaking analysis of available data from a range of destination countries, both Cohen (2015, 210–26) and Lunt et al. (2011, 35–36) arrive at conclusions that are equivocal. They agree that, in a number of countries, there is anecdotal evidence that medical tourism causes poor people in the destination country to have worse medical care as a result, for example, when there is brain drain of medical professionals—plus reallocation of money, medical centers, and equipment—to serve medical tourists instead. However, they determine that the best available evidence is as yet inconclusive. Even if poor people's medical care is getting worse, other factors may be the cause—such as medical resources and personnel being "drained" away to serve the wealthy of their own country. Cohen (2015, 226) ultimately concludes that while he "cannot prove" the causal connection in any country, there is "sufficient evidence" to show "that the claim is plausible enough" to examine the moral objection to medical tourism based on injustice.

I distinguished different versions of the conclusion (4a, 4b, 4c) since, even if poor people in destination countries are suffering an injustice because their right to basic health care has been eroded due to medical tourism, it can still be debated exactly who—or what institution—is morally responsible for that injustice. The more we ponder specific responsibility for such injustice, the more complexities emerge, as follows.

Regarding (4a), deciding whether it is unjust for *medical tourists* from the United States to choose to go to countries where poor people are caused to have worse health care as a result is complicated. US medical tourists, in particular, may have extreme financial problems that prevent them from getting good medical care at home (Cohen 2015, 257). They may have no health insurance, or they may be underinsured—with high copays and annual deductibles, especially for a family. While US patients are not often as poor as poor people in low-income destination countries, it is hard to find them guilty of injustice if medical bankruptcy looms or their medical condition is life threatening (e.g., requiring heart surgery). Arguably, the wealthier or better insured that US patients are, the more blameworthy they may be (Cohen 2015, 259). While the Affordable Care Act (ACA) greatly improved access and lowered costs for many in the United States, much more must be done to guarantee the right to basic health care for all.

This remaining injustice in the US health care system may contribute to injustice in destination countries. Overall, it is necessary to confront the economic and political power affecting health care systems in order to help more people to fulfill their right to basic health care—both in the United States and in destination countries—thereby helping justice be better served.

Regarding (4b), the situation for physicians, nurses, and other medical professionals who grew up—and often trained—in destination countries with significant poverty is difficult to unravel, as well. These professionals' decisions about where to work, whether to specialize, and which patients to serve are often freer choices than those of the medical tourists we just discussed. Of course, destination countries (and medical centers) could give inducements for medical professionals to serve more of their own poor. We miss the big picture if we look only at individuals and not at the policies and practices of institutions—including financial rewards for general practice versus various specialties; the funding sources for major hospitals that influence where they locate; money donated to politicians who vote on health care policies; and policies about medical student debt. An example of the latter comes from California, which has begun a program for medical school loan forgiveness for physicians who serve low-income California patients (Gutierrez 2019).

I added (4c) to ask whether, if medical professionals opt out of serving poor patients in their own countries, there is a moral difference that depends upon where they practice. That is, is there a moral difference between medical professionals staying in their own country to serve medical tourists (4b) and leaving to work in another country (4c)—as long as the patients they serve are similarly well off? Either way, it is brain drain away from serving their poor. While admittedly unlikely, medical professionals in destination countries might leave to serve poor people in another country. That brain drain does not strike me as wrong overall.

To press the point further, if they left their country to work at the world-renowned Mayo Clinic in Minnesota in order to do research on a disease affecting poor people in their own country (again unlikely), that decision strikes me as praiseworthy. In the Mayo Clinic case, the "brain" has not drained away; it has relocated in order to help from afar. We can also imagine that they chose to work at the Mayo Clinic in order to do more total good for the entire world's poor by researching a disease that does not affect their country of origin. This case, although brain drain, seems praiseworthy too. At issue may be a mixture of moral considerations: one's motive (self-regarding or altruistic), commitment to one's country (if one judges this morally relevant), the degree of harm to the health care of poor individuals, and other moral factors (including other justice issues) that may outweigh brain drain.

In sum, even if a country's poor people are treated unjustly because of medical tourism—due, in particular, to brain drain of medical professionals—assigning moral responsibility for that specific injustice is complex. And similar moral issues arise in the United States. Brain drain of medical professionals within the United States—away from poorer areas toward wealthier areas or specialized medical centers—should elicit similar debate.

CONFRONTING POWER IN HEALTH CARE

I was initially put off by the "medical tourist" label. I preferred "cross-border medical traveler" or "international medical traveler." However, since reconciling economic interests with the well-being of patients is one of the larger issues in US health care, I have come to view the term "medical tourist" as a helpful reminder of the general conflict between money and the best interests of patients.

Money from drug, medical device, and private insurance companies infiltrates US health care decisions, sometimes with disastrous results. For example, physicians freely prescribe pain-killing opioids, but most have little or no training in how to get patients safely off them (Rieder, 2019). Drug companies get rich, patients get addicted and die at alarming rates, and federal reporting law is ignored. "For years, long after the opioid crisis began, the giant pharmacy chains, including Walgreens and CVS, and Walmart did almost nothing to fulfill their legal duty to monitor suspicious orders, the plaintiffs' lawyers claim. While they were supposed to block such orders and alert the Drug Enforcement Administration, they did so rarely" (Hoffman et al. 2019).

Another big problem is that transparency of US health care prices is often woefully lacking (Lazarus 2019). Knowing more about costs would help patients save money by knowing their options, and at least some pressure might be exerted to lower prices. A study showed that almost 70 percent of patients who tried to get cost information ahead of time from providers had trouble doing so (Hamel et al. 2016, 26–28). Even medical bills received afterward are designed to be difficult to decipher. Could the US government force transparency and require lower health care prices? Certainly—as governments in many other countries do; but it appears unlikely now. Money's influence on health care and US politics will remain until power is met with power.

In response to the objections raised above to medical tourism—including when patient autonomy is undermined, when patients and others risk harm from lower-quality medical treatment and from drug-resistant bacteria, and when poor people are treated unjustly—many solutions have been offered, and more could be devised.

Let us take determining the quality of health care in destination countries as an example. As we saw above, Cohen (2015, 76) concludes that attempts at accreditation, such as through the JCI, do not guarantee rigorous quality internationally. Cook et al. (2013, 65) concur: "Despite the interest in accreditation, however, there is no effective global regulation of the medical industry," and individuals are largely left to fend for themselves when trying to assess the quality of medical care abroad.

Cook et al. (2013) then recommend seeking institutional support outside of the medical world—both to raise the quality of health care for medical tourists and to give them more reliable information upon which to base their decisions. They speculate that NGOs might help medical tourists to become more effective consumers: "it is possible to imagine that in a context of lax global regulation, non-governmental organisations (NGOs) will take on a global quasi-regulatory role. Being unencumbered by the market forces to which national medical and regulatory actors are subject, . . . NGOs will become the 'global police' of risky biomedicine" (71–72). Perhaps so, but only if these NGOs can remain uncorrupted by market forces in the long run.

Cohen (2015, 71–77) offers a different way for medical tourists to lower their risk of getting poor-quality medical care, while retaining much of their autonomy. He proposes that patients' choices be "channeled" by their private health insurance companies. Well-researched, safer options of destination countries (or specific medical centers) would be designated as the default (or cheaper) choice for medical tourists. Thus, patient autonomy would be respected as much as possible, consistent with protecting both patients and the general public from harm (e.g., from drug-resistant bacteria). Again, I wonder whether those devising and implementing the channeling protocol will remain uncorrupted over time.

I am less fond of another of Cohen's proposals. Instead of making it illegal for US physicians to get referral fees from medical tourist destinations—a clear conflict of interest—Cohen

(2015, 134) proposes that these fees must simply be disclosed to patients considering medical tourism. However, even if paid trips to that country and other inducements were also disclosed, unconscious bias is real, and patient trust may erode.

In sum, these solutions and others run the risk of corruption. A fundamental force works against these solutions being made into policy or law or later being fully enforced: the power of money, which also impacts political power. Little will change until power is met with power.

EXPANDING THE MORAL TOOLBOX: FROM AUTONOMY TO EMPOWERMENT

I offer an approach to bioethics that directly addresses power in health care in two ways. In this section, I expand the discussion of autonomy to include empowerment and later advance this principle: *the duty to confront power, often in coordination with others, in order to further other important moral principles and values.*

The bioethics literature shines a light on respecting the right of individual patients to make decisions that are autonomous, to be fully informed and neither pressured nor coerced. Before patient autonomy gained widespread acceptance in US health care in the 1970s, the term "following doctor's orders" was commonplace. And families of terminal patients were often encouraged not to tell their dying relatives that they were terminal in order not to ruin that person's last days on earth. Patient autonomy was always about power: the power of physicians (and family members) was significantly reined in by competent patients' right to make informed decisions for themselves. A historical note: a secondary, self-interested, financial motive helped propel patient autonomy into its current pivotal place in medical practice. Since the patient, once informed of the risks and alternatives, chose this treatment, then, if the medical results went badly, the threat of a medical malpractice suit being brought against the physician was reduced. Physicians present; patients choose.

While recognizing patient autonomy as a massive, positive cultural shift that does empower patients in some basic respects, I claim that we need to debate how bioethics might go further. I propose expanding the discussion of autonomy, as usually understood in health care, to include empowering patients—as well as health care professionals and the general public—both individually and in partnership with others. A familiar example of empowerment is when patients and their families are encouraged to join support groups around specific medical issues in order to share practical information and give emotional support.

I maintain that the practice of medicine—including, but not limited to, medical tourism—would be enhanced by considering other ways, besides autonomy, of empowering individuals. A wide variety of supportive frameworks could be set up to develop skills, confidence, even courage (hence, there may be some overlap with virtue ethics' concentration on character traits). To advocate for empowerment—of patients, physicians, nurses, and other allied health professionals and to some degree the general public in one's country and beyond—is paradigmatically a social enterprise. This social component is exemplified by many social movements, such as the civil rights struggle for racial equality and the recent #MeToo movement on sexual abuse. Empowerment typically involves changes in the decision-maker, as well as forging connections with people, and striving over time to change institutional policies, laws, and prevailing attitudes and norms.

I offer this *definition of empowerment*: One is empowered when one is (a) involved in long-term projects (b) during which one develops skills and character traits that contribute to shaping one's life and/or furthering social change, (c) often while being supported by—and supporting—others in a group or community effort with which one identifies, (d) thus changing one's view about one's identity and abilities (Warren 2019, 54–55).

In short, autonomy changes what you know; empowerment changes who you are. Autonomy keeps others from interfering with you; empowerment seeks strength through relationships in order to make systemic change over time.

Becoming empowered may help you to act more autonomously—by more assertively requesting information and better resisting outside pressure. However, autonomy—as it is commonly employed in bioethics, and I think of as "tamed autonomy"—is narrower than empowerment, which centrally includes changes to your character traits, skills, self-concept, and relationships over time.

Becoming empowered is explicitly advocated by physicians in a National Public Radio (NPR) essay titled, "Be a Powerful Patient: Take Control of Your Care When You're Seriously Sick" (Schumann et al. 2019). They exclaim: "Figure out what matters to you, and fight for it. . . . Have a frank conversation with your doctor about *your* values and what you want (and don't want!) and you'll be an empowered patient with a doctor as your advocate, not your adversary." A companion NPR essay by Mara Gordon (2019) advocates standing up to a surgeon who pushes you toward surgery before you have fully researched it. She explains how to shop for the best surgeon and how to find out whether a physician is taking money from drug or device companies. You do not simply receive information; you seize power and act to protect yourself from the influence of money.

I would add that setting up actual support groups to empower patients in these ways would jump-start change—reminiscent of feminist conscious-raising groups in the 1960s. Further, we should not only ask how to empower people but also ask how people are currently *dis*empowered—and then change it.

Money—how conveniently hidden from view it is in many discussions of autonomy. The autonomy perspective focuses narrowly on the physician–patient relationship; seeking significant institutional, social, and political change is usually brushed aside. It regularly fails to shine light on the flagrant, intentional, and systemic lack of transparency in US medical costs—including the costs of specific procedures (and how some costs might be reduced), information that autonomous agents certainly need (Lazarus 2019). In the United States, the high cost of medical care is the prime motive for medical tourism.

EXPANDING THE MORAL TOOLBOX: THE DUTY TO CONFRONT POWER

Having explored how the concept of empowerment might change health care for the better, I advance the following principle: *the duty to confront power, often in coordination with others, in order to further other important moral principles and values*. It is not free standing; it concerns how and when one should act to carry out other important moral duties and values. It is the duty that whistle-blowers follow, although I have expanded it—in the age of #MeToo—to accentuate the power of working together, sustained over time, perhaps building a movement to change public opinion or specific policies and laws.

The duty to confront power concerns more than achieving an end. As with empowerment, the process matters: Typically one is changed through carrying out this duty. One stands up and becomes a whistle-blower. If others join in, each gathers strength from the other, as the risk lessens of being attacked or disbelieved. Then there may be progress toward action, including political action, at first within small groups and then within professional organizations.

The key questions then become deciding which specific moral principles or values to promote, and how. A concern for justice might lead to advocating for health insurance for all.

A truly global health concern is mitigating the effects of climate change. Martha Bebinger (2019) reports that the World Health Organization called climate change "the greatest health challenge of the 21st century" and that

> the American Medical Association, American Academy of Pediatrics and American Heart Association were among 70 medical and public health groups that issued a call to action asking the US government, business and leaders to recognize climate change as a health emergency. "The health, safety and wellbeing of millions of people in the U.S. have already been harmed by human-caused climate change, and health risks in the future are dire without urgent action to fight climate change," the coalition statement said.

In addition to direct political advocacy, what else can be done? Bebinger titles her essay, "Has Your Doctor Talked to You about Climate Change?" She considers whether and how physicians should discuss with their patients the ways climate change specifically affects their health. For example, "heat waves, more pollen, longer allergy seasons" worsen symptoms for patients with allergies, asthma, and COPD. We have returned to autonomy: What information should a patient know? Bebinger adds that medical and nursing schools should do better at teaching how the environment—including climate change—impacts patients' health.

CONCLUSION

I examined three reasons for US patients to become medical tourists: to cut waiting time (in particular for kidney transplantations), to get experimental medical treatment as yet unavailable in the United States, and to save money.

Cutting waiting time is rarely a motive for medical tourism from the United States, except to obtain kidneys that are illegally sold by poor people in other countries. Since the people selling are overwhelmingly pressured, lied to, and frequently regret their decision later, this category is ruled out as immoral.

Getting experimental treatment in other countries poses risks to patients over and above the risks of an unproven treatment. The general quality of surgery or postoperative care may be less than in the United States, and it is difficult to get reliable evidence of quality upon which to base an informed decision. Also, both patients and the general public risk drug-resistant bacteria being brought back home. Balancing overall risks and benefits of choosing unproven experimental treatment is based on weighing risks and benefits for the patient, as well as for the public—thus weighing nonmaleficence against beneficence. Moral acceptability will vary with the reliability of the evidence of quality medical treatment in a destination country, how desperate the patient's situation is without the experimental treatment, risk of infection to the general public, and risk of incurring extra costs for follow-up treatment in the United States (which may be borne by others, rather than the patient) from poor-quality treatment.

The primary reason for United States patients to become medical tourists is to save money, and the savings can be considerable. However, the indicators of quality of medical care in other countries are not reliable, including attempts at accreditation. Again, quality may be less than in the United States, and patients may not have reliable information upon which to base comparative judgments. Regarding US patients who are financially desperate, the possible link between injustice in the United States leading to greater injustice in destination countries was considered. That is, when many in the United States who are denied the right to basic, affordable health care become medical tourists, that might lead to poor people in destination countries receiving worse health care—through brain drain of their medical professionals (or draining away other medical resources) in order to treat medical tourists instead. While the causal connection is far from proven, the concern remains.

What is needed? First, there should be lower demand in the United States for medical tourism based on cost—especially for the 27 million people who are uninsured (Kaiser Family Foundation 2018) and millions more underinsured. This is a matter of justice. Second, greater efforts should be made to improve the quality of medical care in destination countries, and to gather and widely release more reliable data, so that patients' decisions are better informed.

The big picture is clear. There is an elephant in the room, and bioethics should be vigilant in calling attention to it: the power of money. Money affects health care throughout the world, and confronting its power should be more central in bioethical discussions.

Many solutions have been offered—and more could be—for raising the quality of medical care in destination countries, for disseminating that information widely, and for treating poor people in destination countries more justly. However, these solutions are, under current conditions, vulnerable to corruption by economic interests and are either not attempted or not carried out effectively.

For example, while destination countries could tax medical tourism and use the money to give their poor people better medical care, no such policies exist to remedy injustice (Cohen 2015, 224–25). As we saw above, the JCI—which accredits the quality of many international medical centers—economically benefits from approving medical centers too easily. I contend that Cohen's (2015) proposal—to channel US patients who are privately insured into better quality destination sites through default selections and rewards—has promise, but would work well only if health care insurers could be trusted to overlook what would benefit them financially. Cook et al. (2013, 71–72) advocate for NGOs to "quasi-regulate" the quality of health care globally precisely because they are not influenced by monetary gain. But I question whether that insulation would long endure if they did begin to regulate.

I propose that we make economic power more central to bioethical debates of all kinds, asking new questions and reframing old ones. We need to empower patients and health care professionals to stand up individually and through professional and political organizations. And the duty to confront power in health care should be actively debated: what is most in need of change and how can it be accomplished, including through political action. Under the right conditions, medical tourism from the United States can be a valuable and morally justified option. Consider the adjoining sister cities of Calexico in California and Mexicali in Mexico. "It is common for residents of Calexico to get dental and medical care in Mexicali, which has first-rate hospitals and a large number of doctors and dentists. Insurance companies routinely send their American patients to Mexicali for care," which is much less expensive (Abcarian 2019). Where we go from here: remember the elephant.

REFERENCES

Abcarian, R. 2019. "Trump's Threat Roils Calexico, Where a Border Closure Could Spell Disaster." *Los Angeles Times*, April 6, 2019. https://www.latimes.com/local/abcarian/la-me-abcarian-calexico-20190406-story.html.

Beauchamp, T., and J. F. Childress. 1979. *Principles of Biomedical Ethics*. 1st ed. New York: Oxford University Press.

Bebinger, M. 2019. "Has Your Doctor Talked to You about Climate Change?" NPR. Published July 13, 2019. https://www.npr.org/sections/health-shots/2019/07/13/734430818/has-your-doctor-talked -to-you-about-climate-change.

Biller-Andorno, N., and Zümrüt Alpinar. 2014. "Organ Trafficking and Transplant Tourism." In *Handbook of Global Bioethics*, edited by Henk A. M. J. ten Have and Bert Gordijn, 771–83. Dordrecht: Springer.

Cohen, I. G. 2015. *Patients with Passports: Medical Tourism, Law, and Ethics*. New York: Oxford University Press.

Cook, P. S., G. Kendall, M. Michael, and N. Brown. 2013. "Medical Tourism, Xenotourism and Client Expectations." In *Medical Tourism: The Ethics, Regulation, and Marketing of Health Mobility*, edited by C. M. Hall, 60–74. New York: Routledge.

Gordon, M. 2019. "Do You Need That Surgery? How to Decide, and How to Pick a Surgeon If You Do." NPR. Published July 19, 2019. https://www.npr.org/sections/health-shots/2019/07/19/743248074/ do-you-need-that-surgery-how-to-decide-and-how-to-pick-a-surgeon-if-you-do.

Gutierrez, M. 2019. "California Doesn't Have Enough Doctors. To Recruit Them, the State Is Paying Off Medical School Debt." *Los Angeles Times*, July 16, 2019. https://www.latimes.com/politics/la-pol -ca-california-doctor-shortage-medical-debt-20190716-story.html.

Hall, C. M. 2013a. "The Contested Futures and Spaces of Medical Tourism." In *Medical Tourism: The Ethics, Regulation, and Marketing of Health Mobility*, edited by C. M. Hall, 203–16. New York: Routledge.

———. 2013b. "Medical and Health Tourism: The Development and Implications of Medical Mobility." In *Medical Tourism: The Ethics, Regulation, and Marketing of Health Mobility*, edited by C. M. Hall, 3–27. New York: Routledge.

Hamel, L., M. Norton, K. Pollitz, L. Levitt, G. Claxton, and M. Brodie. 2016. "The Burden of Medical Debt: Results from the Kaiser Family Foundation/New York Times Medical Bills Survey." https://www.kff.org/wp-content/uploads/2016/01/8806-the-burden-of-medical-debt-results -from-the-kaiser-family-foundation-new-york-times-medical-bills-survey.pdf.

Healy, M. 2017. "FDA's Program to Speed Up Drug Approval Shaved Nearly a Year Off the Process." *Los Angeles Times*, December 5, 2017. https://www.latimes.com/science/sciencenow/la-sci-sn-fda -expedited-drugs-20171205-story.html.

Hoffman, J., K. Thomas, and D. Hakim. 2019. "3,271 Pill Bottles, a Town of 2,831: Court Filings Say Corporations Fed Opioid Epidemic." *New York Times*, July 19, 2019. https://www.nytimes .com/2019/07/19/health/opioids-trial-addiction-drugstores.html.

Kaiser Family Foundation. 2018. "The Number of Uninsured People Rose in 2017, Reversing Some of the Coverage Gains Under the Affordable Care Act." December 10, 2018. https://www.kff.org/un insured/press-release/the-number-of-uninsured-people-rose-in-2017-reversing-some-of-the-coverage -gains-under-the-affordable-care-act/.

Kotikova, H., and E. Schwartzhoffova. 2013. "Health and Spa Tourism in the Czech and Slovak Republics." In *Medical Tourism: The Ethics, Regulation, and Marketing of Health Mobility*, edited by C. M. Hall, 109–22. New York: Routledge.

Lazarus, D. 2019. "Column: Insured Price: $2,758. Cash Price: $521. Could Our Healthcare System Be Any Dumber?" *Los Angeles Times*, July 30, 2019. https://www.latimes.com/business/ story/2019-07-29/column-could-our-health care-system-be-any-dumber.

Lunt, N., R. Smith, M. Exworthy, S. T. Green, D. Horsfall, and R. Mannion. 2011. "Medical Tourism: Treatments, Markets and Health System Implications: A Scoping Review." http://www.oecd.org/els/ health-systems/48723982.pdf.

Lunt, N., S. T. Green, R. Mannion, and D. Horsfall. 2013. "Quality, Safety and Risk in Medical Tourism." In *Medical Tourism: The Ethics, Regulation, and Marketing of Health Mobility*, edited by C. M. Hall, 32–46. New York: Routledge.

Nuremberg Code. 1947. In *Trials of War Criminals before the Nurernberg Military Tribunals under Control Council Law No. 10*. Volume II. Washington, DC: US Government Printing Office, 1949, 181–182. https://www.loc.gov/rr/frd/Military_Law/pdf/NT_war-criminals_Vol-II.pdf. Reprinted in *Journal of the American Medical Association* 276 (1961).

Papanicolas, I., L. R. Woskie, and A. K. Jha. 2018. "Health Care Spending in the United States and Other High-Income Countries." *Journal of the American Medical Association* 319, no. 10: 1024–39. doi:10.1001/jama.2018.1150.

Rieder, T. 2019. *In Pain: A Bioethicist's Personal Struggle with Opioids*. New York: Harper.

Schumann, J. H., M. Gordon, and C. Weiner. 2019. "Be a Powerful Patient: Take Control of Your Care When You're Seriously Sick." NPR. July 10, 2019. https://www.npr.org/2019/07/09/739927857/take-control-of-your-care-when-youre-seriously-sick.

Warren, V. 2019. "Intellectual Disability, Sexual Assault, and Empowerment." In *Analyzing Violence against Women*, edited by W. Teays, 51–61. Cham, Switzerland: Springer Nature Switzerland AG.

5

Impact and Influence of the Institutional Review Board

Protecting the Rights of Human Subjects in Scientific Experiments[1]

Alison Dundes Renteln

ABSTRACT

This chapter offers a critical analysis of the role that Institutional Review Boards (IRBs) play in the research process. It identifies some of the main flaws and biases in the IRB process of evaluating protocols. Particular emphasis is placed on the problem of ensuring that human subjects have given informed consent to participate in scientific experiments. The challenges may include language barriers, lack of familiarity with scientific research protocols, and overt or subtle forms of coercion. Notorious historic examples of failure to obtain informed human subjects in experiments are considered, such as those involving children in institutions, indigent minorities, and the incarcerated. Moreover, when scholars collaborate on projects with colleagues overseas, serious questions arise as to whether the researchers should be required to make occasional on-site visits to monitor compliance with ethics standards, whether failure to fulfill this responsibility should require IRBs to withhold approval for their biomedical or behavioral studies and compels us to ask what approaches institutions should take to achieve compliance with domestic and international standards. As research is becoming more transnational in scope, the special challenges posed by these collaborations across borders deserve much more attention (Carome 2014). To address widely recognized problems in the research process, more and more world conferences on scientific integrity are being convened (Steneck et al. 2018).[2] There is an urgent need to find legitimate ways to protect scientific integrity and human subjects via policies that can be enforced (Annas 2009).

INSTITUTIONAL REVIEW BOARDS: HISTORICAL BACKGROUND AND FUNCTION

The historical record reflects a long-standing lack of concern for the welfare of individuals who have been forced to be subjects in medical and scientific experiments.[3] The infamous

Nazi experiments on Jewish people in concentration camps shocked the conscience of the world (Grodin and Annas 1996; Barondess 1996). These included the notorious hypothermia studies, Mengele studies of 1,500 twins, and other horrendous research carried out in the name of science.[4] In response to these atrocities, after World War II, the Nuremberg Code was drafted. It reflected a global consensus that researchers must obtain informed consent from human subjects in scientific experiments. It states that "the voluntary consent of the human subject is absolutely essential. This means that the person involved should have the legal capacity to give consent." Further, the notion was that such protection should be guaranteed as a fundamental principle; this was subsequently enshrined in the United Nations International Covenant on Civil and Political Rights (ICCPR) in Article 7.[5]

Despite this development, many other research projects, after the horrendous Nazi experiments, also failed to consider the ethical implications of using people as guinea pigs.[6] Studies that violated human rights and created the impetus for the creation of research boards include the Tuskegee and Guatemala syphilis experiments (Edgar 2000; Jones 1981; Reverby 2018), Willowbrook experiments on children, human radiation experiments on indigenous peoples and prisoners (Advisory Committee on Human Radiation Experiments 1996; Johnston 2007), and others.

Not only has biomedical research been called into question, but behavioral studies have been closely scrutinized as well. The conventional wisdom in the United States has been that Stanley Milgram's shock experiments at Yale University,[7] and the trauma students experienced because of them,[8] whether they were subjects or confederates, exerted pressure on the US government to impose new, more stringent requirements on those receiving federal funding.[9]

An in-depth study of the historical development of IRBs attributes the creation of IRBs to the expansion of biomedical research after World War II (Schrag 2010, 24). The Public Health law massively increased the budgets of the National Institute of Health and the Public Health Corporation. In 1953, when the NIH opened the Clinical Center, this was the impetus behind the first US federal policy for the protection of human subjects (Wichman 2012, 53).

Research boards, composed of at least five scholars in various disciplines, are authorized to review a protocol for a study to determine whether the research design meets federal guidelines. Because regulations stipulate that the board consider the impact of research on the larger society, one member must come from the community to represent the interests of society at large (Allison, Abbott, and Wichman 2008). In the United States, research must follow the Federal Policy for the Protection of Human Subjects or the Common Rule.[10] IRBs were mandated to employ a utilitarian approach, a cost-benefit analysis to ensure that the potential risks of involvement in the research project did not outweigh the benefits.[11] Ordinarily, a majority of those present must approve the study. Some projects will be deemed "exempt," that is, not subject to regulation if they involve minimal risk (Petrosino and Mello 2014, 278).

The principles that IRBs employ in evaluating protocols for studies include well-established norms from global bioethics, such as beneficence, respect for persons, and justice.[12] The US federal law is based on the landmark Belmont Study, which provided a comprehensive investigation of research ethics (Wichman 1998).

Inasmuch as IRBs were initially constructed to evaluate biomedical research, policies were not originally formulated with the particular concerns of social scientists in mind.[13] The rules themselves have been modified over the years, so their scope of application has varied. In 2017, the federal government's Department of Health and Human Services Office for Human Research Protections announced that it would propose a significant change in the application of the rules. The new policy would exempt studies involving "benign behavioral interventions"

(Murphy 2017). Some construed this proposed change as giving social scientists license to determine whether their studies would be harmful to human subjects. The changes came into effect in 2018.

Particularly troubling in the reasoning of IRBs is the presumption that a utilitarian calculus is necessarily the appropriate mode of analysis. In general, they weigh risks and balances to judge whether to authorize researchers to proceed. IRBs are advised to approve protocols as long as they do not entail more than minimal risk.[14] Even assuming that it is the appropriate way to judge research, it is hardly clear how best to weigh benefits and risks in a particular study to ascertain the magnitude of the actual harm likely to be involved.

Using the utilitarian calculus may not function well if risks are unknown and researchers have an incentive to downplay them (Manson and O'Neill 2007). Moreover, the risks associated with participation in research may truly be unknown. When research threatens to violate fundamental human rights, even if risks do not appear to be looming on the horizon, then some studies should not be permitted. To be clear, even if individuals appear to be informed and voluntarily give consent, some types of research simply should be prohibited as a matter of principle. According to this rights-based approach, some research should be rejected, even if it may have benefits for the community.[15]

How should one assess benefits to the community and the human subject? It is unclear whether the frame of reference should be within national borders or the world as a whole. Indeed, one of the major challenges of the twenty-first century is the growing trend toward conducting cross-national research. This phenomenon of "outsourcing" data collection raises serious questions about whether it is feasible to enforce the same standards used in North America and Europe to studies carried out in other countries. Not only is there a dire need to harmonize differing national policies, but there also exist explicit rules in international instruments that must be followed.[16] For instance, the International Ethical Guidelines for Biomedical Research Involving Human Subjects state that:

> The investigator must obtain the voluntary, informed consent of the prospective subject [or legally authorized representative]. . . . Waiver of informed consent is to be regarded as uncommon and exceptional, and must in all cases be approved by an ethical review committee.

Nascent research boards abroad may not have the same experience, nor do they necessarily interpret the international standards similarly.[17]

CRITICISMS

IRBs have been criticized on a number of grounds. In what follows, I highlight some of the most common concerns about their enforcement of policies.

Overzealousness and "Overreach"

Research on IRBs has shown dissatisfaction with aspects of the review process deemed overly cumbersome (Ceci et al. 1985, 996). Considerable resistance to IRBs stems from the perception that board members are "overzealous" in their enforcement of research standards; they seem more like a police force than a research board (Rosnow et al. 1993, 821). Much of the literature reflects a sense that these boards engage in censorship, thwarting serious efforts to undertake important studies (Hamburger 2004; Bledsoe et al. 2007). By contrast, others contend that IRBs have proven to be too weak to enforce research standards partly because they do not monitor the process of conducting research (Elliott 2015).

Scope of Authority

That no consensus exists on the scope of authority of IRBs remains a significant problem. Generally, IRBs are not supposed to reject research on the basis of the content because their mandate is to protect human subjects from risk that outweighs the benefit.[18] While the review of biomedical and behavioral studies falls under the purview of IRBs, whether IRBs should also scrutinize research in the humanities and some branches of the social sciences has proven more controversial.

In the late twentieth century, some questioned whether oral histories, journalism, and ethnographic work should be subject to review.[19] With respect to participant observation in anthropology and sociology, for instance, it may not be feasible to obtain informed consent, as it is with other methodologies (Lederman 2009). While some argue that these types of social science should not be covered by IRB regulations, others on IRBs maintain that this research should receive scrutiny because of genuine concern about privacy rights of subjects.[20] Although some types of research were made exempt from IRBs[21] (though researchers must still apply to request exemptions), the issue persists, as with for instance, how to obtain informed consent in studies involving big data. The new US rule mandated a single IRB oversee multi-site research. This has significant implications for conducting transnational research.

Defining and Assessing Risk

Another serious criticism is the inevitable existence of multiple interpretations of rules governing research (Henry, Romano, and Yarborough 2016; White 2007). Partly, this is a consequence of vagueness in the standards that IRBs are expected to apply to the evaluation of research protocols. Inasmuch as IRBs are expected to interpret what line of research involves "minimal risk," this leads to differing interpretations. While this is unavoidable to some extent, this gives the impression that IRBs may be arbitrary and capricious because institutions vary as to what they permit (Stark 2014).

Bias

IRBs also face the challenge that their assessment reflects bias. Since their inception, IRBs have been accused of political bias (Ceci et al. 1973). They have also been charged with the more specific criticism of gender bias on the basis of their treatment of protocols involving reproductive health issues (Barnes and Munsch 2015). The tendency of IRB regulations to reinforce hegemony is part of the critique:

> Consequently, feminist scholars have expressed concern with IRB regulations for imposing strict hierarchical power relations between IRB committees and researchers, and between researchers and human subjects. (Barnes and Munsch 2015, 597–98)

IRBs are accused of "perpetuating historically masculine epistemologies" and "inequality" (Barnes and Munsch 2015, 598). Research demonstrates that IRBs in the United States have

treated male and female researchers differently, particularly, in evaluating gender-related projects, such as infertility studies and gender identity surveys.[22]

An ethnographic study of IRB review noted that board members judged the quality
of research protocols based on the character of researchers. This is problematic because it
"accentuate[s] ad hominem biases in the review process" (Stark 2014, 181–82). A failure of
IRB assessment is also the possibility that IRB members lack sufficient breadth in their knowledge of various types of methodologies.

Handling Deception in Research

Another problematic feature of IRB decision-making is how best to address research that
involves deception. Some psychological studies require that human subjects not know the real
reason for the research project. This premise means it is not possible for human subjects to
give truly informed consent.

To handle this matter, IRBs often have asked researchers to "debrief" subjects, after the
conclusion of the study. When, however, the project is longitudinal, this renders such a
compromise approach impractical. If the study depends on subjects not being aware of the
true purpose of the research, debriefing while the study is ongoing would undermine the
project. Debriefing can occur only at the conclusion of what may be multiyear data collection. This means the potential damage caused by deception can be intensified because of its
duration.

VULNERABLE POPULATIONS AND INFORMED CONSENT

In reality, the primary concern of IRBs is to protect human subjects, particularly those
belonging to vulnerable communities. This includes children, especially if institutionalized,
pregnant women, active duty military personnel, prisoners, individuals with intellectual
and developmental disabilities, individuals at an educational or economic disadvantage, and
indigenous peoples.[23] Given the controversies raging over research of this kind, views differ
as to whether it should be entirely prohibited, allowed unconditionally, or partially permitted
(Beauchamp and Childress 2009, 90).

As mentioned above, there is cause for alarm when individuals are not informed about the
nature of the research or coerced into participation in studies because of the long history of
abuse in human experimentation. As one scholar puts it succinctly when he says: "Throughout
history, it has been marginalized people in society, including racial minorities, prisoners,
and slaves, who have been most experimented on. These experiments attracted little criticism within 'educated' society of prevailing attitudes" (MacNeill 2009, 4710; Moreno 2001,
29–36, 226–28).

Many of the researchers in the infamous studies showed utter disregard for the requirement
that they obtain informed consent from participants in their experiments. For instance, the
US government funded research in Tuskegee, Alabama, and abroad in Guatemala (Reverby
2018; McNeil 2010) that followed individuals infected with syphilis who were left untreated
for years, even when an effective cure was known to exist. To study the long-term effects of the
disease, scientists at the Tuskegee Institute misled African American men in Macon County,
Alabama, about the purpose of the research. The men did not know that they were receiving
only aspirin, even after penicillin was readily available.

After this came to light, because a journalist published an article about it, the Tuskegee experiments became known as one of the most notorious violations of the rights of individuals as human subjects in US history. It was the longest-running such experiment, lasting over three decades from the 1930s to 1972. Critics acknowledge that the data had medical value and helped develop "more reliable tests for syphilis" (Duke 2013, 116; Washington 2006, 117–18). President Clinton offered an apology May 17, 1997, twenty-five years after the study was publicly acknowledged (Reverby 2018, 38; McNeil 2010). Before the eight men who were still alive, Clinton said that the shameful study "diminished the state of men by abandoning the most basic ethical principles." Paltry reparations were paid to those still alive, but only survivors of the experiments and not their relatives.[24]

It is noteworthy that many of the most egregious violations of the human rights of participants in research experiments have been violations of the rights of persons of color, often who were indigent. Indeed, Tuskegee has become a metaphor for historic injustices against African Americans (Reverby 2018).[25] The furor over the extraordinarily cruel violation of human rights also created the impetus for new laws to protect human subjects (McNeil 2010).

What transpired in the Tuskegee experiments is entirely unacceptable because it violates the basic principle that human subjects should give informed consent. The deception used is entirely incompatible with the principle of autonomy (i.e., that individuals should decide whether to participate in research).

CHILDREN WITH INTELLECTUAL DISABILITIES

Children pose a different problem. The presumption is usually that those held in institutions are unable to give informed consent because the institutional setting induces them to agree to participate in research, even if it is actually not in their self-interest to do so. Much ink has been spilled on the matter of informed consent in these particularly coercive contexts. Furthermore, as the Nuremberg Code stipulates that voluntary consent must be given by those with legal capacity, it is unclear whether children should ever participate in experiments.

In some instances, parents may give proxy consent to have their children participate in nontherapeutic research (McCormick 1974). Whether the bioethics standards permit or require this is open to debate (Ramsey 1976; Bartholome 1976). Oftentimes, children have been part of biomedical and behavioral science experiments while living in institutions.

One of the most infamous examples of parents consenting to the participation of their children in studies with no benefit to them is the sinister Willowbrook School case. Over a few decades in the mid-twentieth century, several thousand children institutionalized there were deliberately given hepatitis to study its effects. These studies were conducted by two prominent scholars, NYU Chair of Pediatrics Dr. Saul Krugman and Dr. Robert Ward, who joined the staff at Willowbrook in 1955. Krugman published papers based on the research and later won accolades based on the data gathered, including the Lasker Prize.[26]

While these scientists conducted experiments that are blatantly unethical by standards past and present, the parents were also complicit. They ostensibly agreed to have children be part of studies in order to have them housed there. Willowbrook actually came to be known as a "dumping ground" for these children.[27] Insofar as parents may not always have the best interests of their children, proxy consent should be viewed with skepticism.

In the 1980s after a national television program exposed the brutal abuses and dilapidated conditions in Willowbrook, plaintiffs filed a class action. After protracted litigation, they prevailed in *New York State Association for Retarded Children v. Carey* (1975); the school was closed, and they received substantial compensation. This research had virtually no scientific benefit and offered no therapeutic benefit to the children. The lawsuit mobilized advocates to sponsor the enactment of legislation to protect children with disabilities.

In another disturbing case, MIT researchers conducted research on the absorption of calcium in children with disabilities at the Fernald School in Waltham, Massachusetts. They gave the youngsters milk containing radiation. The parents were not informed that their children would be ingesting radiation because the consent form only requested permission to have them participate in nutritional studies.

The failure to adhere to informed consent requirement is also evident abroad in the treatment of children in clinical trials conducted by US pharmaceutical companies in Africa. In 2000 the *Washington Post* published a sensational story about a 1996 medical experiment in Kano, Nigeria (Annas 2009). Two hundred children in Nigeria were used in experiments to test Trovan, an antibiotic drug for bacterial meningitis, and also Ceftriaxone. Their families consented to the treatment but were not told that a successful therapy existed. Several children died during the clinical trials—five from Trovan and six from taking a substantially reduced dose of Ceftriaxone (compared to what the FDA recommended).

Other children suffered "brain damage, paralysis or slurred speech" (Smith 2011). When the egregious nature of the research came to light, it sparked controversy and revived discussion about the ethics of outsourcing research. Why had Pfizer chosen to conduct the clinical trials in Nigeria if not to circumvent global bioethics standards?[28]

Families of the affected children sued Pfizer, the world's largest pharmaceutical company, in US federal courts under the Alien Tort Claims Act. Although the district court dismissed the case for lack of subject matter jurisdiction, the US Court of Appeals for the Second Circuit ruled in *Abdullahi v. Pfizer* (2009) that a foreign citizen may bring an action for a tort committed outside the United States involving a violation of that customary law norm that medical experiments may not be performed without obtaining informed consent. Reaffirming this global norm was an important victory.

The state of Kano and the federal government of Nigeria also brought suit against Pfizer. Although the entire litigation continued for fifteen years, the parties eventually agreed to a settlement of $75 million. In late 2014 Pfizer paid compensation to the victims of the 1996 Trovan clinical trial in accordance with the 2009 settlement agreement. Payments were $175,000 to each family (Smith 2011), and a fund of $35 million was created to compensate those affected. Pfizer also agreed to finance community health projects.

THOSE IN DETENTION AND PRISONS

Of special concern here is the treatment of those who are detained by the state because they are out of sight and frequently subject to the most dehumanizing conditions. I turn now to the question of how IRBs address studies in which those in jail or prison are sought as subjects for research (Gostin et al. 2007). This discussion shows how dangerous this research can be for the incarcerated.

Those in total institutions are among those most likely to be abused.[29] Not only are they out of the public eye, but they seldom have the means to challenge policies applied to them. In short, they lack access to justice because of resources and because the state prevents advocates from meeting with them. Prisoners have been brutalized in numerous ways; indeed, human rights advocates usually measure the humanity of a country by the treatment of inmates in its penitentiaries.[30] Furthermore, mass incarceration of individuals has increased dramatically, putting more and more individuals at risk for coercion, including pressure to participate in experiments (Alexander 2010; Simon 2014).

While domestic and international standards clearly guarantee prisoners rights, the question is how they apply to their status as human subjects in scientific research. The Eighth Amendment to the US Constitution protects prisoners from cruel and unusual punishment; yet it is unclear whether participation in experiments should necessarily be deemed a constitutionally proscribed form of punishment. What if prisoners wish to participate as part of rehabilitation and giving back to society?[31] Some maintain, based on US constitutional law, that it would be unreasonable to have an absolute prohibition on research in prison, especially if the study offered a potential therapeutic benefit to the incarcerated. In the United States, the American Bar Association Rules on Standards for Treatment of Prisoners, adopted in 2010, allow for the possibility that prisoners may be part of experiments.[32]

The formulation in international law is broader in scope because it prohibits cruel, inhuman, or degrading treatment or punishment, including experimentation. As mentioned above, Article 7 of the ICCPR specifically provides: "No one shall be subjected without his free consent to medical or scientific experimentation."[33] Some contend this clearly prohibited involuntary human experimentation (Rodley 2009, 413). When prisoners are asked to "consent" to behavioral modification techniques, there is a tremendous potential for abuse "even where prisoners do consent. Where they do not, they are illegal under international law" (414).

The notion that inmates can "consent" is rather dubious. Experts convened by the International Association of Penal Law concluded that "the objective conditions of detention precluded the possibility" that a detained or imprisoned person could ever give "free consent" (Rodley 2009, 414). Thus, medical experimentation on prisoners will almost always be construed as a violation of international human rights law.

Unfortunately, prisoners in the United States have often been used in many different types of experiments.[34] For instance, they were subjects in the notorious human radiation experiments for a decade, from 1963–1973 (Moreno 2001, 144–51). Because the military expressed reservations about operating nuclear-powered airplanes because of their potential threat to male fertility, research was conducted to determine the effect of radiation on testicles. One hundred thirty-one prisoners in Oregon and Washington agreed to be part of experiments to evaluate the effects of radiation, funded by the Atomic Energy Commission. When this came to light, it forced review of the general proposition that prisoners could make "voluntary" decisions. The National Commission for the Protection of Human Subjects of Biomedical and Behavioral Research considered the matter in 1976.[35] Ultimately, the commission recommended banning virtually all research on prisoners (Advisory Committee on Human Radiation Experiments 1996, 263). IRBs had approved very few of the studies undertaken in prisons (Gostin, Vanchieri, and Pope 2007).

As a consequence of the policy of prohibition, scholars who wished to have prisoners as human subjects were compelled to turn to other countries and engage in what might be called "scientific tourism."[36] This raises the question as to whether IRBs have or should have extraterritorial jurisdiction. Sometimes, research committees may exist in places researchers wish to conduct their studies; in this situation IRBs may be expected to defer to the judgment of research committees elsewhere. In other places, such committees may not yet have been established, in which case, IRBs in the United States may have to impose their standards. This is increasingly likely with the 2018 shift to a single IRB scrutiny of multisite research.

For universities lacking the capacity to manage large-scale research projects involving more than several sites, this is likely to lead to the use of independent for-profit IRBs (Craun 2019).[37] It seems, generally speaking, that there is a lack of a global approach to solving this problem of bioethics. This poses a serious challenge because of an increasing trend toward international research collaboration (Appelt et al. 2015).

CROSS-CULTURAL CONSIDERATIONS

If international standards and US federal policy stipulate that informed consent is necessary for research on human subjects, this means researchers and IRBs must demonstrate that studies conducted abroad are consistent with domestic and international requirements.[38] With the new requirement of a single IRB responsible for multisite research projects, this will necessitate more careful attention to compliance by those in charge of projects in other countries.

Admittedly, it may be difficult to ascertain whether human subjects across the globe acquiesce. Philosophers debate whether informed consent can be regarded as meaningful in "developing" countries (Macklin 2004; Aguila et al. 2015). Some worry that language barriers preclude the possibility of obtaining it; in rural settings an analogue to this term may not exist or may be hard to identify. If the individuals are not literate, some fear it may be exceedingly difficult to ensure they have understood the protocol and potential risks of participation.

A researcher apparently encountered this type of cross-cultural barrier when conducting a study of a potential cure for breast cancer in Vietnam (Love and Fost 1997), evidently, because patients were not accustomed to making decisions about their own health. In the literature the claim was that Vietnamese experts who were consulted stated that "application of American standards of informed consent would not be acceptable to Vietnamese physicians, political leaders in Vietnam, or the vast majority of Vietnamese patients" (Love and Fost 1997, 424). The claim was that the paternalistic tradition was not to have patients participate in decision-making about health care.

When the researcher asked the research committee at his American medical school to waive the informed consent requirement, after months of negotiation, they declined to do so, although they did modify the consent form, making it much less detailed (Luna and Macklin 2009, 460–61). In spite of these efforts, the researchers were unsure whether the women in the study understood the risks associated with the clinical trial (Luna and Macklin 2009, 451). Although the women had the capacity to give consent, because of the failure to translate the relevant concepts properly, they lacked the information to make a decision. It remains unclear how to balance the desire to protect international standards with cultural sensitivity (Macklin 2004, 131–62). Luna and Macklin acknowledge the challenge:

> Cultural differences are challenging for research in the international arena and conducted in multicultural settings because of the tension between the ethical requirements of informed consent and the need to remain culturally sensitive, both of which are stated in international guidelines. (2009, 461)

CASE STUDY: STUDY OF DETAINEES IN CHINA

Researchers interested in studying the anatomical structure of brains belonging to those accused of violent criminals awaiting trials in detention decided to conduct research on this subject in China. The motivation for the study was to investigate whether there exists a biological basis for or predisposition to homicide (Yang et al. 2010; Schug et al. 2011). Adrian Raine, a psychologist formerly at the University of Southern California (USC) and subsequently at the University of Pennsylvania, took the lead in this line of research.

Cross-national research of this sort must have raised a red flag for the IRB because of particular features of the Chinese legal system. First, the death penalty is imposed for over a hundred different offenses, including white-collar crimes, and some contend that the presumption of innocence is not firmly established.[39] Second, if a defendant is convicted in China, execution of the inmate occurs quickly, within a few weeks.[40] Third, inmates sometimes have their organs harvested before they gasp their last breath (Doffman 2019). In view of the manner in which capital punishment is administered in China, it is reasonable for IRBs to be concerned about research that might influence the outcome of judicial decision-making.

It is within the realm of possibility that brain scans of those accused of committing violent crimes, if they showed an "abnormality," could be used to win a conviction. The IRB could have legitimately been concerned about ensuring that the brain scans not be acquired by the prosecution and used to win a conviction of the defendants in China.

In these circumstances, what is the proper role of the IRB in the United States? One possibility would be for the IRB to ask the researcher to conduct site visits to ensure that the scans are kept away from government officials. That might prove difficult inasmuch as access to jails and prisons would not be allowed for US researchers. Also, some might consider that excessive interference and suggest that an American researcher simply delegate monitoring to his Chinese colleague. If, however, the IRB permitted the researcher to entrust the colleague abroad with ensuring compliance with research ethics standards, this might conceivably put the university at risk for failure to enforce the law.

Even though the USC IRB withdrew its provisional approval of the study (Wagner 2018), the researcher proceeded to complete the data collection and published the results with a statement that the USC IRB had approved it (Schug et al. 2011, 86). When it came to the attention of USC that the scholar, by then, at another university, had used the data and published it in a journal with a statement that the university IRB had approved the protocol (when, in fact, it had not!), university officials notified the editor of the journal (Craun 2018). The editor responded that the journal would investigate the matter but responded only with an acknowledgment that the submitted materials had been received (Craun 2019).

This case study reveals that recalcitrance on the part of some investigators may block efforts to ensure adherence to international human rights standards and undermine compliance with bioethics rules designed to protect scientific integrity. If scholars and journals both ignore admonitions not to publish research not authorized by the IRB, it will be difficult to safeguard the validity of research processes. The defiant attitude on the part of researchers will likely undermine future efforts of IRBs to enforce standards.

Complicated issues will continue to arise when studies involve cross-national collaborations. This will necessitate more careful consideration of what is at stake, in terms of human rights. Furthermore, given that the reputation of scholars and institutions are on the line, it seems advisable for IRBs not to sanction a "hands-off" approach in this circumstance, despite the perception of research boards as being "overzealous." Protection of the human rights of research subjects, particularly those who are members of vulnerable groups, may require that IRBs take a more proactive approach to cross-national research.

RECOMMENDATIONS

Research involving human subjects must continue to be evaluated carefully in an expeditious manner. Those assessing protocols should have the appropriate expertise. If IRBs do not have members with this background, they should request expert opinions from ethicists. When dealing with multisite projects, the IRB should consult the appropriate research committee in the other countries. If such a research committee does not yet exist, then the researcher abroad should follow the requirements mandated by US regulations and international law.

Because human subjects research in other countries has become a matter of concern for the United Nations, initiatives are under way to develop effective means of ensuring compliance with global bioethics standards. A working group of the CIOMS, set up by the World Health Organization and UNESCO, began meeting in 2017 to formulate policies applicable to clinical trials in resource-limited settings.

It would be ideal if this organization, based on the WHO–UNESCO partnership, resulted in the creation of a global research ethics board to handle disputes associated with transnational research projects. This body could establish panels of certified ethicists to review protocols that appear to jeopardize the rights of human subjects. It is conceivable that appeals could be made via an online system of dispute resolution comparable to that of the World Intellectual Property Organization (WIPO) for appeals of domain name assignment by the Internet Corporation for the Assignment of Names and Numbers (ICANN). There appears to be a trend toward online dispute resolution (Katsh and Rabinovich-Einy 2017).

World conferences on scientific integrity can also formulate new policies to pressure institutions to comply with rules and impose sanctions. By urging professional associations and learned societies can take the lead in promulgating stringent standards. Enforcement of the rules will necessitate the imposition of real sanctions. Researchers who fail to adhere to the requirement to provide informed consent could be fined, denied visas to travel to research sites, or prevented from joining prestigious professional organizations. Journals and presses that publish work that lacks proper certification could also be subject to sanctions.

With regard to prisoners specifically, the United Nations should also play a much more active role in monitoring penal institutions to guarantee the human rights of inmates by protecting them from human experimentation that constitutes an atrocity.[41] Unless there is an obvious therapeutic benefit from participation in an experiment, prisoner research should be almost entirely banned.

Ultimately, the only way to prevent scientific misconduct is to inculcate values that encourage the protection of international human rights standards. If we change the way people think about research so they value the principles of respect for persons, nonmalificence, and justice, then it may be less necessary to insist upon obtaining informed consent. There would be less need to protect those in a weaker bargaining position.

As long as we must rely on obtaining informed consent, it will be crucial to modify the system to make it more effective. Manson and O'Neil (2007), in *Rethinking Informed Consent in Bioethics*, challenge the narrow view of the consent process as merely conveying relevant information to human subjects.[42] In reframing the debate about the interpretation of what constitutes informed consent, they urge us to shift from conceiving of it as disclosure of information to a decision-making process. They offer an imaginative way of strengthening the process of ensuring that individuals give informed consent that takes into account different contexts and, in some situations, proposing use of a series of steps to ensure full understanding. Following this advice, the United Nations should mandate a global consent that requires a series of conversations before individuals sign a written document in their own language. The consent form should be a short, clear document (Cressey 2012).[43]

Interpreters, certified by the United Nations as fluent in the language of the prospective human subjects should be present to answer any questions about the protocol. Although some, like Ruth Macklin, assert that informed consent can be understood universally in substantive terms, that position ignores the reality that there may not necessarily be analogues in other belief systems and informed consent may be conceptualized differently in diverse cultural contexts (Sellos Simoes 2010; Sprumont 2015; Sullivan 2017; Grady 2015).[44] However, if this right to language is afforded protection, then this will increase the chances that human subjects will be informed and make an autonomous decision to participate or not.

The partnership between the WHO and UNESCO should lead to the creation of a research board that provides independent experts to evaluate experiments that may involve unusual techniques and members of vulnerable groups. Eventually this organization might consider setting up an online dispute settlement system modeled after the WIPO arbitration system to handle domain name appeals from ICANN.

When the system breaks down, organizations like Public Citizen and others should receive grants to provide annual reports documenting the behavior of universities and pharmaceutical companies known to have engaged in dubious practices.

CONCLUSION

Although IRBs have come under fire for their aggressive efforts to enforce research standards, they actually struggle to achieve their goals. The lack of clear guidelines, the challenges associated with cross-national research, and the smug attitude of investigators undermine sincere efforts by IRBs to achieve compliance with domestic and international standards.

Balancing the right to scientific inquiry with the rights of human subjects is challenging. The reality that IRBs are confronted with many obstacles does not mean they should cease efforts to promote scientific integrity. It does mean that commentators should offer thoughtful recommendations about how to review studies in a fair, timely manner. Greater support of IRBs combined with clearer rules will help institutions reach the right balance between academic freedom and human rights.

REFERENCES

"The 10 Greatest Cases of Fraud in University Research." 2012. *OnlineUniversities.com* (blog) February 27, 2012. http://www.onlineuniversities.com/blog/2012/02/the-10-greatest-cases-of-fraud-in-university-research/.

Abdullahi v. Pfizer, Inc, 2002 US Dist. LEXIS 17436 at *1 (S.D.N.Y. September 17, 2002) (*Abdullahi I*).

Abdullahi v. Pfizer, Inc., 2005 US Dist. LEXIS 16126, at *23 (S.D.N.Y., August 9, 2003) (*Abdullahi II*)

Abdullahi v. Pfizer, Inc., 2005 US Dist. LEXIS 16126 (S.D.N.Y., August 9, 2005) (*Abdullahi III*).

Addessi, Kristen S. 2017. "How the Willowbrook Consent Decree Has Influenced Contemporary Advocacy of Individuals with Disabilities." Master's thesis, CUNY, New York.

Advisory Committee on Human Radiation Experiments (ACHRE). 1996. *Final Report of the Advisory Committee on Human Radiation Experiments*. Oxford: Oxford University Press https://ehss.energy.gov/ohre/roadmap/achre/report.html.

Aguila, Emma, Maria Dolores Cervera, Homero Martinez, and Beverly A. Weidmer. 2015. Norms and Regulations for Human-Subject Research in Mexico and the United States. In *Developing and Testing Informed-Consent Methods in a Study of the Elderly in Mexico*, edited by Aguila et al. Los Angeles: RAND Corporation.

Alexander, Michelle. 2010. *The New Jim Crow: Mass Incarceration in the Age of Colorblindness*. Cambridge, MA: Harvard University Press.

Allison, Robert D., Lura J. Abbott, and Alison Wichman. 2008. "Nonscientist IRB Members at the NIH." *IRB: Ethics and Human Research* 30, no. 5: 8–15.

Angell, Marcia. 1997. "The Ethics of Clinical Research in the Third World." *New England Journal of Medicine* 337, no. 12: 847–49.

Annas, George. 2009. "Globalized Clinical Trials and Informed Consent." *New England Journal of Medicine* 360, no. 20: 2050–53.

Appelt, Silvia, Brigitte van Beuzekom, Fernando Galindo-Rueda, and Roberto de Pinho. 2015. "Which Factors Influence International Mobility of Research Scientists?" In *Global Mobility of Research Scientists: The Economics of Who Goes Where and Why*, edited by Aldo Geuna, 177–213. Amsterdam: Academic Press/Elsevier.

Associated Press. 2017. "Families of Tuskegee Syphilis Study Victims Seek Leftover Settlement Fund. *New York Times*, July 16, 2017. https://www.nytimes.com/2017/07/15/us/tuskegee-syphilis-study -settlement.html.

Barondess, Jeremiah A. 1996. "Medicine against Society: Lessons from the Third Reich." *JAMA* 276, no. 20: 1647–61.

Bartholome, William B. 1976. "Parents, Children, and the Moral Benefits of Research." *Hastings Center Report*: 44–45.

Beauchamp, Tom L., and James F. Childress. 2009. *Principles of Biomedical Ethics*. 6th ed. Oxford: Oxford University Press.

Bhattacharjee, Yudhijit. 2013. "The Psychology of Lying: Diederik Staple's Audacious Academic Fraud." *New York Times Magazine*, April 26, 2013. https://www.nytimes.com/2013/04/28/magazine/ diederik-stapels-audacious-academic-fraud.html.

Bledsoe, Caroline H., et al. 2017. "Regulating Creativity: Research and Survival in the IRB Iron Cage." *Northwestern University Law Review* 101, no. 2: 593–642.

Brainard, Jeffrey. 2003. "Federal Agency Says Oral-History Research Is Not Covered by Human-Subject Rules." *The Chronicle of Higher Education*, October 31, A25.

Brown, Roger. 1986. *Social Psychology*. 2nd ed. New York: The Free Press.

Carey, Benedict. 2015. "Study on Attitudes toward Same-Sex Marriage Is Retracted by a Scientific Journal." *New York Times*, May 29, 2015, p. A16.

Carey, Benedict, and Pam Belluck. 2015. "Maligned Study on Gay Unions Is Shaking Trust." *New York Times*, May 26, 2015, A1, A11.

Carome, Michael. 2014. "Unethical Clinical Trials Still Being Conducted in Developing Countries." Public Citizen. October 1, 2014. https://www.citizen.org/news/unethical-clinical-trials-still-being -conducted-in-developing-countries/.

Ceci, Stephen J., Douglas Peters, and Jonathan Plotkin. 1985. "Human Subjects Review, Personal Values, and the Regulation of Social Science Research." *American Psychologist* 40, no. 9: 994–1002.

Cressey, Daniel. 2012. "Informed Consent on Trial." *Nature* 482: 16.

Christopher, Paul P., et al. 2016. "Exploitation of Prisoners in Clinical Research: Perceptions of Study Participants." *IRB* 38, no. 1: 7–12.

Cousin-Frankel, Jennifer. 2010. "DNA Returned to Tribe, Raising Questions about Consent." *Science* 328, no. 5978: 558.

Craun, Kristin. 2018. Personal communication from USC director of the University Park Institutional Review Board. January 8, 2018.

———. 2019. Personal communication from the USC director of the University Park Institutional Review Board. July 29, 2019.

De Roubaix, Malcolm. 2008. "Are There Limits to Respect for Autonomy in Bioethics?" *Medicine & Law* 27, no. 2: 365–99.

Diekema, Douglas S. "Conducting Ethical Research in Pediatrics: A Brief Historical Overview and Review of Pediatric Regulations." *Journal of Pediatrics* 149, no. 1: S3–S11.

Doffman, Zak. 2019. "China Killing Prisoners to Harvest Organs for Transplant, Tribunal Finds." *Forbes*, June 18, 2019.

Duke, Naomi. 2013. "Situated Bodies in Medicine and Research: Altruism versus Compelled Sacrifice." In *The Global Body Market: Altruism's Limits*, edited by M. Goodwin. New York: Cambridge University Press.

Edgar, Harold. 2000. "Outside the Community." In Susan M. Reverby, ed., *Tuskegee's Truths: Rethinking the Tuskegee Syphilis Study*. Chapel Hill: University of North Carolina Press, 489–94.

Elliott, Carl. 2015. "Minnesota's Medical Mess." *New York Times*, May 26, 2015, A17.

Emanuel, Ezekiel J., David Wendler, and Christine Grady. "What Makes Clinical Research Ethical?" *JAMA* 283, no. 20: 2701–11.

Flaherty, Colleen. 2017. "Oral History No Longer Subject to IRB Approval." *Inside Higher Ed*, January 20, 2017.

Foucault, Michel. 1978. *Discipline and Punish: The Birth of the Prison*. New York: Vintage Books.

Frezza, Eldo E. 2018. "Clinical Research and Institutional Review Board (IRB)." In *Medical Ethics: A Reference Guide for Guaranteeing Principled Care and Quality*, edited by E. E. Frezza, 203–9. New York: Productivity Press.

Goffman, Erving. 1968. *Asylums: Essays on the Social Situation of Mental Patients and Other Inmates*. Aldine Transaction.

Goode, David, Darryl Hill, Jean Reiss, and William Bronston. 2013. *A History and Sociology of the Willowbrook State School*. Silver Spring, MD: American Association on Intellectual and Developmental Disabilities.

Gostin, Lawrence, Cori Vanchieri, and Andrew Pope, eds. 2007. *Ethical Considerations in Research on Prisoners*. Washington, DC: National Academies Press.

Grady, Christine. 2015. "Enduring and Emerging Challenges of Informed Consent." *New England Journal of Medicine* 372, no. 9: 855–62.

Grodin, Michael A., and George Annas. 1996. "Legacies of Nuremberg: Medical Ethics and Human Rights." *JAMA* 276, no. 20: 1682–83.

Guerrier, Gilles, Didier Sicard, and Paul T. Brey. 2012. "Informed Consent: Cultural Differences." *Nature* 483: 36.

Guerrini, Anita. 2003. *Experimenting with Humans and Children: From Galen to Animal Rights*. Baltimore: Johns Hopkins University Press.

Gunderson, Linda C., ed. 2018. *Scientific Integrity and Ethics in the Geosciences*. Hoboken, NJ: American Geophysical Union and John Wiley & Sons, Inc.

Hamburger, Philip. 2004. "The New Censorship: Institutional Review Boards." *Supreme Court Review*: 271–354.

Harmon, Amy. 2010. "Indian Tribe Wins Suit to Limit Use of Its DNA." *New York Times*, April 21, 2010.

Henry, Stephen G., Patrick S. Romano, and Mark Yarborough. 2016. "Building Trust between Institutional Review Boards and Researchers." *Journal of General Internal Medicine* 31, no. 9: 987–89.

Hill, Darryl B. 2016. "Sexual Admissions: An Intersectional Analysis of Certifications and Residency at Willowbrook State School (1950–1985)." *Sexuality and Disability* 34, no. 2: 103–29.

Hornblum, Allen M. 1998. *Acres of Skin: Human Experiments at Holmesburg Prison*. New York: Routledge.

Human Rights Committee. 1992. "CCPR General Comment No. 20: Article 7 (Prohibition of Torture, or Other Cruel, Inhuman or Degrading Treatment or Punishment)." March 10, 1992. https://www.refworld.org/docid/453883fb0.html.

Johnson, Carolyn Y. 2014. "Coauthor of Retracted Stem Cell Papers Commits Suicide." *Boston Globe*, August 5, 2014.

Johnston, Barbara Rose, ed. 2007. *Half-Lives & Half-Truths: Confronting the Radioactive Legacies of the Cold War*. Santa Fe: School for Advanced Research.

Jones, James H. 1981. *Bad Blood: The Tuskegee Syphilis Experiment.* New York: The Free Press.

Kass, Nancy, Lisa Dawson, and Nilsa I. Loyo-Berrios. 2003. "Ethical Oversight of Research in Developing Countries." *Ethics and Human Rights* 25, no. 2: 1–10.

Katsh, Ethan, and Orna Rabinovich-Einy. 2017. *Digital Justice and the Internet of Disputes.* New York: Oxford University Press.

Kolata, Gina. 2018. "Looking to Prison for a Health Study: Inmate Volunteers May Be the Ideal Subjects for a Look at Salt." *New York Times*, June 5, 2018, D3.

Krimsky, Sheldon. 2017. "The Ethical and Legal Foundations of Scientific 'Conflict of Interest.'" In *Law and Ethics in Biomedical Research: Regulation, Conflict of Interest, and Liability*, edited by Trudo Lemmons and Duff Waring, 63–81. Toronto: University of Toronto Press.

Krugman, Saul. 1986. "The Willowbrook Hepatitis Studies Revisited: Ethical Aspects." *Reviews of Infectious Diseases* 8, no. 1: 157–62.

Lederman, Rena. 2009. "Comparing Ethics Codes and Conventions." *Anthropology News* 50, no. 6: 11–12.

Liang, Bin, Hong Lu, and Roger Hood. 2016. *The Death Penalty in China: Policy, Practice, and Reform.* New York: Columbia University Press.

London, Leslie. 2002. "Ethical Oversight of Public Health Research: Can Rules and IRBs Make a Difference in Developing Countries?" *American Journal of Public Health* 92, no. 7: 1079–84.

Love, R. R., and N. C. Fost. 1997. "Ethical and Regulatory Challenges in a Randomized Control Trial of Adjuvant Treatment for Breast Cancer in Vietnam." *Journal of Investigative Medicine* 45: 423–31.

Luna, Florencia. 2019. "Research in Developing Countries." In *Oxford Handbook on Bioethics*, edited by Bonnie Steinbock, 621–47. New York: Oxford University Press.

Luna, Florencia, and Ruth Macklin. 2009. "Research Involving Human Beings." In *A Companion to Bioethics*, edited by Helga Kuhse and Peter Singer, 2nd ed., 457–48. Chichester: Wiley-Blackwell.

Lurie, Peter, and Sidney Wolfe. 1997. "Unethical Trials of Interventions to Reduce Perinatal Transmission of the Human Immunodeficiency Virus in Developing Countries." *New England Journal of Medicine* 337, no. 12: 853–55.

Macklin, Ruth. 2004. *Double Standards in Medical Research in Developing Countries.* Cambridge: Cambridge University Press.

MacNeil, Paul Ulhas. 2009. "Regulating Experimentation in Research and Medical Practice." In *A Companion to Bioethics*, edited by Helga Kuhse and Peter Singer, 2nd ed., 469–86. Chichester: Wiley-Blackwell.

Manson, Neil C., and Onora O'Neill. 2007. *Rethinking Informed Consent in Bioethics.* Cambridge: Cambridge University Press.

McCormick, Richard A. 1974. "Proxy Consent in the Experimentation Situation." *Perspectives in Biology and Medicine* 18, no. 1: 2–20.

McNeil, Donald G. Jr. 2010. "US Apologizes for Syphilis Tests in Guatemala." *New York Times*, October 1, 2010.

Meeker, Martin. 2012. "The Berkeley Compromise: Oral History, Human Subjects and the Meaning of 'Research.'" In *Doing Recent History: On Privacy, Copyright, Video Games, Institutional Review Boards, Activist Scholarship, and History That Talks Back*, edited by Claire Bond Potter and Renee C. Romando, 115–38. Athens: University of Athens Press.

Milgram, Stanley. 1974. *Obedience to Authority.* New York: Harper & Row.

Moreno, Jonathan D. 2001. *Undue Risk: Secret State Experiments on Humans.* New York: Routledge.

Murphy, Kate. 2017. "Some Social Scientists Are Tired of Asking for Permission." *New York Times*, May 22, 2017.

New York State Association for Retarded Children, Inc, et al. v. Hugh L. Carey, 393 F. Supp. 715 (1975).

New York Times. 1964. "Hospital Accused on Cancer Study; Live Cells Given to Patients Without Their Consent, Director Tells Court." January 21, 1964. https://www.nytimes.com/1964/01/21/archives/hospital-accused-on-cancer-study-live-cells-given-to-patients.html.

Nicols, Lisa et al. 2017. "What Do Revised US Rules Mean for Human Rights? The Updated Common Rule Raises Many Questions." *Science* 357, no. 6352: 650–51.

Nicholson, Ian. 2011. "'Torture at Yale': Experimental Subjects, Laboratory Torment and the 'Rehabilitation' of Milgram's 'Obedience to Authority.'" *Theory and Psychology* 21, no. 6: 737–61.

Petrosino, Anthony, and Daniel Mello. 2014. "Institutional Review Boards." *Encyclopedia of Criminal Justice Ethics*. Los Angeles: SAGE, 476–80.

Ramsey, Paul. 1976. "The Enforcement of Morals: Nontherapeutic Research on Children." *Hastings Center Report* 6, no. 4: 21–30.

Reverby, Susan M., ed. 2000. *Tuskegee's Truths: Rethinking the Tuskegee Syphilis Study*. Chapel Hill: University of North Carolina Press.

———. 2018. "'So What?' Historical Contingency, Activism, and Reflections on the Studies in Tuskegee and Guatemala." In *Bioethics in Action*, edited by Françoise Baylis and Alice Domurat Drege, 32–54. New York: Cambridge University Press.

Rodley, Nigel. 2009. *The Treatment of Prisoners under International Law*. 3rd ed. Oxford: Oxford University Press.

Rothman, David, and Sheila Rothman. 2017. *The Willowbrook Wars*. New York: Routledge. (Originally published 1984 by Harper and Rowe).

Schrag, Zachary M. 2010. *Ethical Imperialism: Institutional Review Boards and the Social Sciences, 1965–2009*. Baltimore: Johns Hopkins University Press.

Schug, Robert A., Yalig Yang, Adrian Raine, Chenbo Han, Jianghong Liu, and Liejia Li. 2011. "Resting EEG Deficits in Accused Murderers with Schizophrenia." *Psychiatry Research: Neuroimaging* 194: 85–94.

Sellos Simoes, Luiz Carlos. 2010. "Informed Consent: The Medical and Legal Challenge of Our Time." *Revista Brasileira de Ortopedia* 45, no. 2: 191–95.

Shweder, Richard A. 2006. "Protecting Human Subjects and Preserving Academic Freedom: Prospects at the University of Chicago." *American Ethnologist* 33, no. 4: 507–18.

Simon, Jonathan. 2014. *Mass Incarceration on Trial*. New York: The New Press.

Smith, David. 2011. "Pfizer Pays Out to Nigerian Families of Meningitis Drug Trial Victims." *The Guardian*, August 12, 2011.

Solovey, Mark. 2013. *Shaky Foundations: The Politics-Patronage-Social Science Nexus in Cold War America*. New Brunswick, NJ: Rutgers University Press.

Sprumont, Dominque. 2015. "Informed Consent: Do Not Be Afraid." *Journal of the Formosan Medical Association* 116: 322–23.

Stark, Laura. 2010. "Closing the Ethics Gap in Medical Research." *Los Angeles Times*, October 8, 2010, A19.

———. 2014. "IRBs and the Problem of 'Local Precedents.'" In *Human Subjects Research Regulation: Perspectives on the Future*, edited by I. Glenn Cohen and Holly Fernandez Lynch, 173–86. Cambridge, MA: MIT Press.

Steneck, Nicholas, H. Tony Maryer, Melissa S. Anderon, and Sabine Kleiner. 2018. "The Origin, Objectives, and Evolution of the World Conferences on Research Integrity." In *Scientific Integrity and Ethics in the Geosciences*, edited by Linda C. Gunderson. Hoboken, NJ: The American Geophysical Union and John Wiley & Sons.

Stern, Judy E., and Karen Lomax. 1997. "Human Experimentation." In *Research Ethics: A Reader*, edited by Deni Elliott and Judy E. Stern, 286–95. Lebanon, NH: University Press of New England.

Subramanian, Sushma. 2017. "Worse than Tuskegee." *Slate*. Published February 26, 2017. http://www.slate.com/articles/health_and_science/cover_story/2017/02/guatemala_syphilis_experiments_worse_than_tuskegee.html.

Sullivan, Laura Specker. 2017. "Dynamic Axes of Informed Consent in Japan." *Social Science & Medicine* 174: 159–68.

Union of Concerned Scientists. 2008. "Scientific Integrity in Policy Making: An Investigation into the Bush Administration's Misuse of Science." July 13, 2008. https://www.ucsusa.org/our-work/

center-science-and-democracy/promoting-scientific-integrity/reports-scientific-integrity.html#.Wx qoPqknZMA.

Union of Concerned Scientists. 2017. "Preserving Scientific Integrity in Federal Policymaking." January 11, 2017. https://www.ucsusa.org/center-science-and-democracy/promoting-scientific-integrity/ preserving-scientific-integrity#.WxqocaknZMA.

US Department of Health and Human Services. 2019. *International Compilation of Human Subjects Research Standards*. Accessed October 17, 2019. https://www.hhs.gov/ohrp/sites/default/files/2019 -International-Compilation-of-Human-Research-Standards.pdf.

Wagner, Marlene. 2018. Personal communication from former chair of the University Park Institutional Review Board. January 8, 2018.

Washington, Harriet. 2006. *Medical Apartheid: The Dark History of Medical Experimentation on Black Americans from Colonial Times to the Present*. New York: Harlem Moon, Broadway Books.

White House. 2009. "Memorandum for the Heads of Executive Departments and Agencies on Scientific Integrity." March 9, 2009. https://obamawhitehouse.archives.gov/the-press-office/memorandum -heads-executive-departments-and-agencies-3-9-09.

White, Ronald F. 2007. "Institutional Review Board Mission Creep: The Common Rule, Social Science, and the Nanny State." *The Independent Review* XI, no. 4: 547–64.

Wichman, Alison. 1998. "Protecting Vulnerable Research Subjects: Practical Realities of Institutional Review Board Review and Approval." *Journal of Health Care Law and Policy* 1, no. 1: 88–104.

———. 2012. "Institutional Review Boards." In *Principles and Practice of Clinical Research*, edited by John I. Gallin and Frederick P. Ognibene, 3rd ed., 53–65. London: Academic Press.

Yang, Yaling, Adrian Raine, Chen-Bo Han, Robert A. Schug, Arthur W. Toga, and Katherine L. Narr. 2010. "Reduced Hippocampal and Parahippocampal Volumes in Murderers with Schizophrenia." *Psychiatry Research: Neuroimaging* 182, no. 1: 9–13.

NOTES

1. This essay will appear in a forthcoming volume *Best Practices in Sciences* coedited by Lee Jussim, Jon Krosnick, and Sean Steven to be published by Oxford University Press. Used with permission.

2. The World Conferences on Research Integrity drafted the Singapore Statement in 2010 and the Montreal Statement in 2013.

3. It is beyond the scope of this essay to provide a survey of all the unethical experiments undertaken. For selected historic examples, see, for example, *New York Times*, 1964, "Hospital Accused on Cancer Study; Live Cells Given to Patients Without Their Consent, Director Tells Court," January 21, 1964, https://www.nytimes.com/1964/01/21/archives/hospital-accused-on-cancer-study-live-cells -given-to-patients.html.

4. The hypothermia experiments exposed Jewish concentration camps to extreme temperatures to find out whether they could be revived after being frozen. This was designed to help the German forces dealing with cold. The twin experiments were gruesome and entailed the killing and dissection of young persons. For the most part, the research yielded results with no scientific value. Even if they had, some contend the data should not be used because of respect for the individuals who died during the experiments.

5. International Covenant on Civil and Political Rights, Article 7: No one shall be subjected to torture or to cruel, inhuman or degrading treatment or punishment. In particular, no one shall be subjected without his free consent to medical or scientific experimentation.

6. Pasteur tried out his rabies vaccine on a child who was violently ill, even though this would now be considered a violation of research ethics. For an interesting account, see Anita Guerrini, 2003, *Experimenting with Humans and Children: From Galen to Animal Rights* (Baltimore: Johns Hopkins University Press), 94–102.

7. Stanley Milgram, 1974, *Obedience to Authority* (New York: Harper & Row). For an interpretation of the significance of the study, see Roger Brown, 1986, *Social Psychology*, 2nd ed. (New York: The Free Press), chapter 1. For a reconsideration of Milgram's legacy that challenges the harsh critiques by Baumrind and others, see Ian Nicholson, 2011, "'Torture at Yale': Experimental Subjects, Laboratory Torment and the 'Rehabilitation' of Milgram's 'Obedience to Authority,'" *Theory and Psychology* 21, no. 6: 737–61. Nicholson comments that Milgram never acknowledged "the full extent of the harm he had inflicted" (11) from data he collected himself from participants.

8. Although not all agree they experienced "trauma," Milgram himself recognized the impact of the experiments. According to Nicholson (2011, 5), Milgram "took steps to minimize the physical and psychological impact of the extreme stress his experiment engendered" and in his publications emphasized that all participates were debriefed or "dehoaxed," as he put it. Most likely, some students were more affected by the experiences than others.

9. Although debate continues about the precise effects Milgram's work had on participants, it appears Milgram downplayed the deleterious potential of his research in his published work but in unpublished material acknowledged his recognition of the ethical questions his studies raised. "In his published work, Milgram hid issues of power, sadism, and self-aggrandizement behind the Holocaust and the pose of disinterested science. However, Milgram's unpublished doubts concerning the ethics and meaning of research suggest that darker personal motivations were an important factor in the study" (Nicolson 2011, 18).

10. The so-called Common Rule was revised in 2017. It exempted certain types of research and added a few requirements.

11. For a brief description of the reasoning process, see Eldo E. Frezza, 2018, "Clinical Research and Institutional Review Board (IRB)," in *Medical Ethics: A Reference Guide for Guaranteeing Principled Care and Quality*, edited by E. E. Frezza, 203–9 (New York: Productivity Press).

12. For the classic work on these, see Tom L. Beauchamp and James F. Childress, 2009, *Principles of Biomedical Ethics*, 6th ed. (Oxford: Oxford University Press).

13. For historical background on how government funding reflected ideological influences, see Mark Solovey, 2013, *Shaky Foundations: The Politics-Patronage-Social Science Nexus in Cold War America* (New Brunswick, NJ: Rutgers University Press).

14. Reference to weighing risks and benefits is the main approach. When exemptions are granted based on a conclusion that a protocol involves minimal risk, that implies use of this utilitarian calculus.

15. It is beyond the scope of this paper to consider the contentious debate about whether data collected via unethical research, when of potential scientific value, should be used.

16. After the Nuremberg Code, the Declaration of Helsinki was adopted, and it incorporated principles to protect human subjects. Subsequently, in 1982, the Council for International Organizations of Medical Sciences (CIOMS) in collaboration with the World Health Organization promulgated another instrument geared to "developing" countries. It has been revised since. https://cioms.ch/revising-2002-cioms-ethical-guidelines-biomedical-research-involving-human-subjects/.

17. For a compilation of national boards and regulations across the globe, see *International Compilation of Human Subjects Research Standards*, compiled by the Office of Human Subjects Research Protection, Department of Health and Human Services, 2019 edition, https://www.hhs.gov/ohrp/international/index.html.

18. Some think that participation in a worthless study should be a factor because a waste of time should count for something.

19. For a discussion of the debate about whether these types of inquiry constitute "research," see Meeker (2012). In 2017 the government revised policy to exclude oral histories from IRB scrutiny beginning in 2018 (Flaherty 2017).

20. In 2003 the federal Office for Human Research Protections issued a letter to the American Historical Association and the Oral History Association saying that oral history interviews need not be regulated by IRBs. Some historians hoped this would influence IRBs across the United States. For more, see Brainard (2003).

21. Nichols et al. (2017).

22. In their provocative analysis, Barnes and Munsch note the dearth of scholarship on the efficacy of IRB protection. They rely on data available from IRB committees (601).

23. The Havasupai tribe in Arizona sued Arizona State University for taking hundreds of blood samples without obtaining informed consent. The lawsuit alleged failure of the ASU IRB. It cost the university almost two million dollars (Harmon 2010). See also Cousin-Frankel (2010).

24. Debate about reparations continues as the heirs have requested that they receive what is left in the settlement fund (Associated Press 2017).

25. Reverby (2018).

26. Krugman (1986) continued to insist that his research was ethical.

27. Goode et al. (2013) mention that the Willowbrook facility had become so notorious as a dumping ground for unwanted children that "children were even left in public places with signs on them saying 'Take Me to Willowbrook.'"

28. Why is it attractive for researchers to engage in "scientific tourism"? Drug companies conduct clinical trials abroad because it is more economical to do so (profit motive). They can circumvent the national policies that exist where they are based. There will be fewer drug interactions because people in "developing" countries cannot afford other medications. They do not have the same worries that they will be under IRB scrutiny. By carrying out clinical trials in other countries, they can avoid dealing with regulatory agencies. It is easier to recruit subjects because the incentives provided can be less.

29. For classics, see Goffman (1968) and Foucault (1978).

30. See reports of the United Nations Special Rapporteurs on Torture or Cruel, Inhuman or Degrading Treatment of Punishment, http://www.ohchr.org/EN/Issues/Torture/SRTorture/Pages/SRTortureIndex.aspx.

31. This issue emerged in the context of a debate over a proposed study about the effects of sodium in diets of prisoners. Although Ruth Macklin notes that, even though "[p]risons are an inherently coercive environment," it doesn't mean informed consent is impossible. She says some prisoners want to give back to society (Kolata 2018).

32. The American Bar Association adopted Standard Rules. See Standard 23-7.11 Prisoners as subjects of behavioral or biomedical research. Researchers claim prisoners do not object or feel exploited (Christopher et al. 2016). Of course, they are in prison (only one correctional facility) when answering questions for these studies as well.

33. In 1992, the Human Rights Committee issued a general comment interpreting Article 7. In paragraph 7, it emphasized the need to protect those under any form of detention or imprisonment. https://www.refworld.org/docid/453883fb0.html.

34. The National Institute of Health supported virus research on federal prisoners during the 1960s at the NIH Clinical Center in Bethesda, Maryland. More than 1,000 prisoners from sixteen penitentiaries had been at the center to be part of the experiments (Stark 2010). See also Hornblum (1998).

35. For detailed discussion, see Advisory Committee on Human Radiation Experiments (1996), chapter 9, "Prisoners: A Captive Research Population," 263–83.

36. The ban is not absolute because research that could benefit inmates (i.e., is therapeutic) might be permitted.

37. University of Southern California has a memorandum of understanding with the Western IRB.

38. A vast literature exists on the subject of ethical issues associated with clinical trials in "developing" countries. Some question on whether it is ethical to use placebo-controlled studies in developing countries are in Lurie and Wolfe (1997). It is beyond the scope of this essay to survey all the commentary. See, for example, Angell (1997) and Kass, Dawson, and Loyo-Berrios (2003).

39. China is considered to be the country with the highest number of executions annually. Although this is treated as a state secret, it is estimated to be in the thousands, according to NGOs such as Amnesty International and Reprieve. Discussion of due process aspects of the legal system can be found in Liang et al. (2016).

40. The NGO, Du Hua, "determined that the average length of time a person sentenced to death waits until execution is two months." https://duihua.org/resources/death-penalty-reform/.

41. Special rapporteurs attempt to gain access to penitentiaries, but states deny it. Members of the United Nations should be required to allow fact finding in prisons.

42. For instance, it should be clear that individuals may refuse and renegotiate the consent (Luna 2019, 626).

43. Bioethics commentators increasingly call for simplified consent forms: "Institutions in developed countries are expanding clinical trials in Africa and Asia and most focus on the signing of the consent form rather than on the exchange of information between researchers and potential participants. Information should be culturally adjusted, taking local factors into account. These might include degrees of illiteracy, native dialects of ethnic minorities, a lack of suitable vocabulary, a preference for communal decision-making, and stigmatization by local authorities if people do not sign" (Guerrier, Sicard, and Brey 2012).

44. Macklin (2004) does concede that informed consent may require contextual analysis for the "procedural" aspects of obtaining consent. This distinction between substantive and procedural aspects of informed consent is not persuasive.

6

Understanding the Concept of Vulnerability from a Western Africa Perspective

Peter F. Omonzejele

ABSTRACT

This paper examines several definitions of vulnerability and found such definitions incapable of sufficiently protecting the interests of vulnerable research subjects in the West African region. Hence, we derived a refined definition of the concept of vulnerability that involves identifying the specific nature of vulnerability of potential research subjects in that region. Some categories of research subjects were indicated in the West African setting, and reasons were advanced why those categories hold a special form of vulnerability in that setting. The indicated categories of potential research subjects in the West African setting were classified into identifiable types (contextual or intrinsic) of vulnerability to demonstrate how our refined definition would apply in practice in that region.

INTRODUCTION

Bioethics is the discipline that addresses ethical issues in medicine and in the life sciences. The ethics of the conduct of medical research (research ethics) among humans is an important aspect of that discipline. This is because medical progress relies on ongoing research on human beings. As a result, an interaction between researchers and research subjects is extremely important even where drugs and treatment already exist. And, clearly, it is even more important in the discovery of treatments for hitherto unmanageable diseases. Without research subjects' participation in medical research, researchers cannot know the efficacy and side effects of a new drug, both of which are essential before one can bring a drug to the market.

However, the conduct of medical research among vulnerable populations raises serious moral concerns. This is because potential research subjects who are perceived to be vulnerable could be taken unfair advantage of as they are usually unable to negotiate genuine informed consent in the research setting. This is often the case when studies are conducted in areas where illiteracy and serious poverty thrives; such circumstances are often responsible for the vulnerability of potential subjects in West African countries in the research setting.

The word "vulnerable" is derived from the Latin word *vulnerare*, which means to wound (Oxford Encyclopedic English Dictionary, 1995), and, as with most etymological derivations, this is inadequate for the purposes of definition. The concept of vulnerability is a complex concept to define. According to the New Oxford Dictionary of English, to be vulnerable means to be "exposed to the possibility of being attacked or harmed, either physically or emotionally." For instance, a European visiting any West African country is vulnerable to malaria attacks in a way the native West Africans are not.

On the other hand, a West African visiting any European country during the winter is vulnerable to the cold-related infections in a way that native Europeans are not. Broadly speaking, as a people, we are all vulnerable one way or another since we are all exposed to one sort of risk or another, from which we cannot protect ourselves.

We shall examine the definition of the concept of vulnerability in the Council for International Organizations of Medical Sciences (CIOMS) document and argue that the application of the concept of vulnerability in the CIOMS document as it currently stands does not sufficiently protect potential research subjects in West African countries due to the prevailing circumstances in that region; hence, there is the need for a refined definition of the concept. This is important if we aim to protect this category of potential research subjects in that region from exploitation and harm in the medical research setting.

WHAT IS VULNERABILITY?

We could preliminarily define vulnerability as follows. To be vulnerable means to be under threat of harm or exploitation leading to harm. If we are dealing with vulnerability in medical research, we are therefore referring to the possible exposure to harm or exploitation within medical research. As already indicated above, vulnerability to harm and exploitation in the research setting is more pronounced in developing (African) countries, often occasioned by social, cultural, and economic circumstances.

To define more precisely what vulnerability means in developing (West African countries) countries, we need to move beyond our preliminary definition. To do so, let us look at the definition used by CIOMS (2002). According to CIOMS, vulnerable research subjects are "those who are relatively or (absolutely) incapable of protecting their own interests because they may have insufficient power, intelligence, education, resources, strength, or other needed attributes to protect their own interests."

This quote implies that to be vulnerable is to be relatively or (absolutely) incapable of protecting one's own interests, or, in other words, of protecting oneself from the threat of harm. An already refined definition would therefore be to be vulnerable means to be incapable of protecting one's interests under threat of harm or exploitation leading to harm.

The CIOMS guidelines appreciate that there are different categories of research subjects: those who are vulnerable and those who are not. Those who are vulnerable cannot protect themselves from harm; hence, there is the need for guidelines to protect such subjects. Vulnerable research subjects can be further categorized into subsectors, based on the nature of protection they require. The above-quoted CIOMS guidelines list insufficient power, intelligence, education, resources, and strength as characteristics that make research subjects vulnerable.

For instance, people with insufficient education and intelligence may be unable to protect their interests because of their inability to refuse or give consent. Insufficient (especially due to severe poverty) resources may limit subjects' capacity to protect their interests because of lack of alternatives. An opportunity for exploitation arises from one party lacking any *alternative* to the solution offered by the would-be exploiter, thereby coercing the exploited (the vulnerable) into acceptance.

Benn (1988, 138) supports this suggestion. An important characteristic of exploiters, he maintains, is that they make an otherwise unattractive offer that the exploited cannot reject because the latter (is vulnerable) has no alternative and is in need of the object or service offered. For instance, if someone offers a woman whose child is dying from pneumonia antibiotics at an exorbitant price knowing that the woman cannot get the needed antibiotics elsewhere, there is no doubt that he is trying to exploit the woman. Where there is an urgent and compelling need and a third party offers the only way of meeting the need, the third party holds the power to coerce.

It is important to identify the possible nature of vulnerability of research subjects. This requires two steps: first, to identify exactly what vulnerability means and, second, to identify which subjects are vulnerable. Going by our working definition of vulnerability as the incapacity to protect one's own interests under threat of harm or exploitation leading to harm, it would then be necessary to understand which categories of research subjects fall under this definition and why. Before we look into categories of vulnerable research subjects, let us further define the concept of vulnerability for the purposes of this paper. In addition to the preliminary definition already given, it is necessary to introduce one more distinction, namely, the distinction between contextual and intrinsic forms of vulnerability.

Contextual forms of vulnerability refer to situations where the inability to protect one's own interests emanates from social, cultural, political, or economic circumstances. The cause of making somebody vulnerable is extraneous. For instance (and, as we shall see below, in our examples), married African women and people who are seriously economically disadvantaged fall into the extraneous category of vulnerability. The lack of choices for access to essential medicines in, for instance, rural Rwanda is a social, political, and economic circumstance affecting Rwandan citizens, rather than vulnerability related to specific people.

If some of the affected citizens were to receive political asylum in the United Kingdom, their access to essential medicines would be guaranteed. Intrinsic forms of vulnerability, on the other hand, exist when the nature of vulnerability is embedded in the research subjects themselves, such as in the case of the incompetent mentally ill[1] or children.

Consequently, the concept of vulnerability can be defined as a contextual or intrinsic state of being incapable of protecting one's own interests under threat of harm or exploitation leading to harm. A proper appreciation of the concept of vulnerability must necessarily take those two forms into reckoning.

THE APPLICATION OF OUR REFINED DEFINITION IN THE WEST AFRICAN CONTEXT: THE INCOMPETENT MENTALLY ILL

The incompetent mentally ill are vulnerable research subjects in ways that competent research participants are not. The most pronounced form of their vulnerability is that of incompetence, the inability to do certain things because of their lack of mental capacity. According to Lott (2005, 42–45), the limitations of using incompetent mentally ill in research revolves around their lacking in the mental faculty required to consent to involvement in clinical research trials.

This makes them vulnerable and exposed to exploitation and therefore requires special protection for them. The incompetent mentally ill do not have the capacity to balance risks and benefits in matters that concern them and are therefore incapable of protecting their own interests under threat of harm or exploitation leading to harm. Hence, the usual protective mechanism of securing informed consent that is to be freely given by research subjects is not helpful in research involving the incompetent mentally ill.

Informed consent, which is a philosophical idea based on the principle of autonomy (Moreno, Caplan, and Wolpe 1998, 690), poses special problems in research involving the incompetent mentally ill because of the subjects' impaired mental faculties. To give informed consent, research subjects are expected to make autonomous decisions. In the West African setting, this may imply securing family or community consent, depending on the ethnic group and the nature of research to be conducted.

Whatever the mode of securing the required consent, an incompetent mentally ill cannot actively participate in the informed consent process, yet it is crucial to secure some form of consent (be it first person, proxy, etc.) from all research subjects, including the incompetent mentally ill.

Proxy consent is normally obtained when the research subjects cannot decide for themselves to participate in research. The inability to decide could be a result of a research subject's being unconscious and a new unapproved drug is thought to be of potential benefit to him or her. Or a research subject is unable to understand or appreciate disclosures in terms of risks and benefits to him or her; such is the case with an incompetent mentally ill person.

Whatever the reason for the incompetence of the research subject, proxy decision-makers need to be those who regard the interests of such incompetent research subjects as paramount. Hence, most proxy decision-makers are family members or those who know such incompetent research subjects well enough to know what the person would have wanted had she or he been able to make the decision herself or himself.

According to Andanda (2005, 16), the moral foundation of informed consent is the moral principle of respect for autonomy. She explains that the requirement for autonomy has two aspects:

> firstly, the requirement that those who are capable of deliberating on their personal choices should be treated with respect for their capacity for self-determination; and secondly, persons with diminished or impaired autonomy, or those who are in dependent or in vulnerable positions, should be protected against harm and abuse.

What is special about involving mentally incompetent research subjects in West Africa? In other words, where are special vulnerabilities, if there are any? We shall restrict ourselves to Nigeria, where I have previously undertaken research on the subject (Omonzejele 2004).

In Nigeria, the causes of mental health problems can be regarded as those prevalent in the West, but they can also be said to be caused by evil casting and machinations. Based on this view, traditional healing, which could involve the use of oracles and divination, are used side by side with Western therapies. In many cases, patients, or, better put, relatives, of such patients prefer to use traditional medicines for mental health care, which they regard as more effective than the Western option. This preference is responsible for the engagement of the services of traditional psychiatrists by many state governments in Nigeria and other West African countries.

Suggested cures tend toward spiritualism in combination with Western treatments. Mental ill health is stigmatized and so constitutes embarrassment to family members and the community of the sufferer (Omonzejele 2004, 165–68). This brings about conflicts of interest between the incompetent mentally ill and their family members and community, which are supposed to give proxy consent on their behalf to participate in research or not. For instance, they could consent on the incompetent mentally ills' behalf more willingly to enlist in research than they would do with those who are not mentally incompetent, whom they perceive to be of more value to the family and the community.

This means that the incompetent mentally ill, who are already vulnerable, have the potential for further damage in a marginalized region, such as West Africa, where they are perceived to be "an embarrassment" to family members. Within the African context, they would have to be regarded as specifically vulnerable and therefore needing further protection according to our definition of intrinsic vulnerability.

To summarize, the incompetent mentally ill are vulnerable research subjects for medical research because they are intrinsically unable to protect their own interests through the channel of giving first-person voluntary informed consent. In West African countries, they are additionally at risk of being volunteered for potentially harmful research by proxy consent given the heavy stigmatization of mental illness in the region.

CHILDREN AS RESEARCH SUBJECTS

In like manner with the incompetent mentally ill in the research setting, it is impossible to secure first-person consent from children (minors) when they are required to enlist in a study. The reason is that, by their very nature, they cannot evaluate risks. Nevertheless, it is important to enlist children into research when there is the need to develop drugs that are exclusively meant to ameliorate children's medical conditions. In such circumstances, their parents make the needed decision for them. For instance, that was the case in the Kano meningitis trials.

In 1996, Pfizer, a big multinational pharmaceutical company, conducted a meningitis study in Kano, Nigeria. According to Stephens (2000), Pfizer tested trovafloxacin (trade name Trovan), an antibiotic, "amid a terrible epidemic in a squalid, short-staffed medical camp lacking basic diagnostic equipment." Macklin explains that the said trial resulted in the death of eleven children, and 200 became deaf, blind, or lame as a result of the trial (Macklin 2004, 99).

The study resulted in litigation between Pfizer and the Federal Republic of Nigeria. The Nigerian government, on behalf of the subjects, argued that the vulnerability of the research subjects in the study was taken advantage of by Pfizer. Pfizer, on the other hand, claimed that it secured proxy (substituted) consent from the guardians of the children involved in the study, but it (Pfizer) could not substantiate its claim.

Besides, it is very likely that the children's parents or guardians may not have been sufficiently aware of the risks involved in the trial (that is, if they were even aware that their wards were involved in a study in the first place) since Kano is located in northern Nigeria, where illiteracy levels are very high. This brings the quality of proxy consents given on behalf of minors to participate in research to question in the West African setting.

How does this state of affairs pose special vulnerability for children in the research setting in West African countries? Let us use the Pfizer study to address this question. Minors by their nature suffer from intrinsic vulnerability and so cannot (and are usually not expected to) sensibly access risks and benefits in most important matters. Most people would agree that the decision to enlist in a study is an important issue (sometimes) with far-reaching consequences.

This implies that investigators have to rely on their guardians or parents to give proxy consent on behalf of their wards after evaluating the risks and benefits associated with a study before giving consent (or otherwise) for their wards' participation in research. In this way, guardians or parents are able to protect their wards from being recruited into harmful and exploitative research. But this line of reasoning works well only in affluent countries where there is easy access to basic health care, with high literacy levels and low poverty levels.

But, in West African countries, the reverse is the case due to lack of access to basic health care and high illiteracy and poverty levels. For instance, in the Pfizer Kano meningitis study, the parents of the children had no alternative to what Pfizer had to offer to their children who suffered from the medical condition. This means that, whatever risks are involved in a study, parents whose children are afflicted with a condition for which they cannot access care elsewhere would consent to enlist their children into a study, irrespective of associated risks, as the only way of accessing care.

Additional risk with recruiting children into research in the West African region is that of the high poverty levels in that region, which could result in guardians or parents placing their own interests before those of their children in the research context. For instance, guardians or parents could give substituted consent for their wards to enlist in risky research if investigators promised to reward such parents or guardians with monetary incentives.

To sum up, children are vulnerable research subjects in the research context because, as with the incompetent mentally ill, they (children) are intrinsically unable to protect their own interests in terms of giving voluntary first-person consent. In the West African context, they are further at risk because those who are in a position to give substituted consent on their behalf may consider their own interests over those of the children they are supposed to protect (in terms of making sure they do not come to harm).

THE POOR AS RESEARCH SUBJECTS

Medical research is generally conducted across different economic groups, at least in most cases. However, undertaking clinical research among poor people raises ethical problems not usually associated with those who are relatively well-off. This is because the poor often volunteer to participate in research as the only way of accessing drugs that they cannot afford otherwise.

Poverty is pandemic and, thus, is not restricted to any continent. But the density of poverty differs from one continent (region) to another. For instance, poverty is much more pronounced in developing (West African) countries; hence, conducting medical research in such regions poses special moral concerns because of the vulnerability of such research populations. According to Dickens and Cook (2003, 79–86):

> Concerns have arisen with special regard to developing countries, however, that commercially-inspired sponsors of studies from developed countries may take advantage of them as host sites to test products intended for sale in affluent markets. These countries may allow studies that recruit suitable participants who are more willing to participate, perhaps for inexpensive inducement, less understanding of study risks, and for instance, less likely and able to pursue grievances and litigation in the event of injury, than developed-country residents.

Economic depravity responsible for the vulnerability of research subjects in developing countries is sometimes not appreciated in its entire ramification. In African countries, most research subjects participate in research for goods they cannot access otherwise, including money. For instance, if money is offered to a research subject in a West African country where draught and hunger thrive, such a subject might not properly evaluate risks associated with a study.

Rather, the subjects would be more interested in the money they are offered to meet some of their urgent needs than in the evaluation of risks. This is because their economic circumstances potentially expose them to exploitation because money offered to them can serve as undue inducement for them to participate in risky research.

Current statistics of the level of poverty in developing countries are worrisome. According to a United Nations Development Programme (UNDP 2005) report, about 850 million people are undernourished, most of whom reside in developing countries. The report goes on to state that, a significant number of deaths in developing countries were linked to poverty. Specifically, UNDP statistics indicate that sub-Saharan Africa accounts for 20 percent of births but 44 percent of child deaths:

> Almost all childhood deaths are preventable. Every two minutes four people die from malaria alone, three of them children. Most of these deaths could be prevented by simple, low-cost interventions. Vaccine preventable illnesses—measles, diphtheria and tetanus—account for another 2–3 million childhood deaths. For every child who dies, millions more will fall sick or miss school, trapped in a vicious circle that links poor health in childhood to poverty in adulthood. Like the 500,000 women who die each year from pregnancy related causes, more than 98% of children who die live in poor countries. They die because of where they are born.

Using World Health Organization statistics, Pogge (2002, 98) captures the situation quite clearly when he states that one-third of all human deaths are poverty related. Diseases such as pneumonia, starvation, and tuberculosis "could be prevented or cured cheaply through food, safe drinking water, vaccinations, dehydration packs and medicines." This state of affairs has serious moral implications for conducting medical research in developing countries, especially as it relates to securing voluntary informed consent. This is because research subjects in poor nations could be easily induced into participating in risky research when offered incentives.

Incentives could be offered to research subjects in poor countries through several ways. For instance, incentives could be the prospect of financial compensation. But incentives could also be offered in nonfinancial form. According to Lott (2005, 45–46):

> Non-financial rewards that could potentially improve the standard of living of impoverished individuals may also be overly coercive. These rewards might include food, shelter, clothing, medical treatment, etc. Again, the depressed level of economic subsistence characterizing the developing world may turn these simple rewards/basic entitlements into forceful incentives for the poor. Researchers conducting trials among the poor of the developing world must not assume that the incentives structure characterizing the poor of their home (developed) countries applies as equally to the poor in the developing world.

It is worthy of note that, though there are poor people in developed countries, the pressure on people in developing countries in terms of providing voluntary informed consent is radically different. For instance, access to essential drugs is not an incentive for the poor in the United Kingdom because a national health system exists. But access to essential drugs is a strong incentive for the poor in West African countries, such as Nigeria, Ghana, Mali, Liberia, Sierra Leone, and Togo.

Though there are people in some developed countries who have no access to essential drugs, poverty in developing countries is much more prevalent, especially, where such developing countries are on the African (West African) continent. This implies that the problem of lack of access to medication is more prevalent in poor nations.

To reiterate, the poor in Britain (and in many developed countries) can access most essential drugs through their public health systems and are therefore not under pressure to participate in medical research in order to access those drugs. The same cannot be said for research subjects in West African (developing) countries, who may enlist in a study as the only way of accessing essential medicines. This means potential research subjects in the West African region are vulnerable in a way potential subjects in developed countries are not.

Hence, the need for a refined definition of the concept of vulnerability is necessary in order to fully capture and appreciate the nature of the specific form of vulnerability of potential research subjects in the West African region. For instance, there is the possibility that pregnant women in West Africa may wish to enlist in research as the only way of receiving free antenatal and postnatal care, irrespective of potential risks to themselves. Because they are responsible for two lives, their own and their babies', this imposes an additional burden.

As already stated, oftentimes, people in poor (West Africa) nations enlist in medical research as the only way to access essential medicines, irrespective of risks associated with such research. This has significant implications for securing genuine and voluntary informed consent because it exposes research subjects in West African (developing) countries to potential exploitation. When there is no alternative, one can easily be induced into research studies with high risks. This form of vulnerability could be subsumed into our definition of contextual vulnerability.

PRISONERS IN WEST AFRICA AS RESEARCH SUBJECTS

Prisoners are people who have been stripped of their freedom and confined to particular surroundings, where their day-to-day activities are monitored by those responsible for their care. In terms of involvement in research studies, they are vulnerable subjects due to their restricted autonomy.

According to Lott (2005, 37), due to their confinement for whatever punitive or rehabilitative reasons, prisoners stand in an unequal power relationship with prison authorities, which could be described as coercive. DeCastro (2003, 171–75) states that coercive conditions make prisoners vulnerable as clinical research subjects because their circumstances militate against voluntary decision-making.

One reason for this is that most prisoners can only get parole based on the recommendations of those who look after them. This is an important factor when prisoners are confined in unhealthy and deplorable prison situations because it is often the case in most African prisons due to shortage of resources for maintaining prisons and prisoners.

Lott (2005. 37–39) advanced several reasons consent given by prisoners to participate in clinical trials may not be considered as voluntary, the most relevant of which is the prospect of reward. Lott (2005, 38) also states that one of the reasons for the vulnerability of prisoners as research subjects is their belief that, if they cooperate in clinical research, they might get rewards for their consent. According to Lott:

Prisoners may be unduly influenced by potential gains offered by research participation, such as reduced prison time or "extra" perks (more/better food, increased access to entertainment or exercise facilities, increased free time, etc.). These rewards can easily cloud prisoners' judgements and prevent them from adequately assessing the potential risks involved in the proposed research, leaving them unable to give informed consent.

He argues further that, although populations who are not confined could be affected by prospects of rewards as well, prisoners are at a higher risk and more vulnerable to abuse. This is because what nonprisoners normally take for granted could be considered as a reward to prisoners for being "good" prisoners.

The prospect of reward may be an even stronger inducement for prisoners to participate in research when such prisoners are imprisoned in Nigeria (Africa). This is because funding for prison services is limited and prisoners often live in deplorable conditions. Hence, if a prisoner thought he could have regular access to bathing soap, instead of one bar a month, or if he thought he could have three meals a day, instead of the usual one or two, he is very likely to be induced to participate in risky research even when he is conscious of the potential harm of the research to him.

This further exposes already vulnerable research subjects to potential damage in a way prisoners in wealthy nations tend not to be. Monetary and nonmonetary advantages derived from pleasing authorities or researchers influence their decision-making on whether a clinical trial is a risk to their health and well-being or not. We could subsume this sort of vulnerability in the research setting within our definition of contextual vulnerability.

WEST AFRICAN MARRIED WOMEN AS RESEARCH SUBJECTS

In most African countries, marriages are recognized only on the payment of the so-called bride price, known as "labola" in South Africa, "roora" in Zimbabwe, "mahari" in East Africa, and "head money" in West African countries. The bride price is the payment either in cash or kind that family members of the groom make to the family members of the bride in order to marry the latter's daughter; the bride price is the last and most important marriage rite, which takes place only after all other rites (such as consultations, "wine carrying," etc.) have been performed to the satisfaction of both families.

The execution of the bride price "ranges from a mainly ritualistic transfer of tokens of esteem to an outright purchase in which the man reserves a right to ask for a refund from the woman's parents if he backs a claim that her behavior is unsatisfactory" (Bishai et al. 2009, 147).

West African women who live with their men in a "marriage-type" union without the payment of the bride price are regarded as concubines to such men. Their families do not consider themselves as in-laws. And neither are such women treated respectfully; they are usually not invited to nor partake in traditional functions, at least not in the capacity of a married woman.

Most West African women would not opt for the nonpayment of their bride price due to its traditional and social implications, not even by women who want to use this as a way of asserting their individuality and autonomy. In any case, women are not in a position to determine whether they want the bride price to be paid or not because it is paid to the bride's kindred.

The payment of the bride price is taken so seriously that, when a couple lived together (and perhaps had children) and the woman died before the payment of her bride price, the price has to be paid even in death; otherwise, she will not receive befitting burial rites as accorded to married women. The payment of the bride price gives husbands and husbands' family members controlling influence over married West African women. This is because the payment of the bride price gives husbands and husband's family members the impression of having "purchased" their wives. Hence, the bride price places West African women in an inferior power relationship in marital unions, and the linked male superiority is supported by native laws and customs tenable in West African countries.

This unequal relationship means that West African women are marginalized in terms of giving first-person voluntary informed consent because they are required to get approval from their husbands before they can enlist in medical research. This state of affairs could also work the other way around where the husband may make his wife partake in a risky clinical research in order to get the money.

West African married women can be considered vulnerable research subjects in the medical research setting because they are unable to protect their own interests through the channel of giving first-person voluntary informed consent. The reason for this is extraneous (that is contextual); through customs and laws expressed in bride-price payments, husbands and their families "buy" the bride and her rights to, for instance, take part in clinical trials.

Consequently, what is clear is that West African women who fall under the bride-price tradition usually require the consent of their husbands or other male members of his family before enrolling in medical research (Omonzejele 2008, 124). This means that at least two people need to consent before a West African woman can participate in a study. This sort of vulnerability falls within our definition of contextual vulnerability.

CONCLUSION

What we have achieved in this essay is to refine the definition of the concept of vulnerability in the research context in order to identify specific forms of vulnerability in the medical research setting. This in turn we believe would potentially assist investigators to devise an appropriate mode of protection required by subjects who fall within an identifiable (contextual or intrinsic) form of vulnerability in order to prevent exploitation and harm in the medical research setting.

To demonstrate how our refined definition (which is a contextual or intrinsic state of being incapable of protecting one's own interests under threat of harm or exploitation leading to harm) works in practice, we applied it to circumstances in the West African region, where we categorized subjects who are unable to protect their own interests, such as the poor, prisoners, and married African women in that region as contextually vulnerable, while the incompetent mentally ill in that region were categorized as being intrinsically vulnerable.

REFERENCES

Andanda, P. 2005. "Informed Consent." *Developing World Bioethics* 5, no. 1.

Benn, S. 1988. *A Theory of Freedom*. Cambridge. Cambridge University Press.

Bishai, D., K. Falb, G. Pariyo, and M. Hindin. 2009. "Bride Price and Sexual Risk Taking in Uganda." *African Journal of Reproductive Health* 13, no. 1.

Council for International Organization of Medical Sciences. 2002. "International Ethical Guidelines for Biomedical Research Involving Human Subjects." Accessed December 15, 2006. https://cioms.ch/wp-content/uploads/2016/08/International_Ethical_Guidelines_for_Biomedical_Research_Involving_Human_Subjects.pdf.

DeCastro, L. D. 2003. "Human Organs from Prisoners: Kidneys for Life." *Journal of Medical Ethics* 29.

Dickens, B. M., and R. J. Cook. 2003. "Challenges of Ethical Research in Resource-Poor Settings." *International Journal of Gynaecology and Obstetrics* 80.

Lott, J. 2005. "Vulnerable/Special Participant Populations." *Developing World Bioethics* 5, no. 1.

Macklin, R. 2004. *Double Standards in Medical Research in Developing Countries.* Cambridge: Cambridge University Press.

Moreno, J. D., A. L. Caplan, and P. R. Wolpe. 1998. "Informed Consent." In *Encyclopedia of Applied Ethics.* San Diego: Academic Press.

Omonzejele, P. 2004. "Mental Healthcare in African Traditional Medicine and Society: A Philosophical Appraisal." *Eubios Journal of Asian and International Bioethics* 14, no. 5.

Omonzejele, P. F. 2008. "African Women as Clinical Research Subjects: Unaddressed Issue in Global Bioethics." *Studies on Ethno-Medicine* 2, no. 2.

Pogge, T. 2002. *World Poverty and Human Rights.* Cambridge: Polity Press.

United Nations Development Programme. 2005. "Statistics." http://hdr.undp.org/reports/global/2005/pdf/HDR05_chapter1.pdf.24.

NOTE

1. Those incompetent mentally ill for whom treatment would be available but is not under current circumstances (due to severe poverty, for instance) fall into both categories.

7

Ethics of Aboriginal Research[1]

Marlene Brant Castellano

ABSTRACT

This paper proposes a set of principles to assist in developing ethical codes for the conduct of research within the Aboriginal community or with external partners. It places the discussion of research ethics in the context of cultural worldview and the struggle for self-determination as peoples and nations. It affirms that Aboriginal Peoples have a right to participate as principals or partners in research that generates knowledge affecting their culture, identity and well-being. To provide context and rationale for the principles presented, the paper outlines features of the current public dialogue on research ethics, how ethics are framed in Aboriginal cultures, and how Aboriginal perceptions of reality and right behavior clash with norms prevailing in Western research. Current initiatives of Aboriginal communities and nations, research-granting councils, and institutions to establish ethical guidelines for Aboriginal research are highlighted as evidence that the development of workable ethical regimes is already well begun.

INTRODUCTION

In September 1992, the Royal Commission on Aboriginal Peoples (RCAP) brought together about 80 Aboriginal Peoples who were involved in research as academics, lawyers, graduate students, project staff and consultants, community leaders, and Elders. We met at a workshop at Nakoda Lodge in Alberta to shape the emerging research agenda of RCAP. As Co-Director of Research, I was the chairperson of the initial session in which numerous participants voiced harsh criticism of past research and serious skepticism that RCAP research would serve them any better. "We've been researched to death!" they protested. The workshop was not off to a promising start, until an Elder who had opened the meeting spoke quietly from a corner of the room. "If we have been researched to death," he said, "maybe it's time we started researching ourselves back to life."

That piece of wisdom has been repeated often in the past 10 years. It was prophetic of the change that would gather remarkable momentum in just a decade. Aboriginal knowledge has always been informed by research, purposeful gathering of information, and thoughtful distillation of meaning. Research acquired a bad name among Aboriginal Peoples because the purposes and meanings associated with its practice by academics and government agents were usually alien to the people themselves and the outcomes were, as often as not, misguided and harmful. Aboriginal Peoples in organizations and communities, as well as universities and colleges and some government offices, are now engaged in transforming Aboriginal research into an instrument for creating and disseminating knowledge that once again authentically represents us and our understanding of the world.

Researching ourselves may mean self-initiated action or it may mean entering into effective partnerships. In either case, the ground rules that should guide new practices are not immediately evident. Where Aboriginal expectations diverge from past practice, resistance from the academic research establishment is to be expected.

This paper proposes a set of principles to assist in developing ethical codes for the conduct of research internal to the Aboriginal community or with external partners.[2] The context and rationale for these principles is developed in early sections outlining the current dialogue on research ethics, how ethics are framed in Aboriginal cultures, and how Aboriginal perceptions of reality and right behavior clash with prevailing norms of western research. Efforts of Aboriginal communities and nations, as well as research granting councils and institutions, to establish ethical guidelines for Aboriginal research are highlighted as evidence that the development of workable ethical regimes is already well begun.

In this paper: research means activity intended to investigate, document, bring to light, analyze, or interpret matters in any domain, to create knowledge for the benefit of society or of particular groups. Aboriginal refers to First Nations, Inuit and Métis Peoples as referenced in the Canadian Constitution. Indigenous is used interchangeably with Aboriginal, usually in international contexts. Where sources refer to specific groups, such as First Nations, the terminology of the source is retained.

Aboriginal research means research that touches the life and well-being of Aboriginal Peoples. It may involve Aboriginal Peoples and their communities directly. It may assemble data that describes or claims to describe Aboriginal Peoples and their heritage. Or, it may affect the human and natural environment in which Aboriginal Peoples live. Ethics refers to rules of conduct that express and reinforce important social and cultural values of a society. The rules may be formal and written, spoken, or simply understood by groups who subscribe to them.

The language, images and perspectives in this paper are those of a Mohawk woman and academic of a certain generation. I suggest that the principles I articulate are relevant more broadly to Aboriginal research, though readers from other cultures, particularly Métis and Inuit colleagues, will undoubtedly need to do some translation to connect my words with their own worldviews and experiences.

AN ACTIVE DISCOURSE ON RESEARCH ETHICS

International concern about research ethics arose from revelations in the Nuremburg trials of atrocities committed in experimentation on humans by the Nazis during the Second World War. To prevent future violations of human rights in the name of science, western nations developed the Nuremburg Code representing broad international agreement on ethical standards in medical research. The Nuremburg Code was replaced by the Helsinki Declaration, which was adopted in 1964 and subsequently updated.[3] Ethical codes place emphasis on informed consent and are intended to strike a balance between the risk incurred by participants and the potential benefit of the research to society.

The federal government is a major funding source, directly and indirectly, of research involving human subjects. It relies on other agencies to ensure that an ethical balance between benefit and risk is maintained in much of the research that it funds. This leaves open questions about the adequacy of safeguards of the public interest.

Aboriginal Peoples interested in research share the concerns cited above and welcome the current review of principles and processes for governing research involving human subjects. However, even if ethical oversight of research sponsored by public institutions is made more consistent, up-to-date and enforceable, there is a danger that concerns particular to Aboriginal Peoples will be neglected or made subject to inappropriate regulation.

It is essential that Aboriginal Peoples and their organizations put forward, not only concerns, but also solutions to the ethical problems that too often have made research affecting them inaccurate and irrelevant. Reframing ethical codes and practice is necessary to ensure the social benefit that motivates research also extends to the Aboriginal Peoples whose universe is being studied.

AN ABORIGINAL PERSPECTIVE ON ETHICS

Descriptions of Aboriginal societies seldom speak of the ethics that support order, cohesion, and personal responsibility in those societies. Anthropological studies document customs that sometimes have the character of law. Dr. Clare Brant, a Mohawk physician who became the first Aboriginal psychiatrist in Canada, wrote an influential paper entitled Native Ethics and Rules of Behavior. In it, he used the language of ethics to illuminate some powerful, unspoken assumptions that guide behavior he observed in his Iroquoian, Cree and Ojibway patients.

Brant's elaboration of the ethic of non-interference, which inhibits argument and advice-giving as normal means of communication, is particularly relevant for researchers and professionals offering services to Aboriginal Peoples. While non-interfering behavior may be perceived as passive and irresponsible, Brant points out that it is consistent with teaching based on non-intrusive modeling rather than direct instruction that attempts to shape the behavior of the learner.[4] Elder Peter Waskahat [speaks] of the foundations of knowledge and the connections between land, family, spirituality, values, and everyday living:

> We had our own teachings, our own education system, teaching children that way of life was taught by the grandparents and extended families; they were taught how to view and respect the land and everything in Creation. Through that the young people were taught how to live, what the Creator's laws were, what were the natural laws, what were these First Nations' laws, and so on, the teachings revolved around a way of life that was based on their values.[5]

When Aboriginal Peoples speak about maintaining and revitalizing their cultures, they are not proposing to go back to igloos and teepees and a hunter-gatherer lifestyle. They are talking about restoring order to daily living in conformity with ancient and enduring values that affirm life. The relationships between individual behavior, customs and community protocols, ethics, values, and worldview are represented [by] the symbol of a tree.

The leaves represent individual behaviors. Protocols and community customs are small branches while ethics, the rules governing relationships, are the large branches. Values, deeply held beliefs about good and evil, form the trunk of the tree. The worldview or perception of reality underpinning life as it is lived, like the roots of the tree, is not ordinarily visible. The whole of the tree is rooted in the earth that supports us. In this symbolic representation, I suggest that the earth is like the unseen world of spirit vast, mysterious, and friendly if we learn how to respect the laws that govern it.

Some nations have codified their ethical systems. The Iroquois Great Law of Peace teaches the importance and the requirements of cultivating a "good mind" in order to live well and harmoniously in the world. The potlatching ceremonies of West Coast nations were public means of validating genealogies, family responsibilities, inheritance rights, and land tenure. Many other nations transmitted their ethical codes orally and non-verbally through family and community relationships. Public ceremonies reinforce the community's worldview and provide instruction for living. Skills for decoding complex messages from the social and natural environment are embedded in traditional languages.

The persons most knowledgable about physical and spiritual reality, the teaching and practice of ceremonies, and the nuances of meaning in Aboriginal languages, are Elders. Elders typically have been educated in the oral tradition, apart from the colonizing influence of the school system. They carry credentials that are recognizable within Aboriginal society, but invisible to those who assess expertise on the basis of formal education. They enjoy respect as sources of wisdom because their way of life expresses the deepest values of their respective cultures. In many cases, they have exceptional skills in transmitting these values to those who seek their counsel.

Within Aboriginal communities, the struggle has gone beyond survival as small enclaves set apart from non-Aboriginal Canada. The struggle now extends to applying cultural ways in the management of lands and economic activity; the structures of governance; the provision of health, education, justice, and other human services; and relations with the larger Canadian society and the world community. The struggle is to live and thrive as peoples and nations maintaining and expressing distinctive worldviews and contributing uniquely to the Canadian federation. In the language of the United Nations Working Group on Indigenous Populations, this is the pursuit of self-determination.

Indigenous peoples have the right of self-determination. By virtue of that right they freely determine their political status and freely pursue their economic, social, and cultural development.[6] Fundamental to the exercise of self-determination is the right of peoples to construct knowledge in accordance with self-determined definitions of what is real and what is valuable. Just as colonial policies have denied Aboriginal Peoples access to their traditional lands, so also colonial definitions of truth and value have denied Aboriginal Peoples the tools to assert and implement their knowledge. Research under the control of outsiders to the Aboriginal community has been instrumental in rationalizing colonialist perceptions of Aboriginal incapacity and the need for paternalistic control.

Aboriginal scholars who have been educated in Western universities and who are conversant with Aboriginal ways of knowledge-seeking are challenging Western assumptions and methodologies of research. In the study of Elders' language referred to earlier, the authors explain:

The Elders' comments allude to formal and long-established ways, procedures, and processes that First Nations persons are required to follow when seeking particular kinds of knowledge that are rooted in spiritual traditions and laws. The rules that are applied to this way of learning are strict, and the seekers of knowledge are required to follow meticulous procedures and processes as they prepare for and enter the "quest for knowledge journey."

In the world of Aboriginal knowledge, a discussion of ethics cannot be limited to devising a set of rules to guide researcher behavior in a defined task. Ethics, the rules of right behavior, are intimately related to who you are, the deep values you subscribe to, and your understanding of your place in the spiritual order of reality. Ethics are integral to the way of life of a people.

The fullest expression of a people's ethics is represented in the lives of the most knowledgable and honorable members of the community. Imposition of rules derived from other ways of life in other communities will inevitably cause problems, although common understandings and shared interests can be negotiated. This is the ground on which Aboriginal Peoples stand as they engage in dialogue about research ethics that will limit the risks and enhance the benefits of research affecting their lives.

"JAGGED WORLDVIEWS COLLIDING"

Leroy Little Bear coined the phrase "jagged world-views colliding" to describe the encounter of Aboriginal philosophies and positivist scientific thought.[7] Aboriginal worldviews assume that human action, to achieve social good, must be located in an ethical, spiritual context as well as its physical and social situation. Scientific research is dominated by positivist thinking that assumes that only observable phenomena matter.

Little Bear points out that much externally-sponsored research has documented customs, but missed the deeper significance of those customs: [anthropologists] have done a fairly decent job of describing the customs themselves, but they have failed miserably in finding and interpreting the meanings behind the customs. The function of Aboriginal values and customs is to maintain the relationships that hold creation together.[8]

Research was defined earlier in this paper as knowledge creation for social benefit. If researchers and those researched have vastly different notions of what constitutes social benefit and how it is achieved, the research is unlikely to satisfy the needs and expectations of participants on both sides of the divide. This section outlines some of the issues that arise in devising ethical regimes that are appropriate for Aboriginal research.

SHOULD ETHICS BE RESTRICTED TO RESEARCH ON HUMAN SUBJECTS?

In Aboriginal knowledge systems, the boundary between material and spiritual realms is easily crossed. Similarly, the boundaries between humans, animals, plants, and natural elements are also permeable. This is represented in traditional stories of communication between humans and other beings and transformation of persons into animals and sea creatures, or vice versa.

Because many Aboriginal societies maintain primary dependence on a healthy natural environment to meet their needs, industrial development that sacrifices environmental values directly infringes on their well-being and human rights. Ethical regimes for Aboriginal research must therefore extend beyond current definitions of research involving human subjects to include research that affects Aboriginal well-being. This includes environmental research that will impact their physical environment or archival research that may perpetuate negative or inaccurate representations of Aboriginal Peoples.

MAINTAINING A BALANCE BETWEEN
REDUCTIONIST ANALYSIS AND HOLISTIC VISION

The prevailing model of scientific inquiry reduces the scope of analysis to smaller bits of reality that can then be analyzed with greater specialization. This is referred to as a reductionist approach. Research that takes measures to exclude variables or influences from the environment that might contaminate cause-effect sequences is applauded as more reliable than data about complex and unexplainable lived experience.

Social sciences exploring human experience have adopted scientific method as the hallmark of their credibility even though human behavior is subject to many variables that interrupt linear cause-effect sequences. The science of ecology has emerged as an approach to understanding the interdependence of elements and processes in the natural world, to some extent countering the dominance of reductionist research. However, the role of intuitive insight or vision in scientific breakthroughs is regularly downplayed in Western disciplines and institutions.

In contrast, the heart of Aboriginal science acknowledges the spirit of the plant, animal, or the land and the importance of relationships in supporting life. Gregory Cajete, a Tewa educator, writes:

> Native peoples through long experience and participation with their landscapes have come to know the language of their places. In learning this language of the subtle signs, qualities, cycles and patterns of their immediate environments and communicating with their landscapes Native people also come to know intimately the "nature" of the places which they inhabit. Learning the language of place and the "dialects" of its plants, animals, and natural phenomena in the context of a "homeland" is an underlying foundation of Native science.[9]

Aboriginal science does not ignore analysis of the particular. In fact, the perception of patterns is synthesized from multiple keen observations. Holistic awareness and highly focused analysis are complementary, not contradictory. There are examples of effective partnership between communities and scientists. The Sandy Lake Health and Diabetes Project in northwestern Ontario has brought together clinical treatment, community-based prevention strategies, and participation in genetic studies.[10]

The Akwesasne Mohawk community enlisted scientists from Cornell University to assist in verifying the nature and degree of pollution that was destroying the health of their crops and animals. Too often, however, perceptions and concerns at the community level are dismissed as anecdotal while priority setting for research proceeds on a different track. The Aboriginal ethic is that all aspects of the world we know have life and spirit and that humans have an obligation to learn the rules of relating to the world with respect. We enter into mutual dialogue with the many people and other beings with whom we share the world.

Knowledge is not a commodity that can be purchased and exploited at will. Information can be gathered by individuals to shape personal perceptions. Aboriginal societies traditionally were respectful of the unique vision of individuals. However, individual perceptions had to be validated by community dialogue and reflection before they became collective knowledge, the basis of collective action. This was the function of the many councils responsible for family, clan, village, or nation affairs. Research that seeks objectivity by maintaining distance between the investigator and informants violates Aboriginal ethics of reciprocal relationship and collective validation.

If the researcher assumes control of knowledge production, harvesting information in brief encounters, the dialogical relationship with human and nonhuman sources is disrupted and the transformation of observations or information into contextualized knowledge is aborted. Attempts to gain an understanding of Aboriginal life and concerns from an objective, short-term, outsider vantage point have produced much research that Aboriginal Peoples reject as distortions of their reality.

Where Aboriginal Peoples control access to research sites, for example research on First Nations territories, organizations and local governments are increasingly insisting on community control. This may mean assuming full responsibility for conducting the research or it may mean collaborative research in which the respective responsibilities of community and outside researchers are set out in a contract. Some initiatives to achieve balanced, mutually-respectful partnerships between Aboriginal communities and researchers are described in a later section of this paper.

VOLUNTARY CONSENT

In many cases, research in Aboriginal communities and on Aboriginal matters is initiated by agencies that Aboriginal Peoples receive essential services from. The research is often funded by governments that control the resources on which the community depends. Rightly or wrongly, many Aboriginal Peoples fear that refusing to consent to research may result in loss of funding for essential needs. They are at a disadvantage in negotiating conditions that would alter the imbalance in power between researchers and the community and give adequate recognition to community priorities and approaches to knowledge creation.

Privacy of health data collected routinely in the delivery of services has become a major concern in health research, especially with the possibility of sharing masses of data electronically across borders. Once information is transferred, it becomes difficult to monitor the secondary or tertiary purposes for which it is used.

FROM GUIDELINES TO GOVERNANCE

The discussion on ethics of Aboriginal research over the past decade has clearly demonstrated that more appropriate and enforceable protection of Aboriginal Peoples' interests in research activities is required. Aboriginal Peoples are wary, however, of regulations that seek to include them as an addendum to protocols based on Western assumptions about the construction and distribution of knowledge. This section proposes some principles flowing from the previous discussion that could guide the development of appropriate ethical regimes.

CREATING KNOWLEDGE: AN ABORIGINAL RIGHT

Aboriginal Peoples in Canada enjoy Constitutional protection of rights to maintain their identity and participate as collectives in Canadian society. Creating and sharing knowledge that authentically represents who you are and how you understand the world is integral to the survival of a people's identity. The Royal Commission on Aboriginal Peoples, in its analysis of the foundations and exercise of self-government, proposed that, "All matters that are of vital concern to the life and welfare of a particular Aboriginal people, its culture and identity" fall within the core of Aboriginal jurisdiction.[11]

The Government of Canada has acknowledged the inherent right of self-government, although the substance of the right has not been defined. This leads to the first principle in devising an ethics regime for Aboriginal research.

Principle 1: Aboriginal Peoples have an inherent right to participate as principals or partners in research that generates knowledge affecting their culture, identity, and well-being. This right is protected by the Canadian Constitution and extends beyond the interests that other groups affected by research might have.

FIDUCIARY OBLIGATIONS

The restricted capacity of Aboriginal nations and communities to protect their interests and rights in the face of more powerful governments and institutions has led to case law defining fiduciary obligations of Canadian governments. A duty to consult, which could affect how research is conducted, has been recognized in decisions of the British Columbia Court of Appeal. NAHO (National Aboriginal Health Organization) is currently preparing a paper exploring related issues in Federal Government Fiduciary Obligations to Aboriginal Peoples and Health.[12]

Principle 2: The Government of Canada has a fiduciary obligation to guard against infringement of Aboriginal rights in research activities, particularly in institutions and activities for which it is responsible. The appropriateness of particular safeguards must be endorsed by Aboriginal Peoples through their representative organizations.

DIVERSITY OF ABORIGINAL CULTURES

In the speech from the throne September 30, 2002, Governor General Adrienne Clarkson announced the Government of Canada's intent to "work with provinces to implement a national system for the governance of research involving humans, including national research ethics and standards." Ethical codes developed by Aboriginal Peoples recognize the diversity of Aboriginal communities and the primacy of community authority in deciding what matters are appropriate for research, the protocols to be respected, and how resulting knowledge should be distributed.[13]

The situation of the Métis deserves specific attention. Although they are recognized in the Constitution as one of the Aboriginal Peoples of Canada, they are excluded from federal and most provincial legislation protecting their Aboriginal rights and access to culturally specific services. They generally lack resources to develop organizational and governance infrastructure and to conduct or partner in research undertakings. A search for examples of community-based research protocols did not turn up examples of Métis-specific documents.

Principle 3: Action by the Government of Canada to establish ethical standards of research should strike a balance between regulations that restrict infringement of Aboriginal rights and those that respect the primacy of ethical codes originating in affected communities, including Métis communities.

THE SCOPE OF ETHICS REGIMES

Ethics that govern research only on human subjects is too restricted to provide the protections sought by Aboriginal Peoples. The report to the Commission on Human Rights from the seminar on draft principles and guidelines for the protection of the heritage of Indigenous People provides a useful model for defining the scope of ethical regulation. The report proposes that heritage broadly defined should be the object of protective measures.

Principle 4: Ethical regulation of research affecting Aboriginal Peoples should include protection for "all knowledge, languages, territories, material objects, literary or artistic creations pertaining to a particular Aboriginal Peoples, including objects and forms of expression which may be created or rediscovered in the future based upon their traditions" as cited in emerging international norms.

HARMONIZATION OF ETHICAL PROTECTION AND INTELLECTUAL PROPERTY LAW

A study of intellectual property and Aboriginal Peoples sponsored by Indian and Northern Affairs Canada underlines the inadequacy and inappropriateness of existing intellectual property regimes in protecting traditional Aboriginal knowledge. National and international rules governing copyright, trademarks, patents, and licensing procedures consistently conflict with Aboriginal culture norms or are practically inaccessible. Canadian rules are designed to conform to international standards

Principle 5: "The federal government, in collaboration with Aboriginal peoples, [should] review its legislation on the protection of intellectual property to ensure that Aboriginal interests and perspectives, in particular collective interests, are adequately protected."[14]

ADMINISTRATIVE INFRASTRUCTURE

Implementation of an ethics regime in Aboriginal research requires more than the clear statement of principles. Legislation at best sets out boundaries for protection of heritage rights. As noted earlier, the administration of existing guidelines is in the hands of research ethics boards (REBs) located in universities and research institutes from which Aboriginal communities are generally distant socially and culturally. The Indian Act, which sets parameters for program funding for registered Indians, makes no provision to support research administration or ethics enforcement in its administrative regimes.

In its submission to Health Canada on Governance of Research Involving Human Subjects, NAHO recommended the creation of a system of Aboriginal research ethics boards (AREBs) to address local, regional and national Aboriginal concerns. The brief further recommended that a national committee be formed consisting of Aboriginal experts who would develop ethical standards that could provide a reference point for AREBs and minimum standards for institutional REBs.[15]

Principle 6: Development and implementation of ethical standards for Aboriginal research should be in the hands of Aboriginal Peoples, as experts in devising minimum standards for general application and as majority members on Aboriginal-specific research ethics boards serving local, regional, and national communities.

COSTS OF IMPLEMENTING AN ETHICAL REGIME

Briefs submitted in 2002 noted that establishing the relationships and ground rules for research in Aboriginal communities required time and effort prior to finalizing a research proposal.[16] Granting councils generally do not fund up-front costs of developing a research plan, thereby placing serious limitations on respectful, that is, ethical research practice in or with Aboriginal communities.

Aboriginal involvement in research to support evidence-based decision-making in service planning is generally not recognized in the administration budgets of Aboriginal communities and organizations.

Principle 7: The costs of community consultation, development of research plans, negotiation and implementation of ethical protocols, and skills transfer should be recognized in budget formulas for research grants and project planning whether conducted by researchers internal or external to Aboriginal communities.

EDUCATION FOR ETHICAL PRACTICE

Ethics of consent, safety, and social benefit in research has evolved over decades. Ethical practice is advanced through a combination of institutional regulation, peer monitoring, and communication in the venues where researchers meet and confer with one another. Establishing research practices that respect Aboriginal worldviews, priorities, and authority will also be an evolving process.

Aboriginal communities that have taken up the challenge of conducting and monitoring research have promoted a broad base of local involvement in field research, management committees, and board governance. By their actions, they have demonstrated that research is too important to be left to a small group of academics, even if the experts are Aboriginal. Aboriginal community researchers, in concert with their peers in graduate schools and universities, are now talking about reinstating Aboriginal research methodologies to explore processes that have been neglected or poorly represented in past research. The terminology used for this process is community control, borrowing the language that has driven parallel moves to assert Aboriginal authority over government institutions, education, health, and social services.

Aboriginal initiative is essential to reform research practice and bring it into conformity with Aboriginal notions of ethical behavior. Aboriginal assertiveness is already evident in the surge of activity devising community research codes and the demands for effective partnership in major research undertakings.

Principle 8: Responsibility for education of communities and researchers in ethics of Aboriginal research rests with Aboriginal communities and organizations, government funders, granting agencies, professional associations, research institutions, and individual researchers working collaboratively.

CONCLUSION

This paper places the discussion of ethics governing Aboriginal research in the context of cultural worldview and the struggle for self-determination as peoples and nations. Self-determination has been seen as a political goal expressed most notably in self-government that recognizes a degree of autonomy in relation to Canadian state institutions. The language of self-government has obscured the reality that Aboriginal Peoples are engaged in a struggle to re-establish ethical order in their communities and nations.

This order re-affirms fundamental values that are rooted in their traditional construction of reality, sometimes called a worldview. Efforts to regain control of education, health, justice, etc. are only in part about the power to govern. They are fundamentally about restoring order to daily living in conformity with ancient and enduring principles that support life.

Aboriginal Peoples are digging deep into their traditional teachings, reviving their ceremonies, and working to conserve their languages. As they take control of community services and institutions, they are proving that traditional teachings offer a sturdy ethical framework for restoring vitality to community life. Aboriginal academics, professionals, service providers, and political leaders are rediscovering and updating traditional values in the practice of education, the arts, health services, justice, and government. They are also challenging the assumptions of research rooted in a scientific worldview that clashes with their concepts of reality and right relationships.

It would be wrong to suggest that all Aboriginal Peoples hold traditional worldviews with the same degree of tenacity. However, applied research, going on spontaneously and autonomously in Aboriginal communities and organizations, is demonstrating that when learning, healing, or rehabilitating is aligned with traditional ethics and values, it takes on astounding energy. The leaves of a tree, connected to their vital source, display health and vigor.

The active discussion of research ethics now going on in government and in granting councils opens up an opportunity for Aboriginal Peoples to engage in dialogue on how research can be adapted to achieve social benefit as they define it. The principles proposed in this paper start with an affirmation of the right of Aboriginal Peoples to generate and disseminate knowledge for and about themselves. This is not to say that all dialogue should halt until complex questions about rights and responsibilities are definitively resolved. Starting with such an affirmation simply underlines that governance of research touches on fundamental issues of Aboriginal culture, identity, and well-being.

Establishing and enforcing ethical practice in Aboriginal research will require a continuing commitment to implementing protective legislation, administrative infrastructure and education of the many participants in research. It is my hope that the articulation of issues and principles in this paper will advance the dialogue that is already underway.

UPDATE (WANDA TEAYS)

At the author's request, we have added an update on recent changes.

In December 2010, three major research agencies of the Canadian federal government adopted an updated policy statement, *The Tri-Council Policy Statement: Ethical Conduct For Research Involving Humans (TCPS)*.[17] The revised guidelines include a chapter titled "Research Involving the First Nations, Inuit and Métis Peoples of Canada."

Aspects of this policy statement are relevant to the discussion on research protocol involving Aboriginal peoples and are worthy of mention. From what is set out below, we can see that steps have been made to address the concerns raised in this chapter and better appreciate the concerns Marlene Brant Castellano has raised.

The key points of the TCPS guidelines for research involving the First Nations, Inuit, and Métis Peoples of Canada include the following:

- The *Principle of Concern for Welfare* is broader, requiring consideration of participants and prospective participants in their physical, social, economic, and cultural environments, where applicable, as well as concern for the community to which participants belong.
- This policy acknowledges the important role of *Aboriginal communities* in promoting collective rights, interests, and responsibilities that also serve the welfare of individuals.
- Aboriginal peoples are particularly concerned that research should enhance their *capacity to maintain their cultures, languages, and identities* as First Nations, Inuit, or Métis peoples and to support their full participation in, and contributions to, Canadian society.
- The interpretation of Concern for Welfare in First Nations, Inuit, and Métis contexts may therefore place strong emphasis on *collective welfare* as a complement to individual well-being.
- *Justice* may be compromised when a serious imbalance of power prevails between the researcher and participants.
- In the case of Aboriginal peoples, *abuses stemming from research* have included misappropriation of sacred songs, stories, and artifacts; devaluing of Aboriginal peoples' knowledge as primitive or superstitious; violation of community norms regarding the use of human tissue and remains; failure to share data and resulting benefits; and dissemination of information that has misrepresented or stigmatized entire communities.

The TCPS guidelines acknowledge that mutual trust and communication take time, not to mention mutually beneficial research goals, collaboration in research, and the assurance "that the conduct of research adheres to the core principles of Respect for Persons, Concern for Welfare—which in this context includes welfare of the collective, as understood by all parties involved—and Justice."

Among the new requirements is the "Recognition of the Role of Elders and Other Knowledge Holders." Such knowledge holders should participate in the design and execution of research and the interpretation of research results. In this way, research will be understood within the context of cultural norms and traditional knowledge. Moreover, "Community advice should also be sought to determine appropriate recognition for the unique advisory role fulfilled by these persons" (Article 9.15).

The TCPS guidelines also recognize the importance of privacy and confidentiality. Article 9.16 sets out the specifics and emphasizes that "Researchers shall not disclose personal information to community partners without the participant's consent." To examine the entire document to get a more detailed presentation of the changed policies, see the Council Policy Statement: Ethical Conduct for Research Involving Humans, December 2010. This is available online at http://www.pre.ethics.gc.ca/eng/resources-ressources/news-nouvelles/nr-cp/2010-12-07.

ACKNOWLEDGMENT

I wish to thank the National Aboriginal Health Organization (NAHO) for providing the stimulus and the forum for exploring these important matters.

NOTES

1. © 2004 National Aboriginal Health Organization and on Creative Commons. Reprinted with permission of the author.

2. This paper was commissioned in 2002 by the National Aboriginal Health Organization to assist in developing an organizational position on research ethics. Documentary research and conceptual development were substantially advanced by conversations with NAHO staff, particularly Richard Jock, Yvonne Boyer, and Gail McDonald. Analysis and interpretation, errors and omissions are entirely the responsibility of the author.

3. Boyer, Yvonne (2003). "Aboriginal Health - A Constitutional Rights Analysis." *Ottawa: National Aboriginal Health Organization*. Available online at: http://www.naho.ca/documents/naho/english/publications/DP_rights.pdf

4. Brant, Clare C. (1990, August), "Native Ethics and Rules of Behavior," *Canadian Journal of Psychiatry*, Vol. 35, p. 534-539.

5. Cardinal, Harold and Walter Hildebrandt, *Treaty Elders of Saskatchewan* (2000). Calgary: University of Calgary Press, p. 6.

6. United Nations, Economic and Social Council, Draft Declaration on the Rights of Indigenous Peoples (1994) E/CN.4/Sub.2/1994/2/Add.l.

7. Leroy Little Bear (2000). "Jagged Worldviews Colliding" In Battiste, Marie (Ed.) *Reclaiming Indigenous Voice and Vision* Vancouver: University of British Columbia Press, p .77.

8. Ibid. p. 81.

9. Cajete, Gregory (2000). *Native Science, Natural Laws of Interdependence*. Santa Fe, NM: Clear Light Publishers, p. 284.

10. National Council on Ethics in Human Research (NCEHR) (2001). Research Involving Aboriginal Individuals and Communities: Genetics as a Focus, Proceedings of a workshop of the consent committee, November 19 to 21, 1999 Ottawa: NCEHR, p. 51.

11. Royal Commission on Aboriginal Peoples (RCAP) (1996). *Report of the Royal Commission on Aboriginal Peoples, Vol. 2, Restructuring the Relationship*. Ottawa: Canada Communications Group, p. 215.

12. Boyer, Yvonne (2003). "Aboriginal Health - A Constitutional Rights Analysis." Ottawa: National Aboriginal Health Organization, Available online at: http://www.naho.ca/documents/naho/english/publications/DP_rights.pdf

13. Mi'kmaw Ethics Watch, Principles and Guidelines for Researchers; Kahnawake Schools Diabetes Prevention Project, Code of Research Ethics; and Schnarch, "Ownership, Control, Access and Possession (OCAP)."

14. Royal Commission on Aboriginal Peoples (RCAP) (1996). Report of the Royal Commission on Aboriginal Peoples, Vol. 3, Gathering Strength, p. 601.

15. National Aboriginal Health Organization (NAHO), "Governance of Research Involving Human Subjects, Research Brief." Ottawa: National Aboriginal Health Organization.

16. Social Sciences and Humanities Research Council (SSHRC) (2002, November 29). A Discussion Paper for the Roundtable Consultation. Ottawa: SSHRC.

17. Canadian Institutes of Health Research, Natural Sciences and Engineering Research Council of Canada, and Social Sciences and Humanities Research Council of Canada, Tri-Council Policy Statement: Ethical Conduct for Research Involving Humans, December 2010. Available online at http://www.pre.ethics.gc.ca/eng/resources-ressources/news-nouvelles/nr-cp/2010-12-07.

Part II Discussion Topics

Wanda Teays

1. What should we do when there are human rights violations that are not recognized or addressed by the government and/or ruling parties of a particular country?
   - Can you think of examples to illustrate your suggestions?

2. In setting out a historical perspective on human rights, Robert Baker asserts that "Pandemics leap from continent to continent, companies peddle their cures around the world, biomedical experiments sponsored in the developed world are conducted in the developing world, and, in all corners of the globe. . . . Thus, to meet the challenges of global bioethics, we need to turn to the more cosmopolitan concept of human rights."
   - State four or five examples of biomedical issues that are fundamentally international.

3. On its website on September 15, 2013, Amnesty International praised the Canadian government for apologizing to Canadian citizen Maher Arar. This was for Arar's torture while a victim of mistaken identity as a terrorism suspect in the war on terror. Amnesty International called for the United States to apologize as well. This has yet to happen.
   - What should professional organizations (the AMA, WMA, etc.) do by way of a response when physician members enable or assist in torture or "harsh interrogation"?

4. Nurses, as well as doctors, have participated in force-feeding (e.g., at Guantanamo Bay). It has been described as brutal and painful and, even if without discomfort, violates informed consent right of refusal under patient autonomy.
   - Besides the public stands against the participation of its members, is there something more professional organizations should be doing?
   - When a hunger striker may be close to death, is life-saving intervention via force-feeding morally acceptable?

5. Disability rights as human rights: According to the UN Statement on Human Rights,

    Persons with disabilities are still often "invisible" in society, either segregated or simply ignored as passive objects of charity. They are denied their rights to be included in the general school system, to be employed, to live independently in the community, to move freely, to vote, to participate in sport and cultural activities, to enjoy social protection, to live in an accessible built and technological environment, to access justice, to enjoy freedom to choose medical treatments and to enter freely into legal commitments such as buying and selling property. (http://www.ohchr.org/EN/Issues/Disability/Pages/Disability Index.aspx).

    *   How could more attention be brought to bear on the sorts of "invisibility" as set out in the quote above?
    *   What needs to shift in terms of attitudes and resources to make an appreciable change for person with disabilities?

6. Do you think it should be morally acceptable to trade, purchase, or barter organs, such as kidneys, that are needed for transplant? Share your thoughts.
    *   What might be done to better protect people from being exploited by international organ brokers?

7. Do you think scientists should use data obtained from experiments that are now seen as immoral, unjust, or exploitative, for example, the Nazi hypothermia studies, the Tuskegee syphilis studies, the Guatemalan studies, the human radiation studies, and so on?
    *   Share your thoughts about using information obtained by means that violate human rights.

8. What role should institutional review boards (IRBs) play in protecting human subjects?

9. In his chapter on human subjects, Peter F. Omonzejele argues that "vulnerability to harm and exploitation in the research setting is more pronounced in developing (African) countries often occasioned by social, cultural, and economic circumstances."
    *   What should Western researchers and pharmaceutical companies do to provide more protection for vulnerable research subjects?
    *   As Omonzejele notes, one condition that makes human subjects more vulnerable is poverty. What sorts of steps could be taken to better protect poor people in developing countries so they are less susceptible to exploitation in research settings?
    *   Omonzejele states that prisoners are another vulnerable research group. They tend not to elicit as much sympathy as the poor. In addition, by their incarceration, the use of prisoners in experimentation is not as easily monitored. What sorts of steps could be taken to address their vulnerability as research subjects?

10. Native Americans, members of First Nations, and other indigenous groups have raised issues around the Human Genome Project, other DNA research of native peoples, and the patenting of genetic material obtained from these research projects.

- How might governments around the world follow the policy guidelines set down by the government of Canada (as discussed in Marlene Brant Castellano's essay in this unit)?
- Castellano shows that there are significant issues in researching Aboriginal people—not to mention major differences in both worldview and values. Would one way to address those to rethink the role and composition of IRBs? Share your thoughts.

11. Should children be allowed to be human subjects in nontherapeutic experimentation?
    - Are there societal or medical benefits that would justify use of children?

12. When the Environmental Protection Agency planned a two-year environmental study using infants and children up to three years old, it offered the families $970, children's clothes, and a camcorder in exchange for using pesticides in their homes.
    - State your major concerns.
    - Respond to this argument for using children in pesticide studies: "It is crucial to study small children because so little is known about how their bodies absorb harmful chemicals."

Part III

LIFE AND DEATH

1

Pediatrics Genomics

Current Dilemmas and a Messy Future

Maya Sabatello

ABSTRACT

Children and adolescents are increasingly exposed to genomic data in nonclinical settings. However, their engagement and power to decide about genomic testing and use of genomic data in such settings is limited. Following the traditional conceptualizations of children as incapable of making medical decisions and the parental prerogative to do so on their behalf, children, and especially adolescents' views, are understudied. In this chapter, I begin with a brief historical summary of the genomic revolution and its scientific challenges. I then explore three key nonclinical settings in which children and adolescents' genomic data are likely to be introduced—genomic research, education, and judicial proceedings—and consider the ethical, legal, and social issues that arise. I argue that the risks associated with such exposure of children's genomic data merit that children, especially adolescents, engage in genomic conversations; indeed, adolescents challenge us to rethink the arbitrariness of age as a determinative factor in genomic decisions, and their exclusion from such conversations runs the risk of betraying the preventive goals of the genomic revolution.

INTRODUCTION

Advances in genomic sequencing technologies and knowledge are developing exponentially—and are entering ever more spaces that are relevant for children. Moving away from the traditional focus on medical settings and diagnosis of genetic conditions among children with disabilities, children today may be exposed to genomic data in a myriad of other nonclinical settings, from research and recreational genomics to education and judicial proceedings.

Whether this knowledge will improve children's well-being is unclear, yet the introduction of genomic data in nonclinical settings raises ethical, legal, and social issues (ELSI) that will need to be addressed. To what extent should children be involved in genomic decisions? For what purposes? What are the acceptable uses of children's genomic data? Who is to determine? Who stands to benefit (or not) from the increased genomic knowledge? And how are we to balance the potential benefits and costs?

This chapter will explore these questions, taking a child-centered perspective; namely, its starting point is of children as subjects of the law, as bearers of human rights, and as rising genomic citizens (Sabatello and Appelbaum 2016). It will start with a brief discussion of the rise of genomic data and technologies and then consider key ELSI challenges in three nonclinical contexts: translational genomic research settings, education, and judicial proceedings. Although pediatrics in its medical connotation applies to all children under the age of eighteen, particular attention will be given to adolescents (ages greater than thirteen). No longer children but not yet adults, this age group challenges us to rethink the boundaries of decision-making and abilities in the genomic era.

THE GENOMIC REVOLUTION IS HERE . . .
AND IT IS HERE TO STAY

The completion of the Human Genome Project in 2003 marks a historical moment, moving from the pre- to the postgenetic revolution. This international effort has been described as a "first glimpse of our own instruction book," "genetic gods" to "figure in our emotional disposition, personality and ethical leanings," and the "book of life" that holds a boom to human health (Nelkin 2001). With this salutary node and a promissory message of conquering knowledge of nature's genetic blueprint, for a time it seemed as though the world's ills would soon be behind us. Of course, this did not happen. Although the number of genetic tests that are performed in clinical and research settings has since increased (American Academy of Pediatrics 2013), it became increasingly clear that the knowledge gained from the Human Genome Project was only the beginning.

Two key forces played a role in this process. First, the increasing knowledge of genetics showed only how much there is yet to learn. As researchers became acutely aware, the common focus on Mendelian inheritance patterns, whereby health conditions are the result of single-gene mutations (e.g., Huntington's disease), is not applicable to most common disorders, such as diabetes, cardiovascular disorders, and most of the psychiatric conditions (McCabe and McCabe 2007). These latter conditions are often genetically complex, involving interaction among multiple genes with each gene having only a small effect on the outcome, as well as interactions between these genes and environments. The realization of the genomic complexity of health conditions called for increased genomic research, development of sophisticated technologies that allow generating extensive genomic data, and ongoing efforts to shift emphasis from treatment to prevention by quantifying health predictions based on genetic data (Katzmarzyk et al. 2014; Lazaro-Munoz et al. 2015).

Another factor that has impacted the scientific revolution is the growing private sector of genomics. Since the completion of the Human Genome Project, direct-to-consumers (DTC) genetic testing companies have sprung up in the United States, offering "off the counter" testing for an array of genetic-based health conditions and lifestyle advice (Caulfield et al. 2015). Despite criticism of the dubious scientific value of their genetic tests (Evans 2008), DTC companies have aggressively marketed "recreative genomics" as a way of "finding ourselves" and as an integral part of the democratization of genomic information (Lee and Crawley 2009). With a strong grounding in individualism, DTC companies have further constructed genomic data as key for consumers' empowerment (Nordgren and Juengst 2009), shifting the responsibility for a healthier future from states to consumers and successfully pushing to the fore personalized or stratified medicine (so-called Me Medicine) as the ultimate path forward (Dickenson 2013) while they engage in a profitable business of selling and conducting research with genomic data of consumers (Niemiec and Howard 2016; Grand View Research 2019).

Discussions about these developments have largely occurred in the adults' world. The focus on autonomy in medical, research, and familial settings has allowed sidestepping the question of whether the underpinning justifications for parents' (and other adults') power over children stands in nonclinical genomic settings. The next sections consider three emerging contexts in which children's genomics data are becoming increasingly important—that is, translational genomic research, education, and judicial proceedings—and highlight the ethical, legal, and social issues that arise.

PEDIATRIC PARTICIPATION IN TRANSLATIONAL GENOMIC RESEARCH

Children are increasingly participating in genomic research (Henderson et al. 2013; Borry et al. 2010); indeed, including them in research is necessary if they are to reap the benefits of genomic research. But children's participation in genomic research evokes ethical and policy dilemmas that are markedly different from those encountered with adults. Below, I discuss two key dilemmas: consent and translational genomics, that is, the application of advances in information technologies, and genomic data to improve clinical care and public health.

Informed consent is widely accepted as an ethical and legal requirement of biomedical research, including genomic research (e.g., Nuremberg Code 1949; ICCPR 1968; Belmont Report 1972). In contrast, children—including adolescents—do not provide consent to participation in genomic research. Rather, their parents are the ones who provide consent on their behalf, while children are only requested to provide an assent (Clayton 2015). Historically, the rationales for this parental prerogative were grounded in notion of family autonomy and assumption that parents are better equipped to make informed decisions about their child's best interests (Capron 1982; King 1984–1985). Although the "best interests" standard does not provide a clear formula, it had been commonly interpreted to mean parents' superior ability to weigh the risks and benefits involved in genomic (and other) research.

Yet these rationales require a pause in the genomic era. With the rise of children's rights worldwide, children can no longer be viewed merely as their parents' passive property. This would apply also in the United States—the only country in the world that has not ratified the Convention on the Rights of the Child—given its commitment, as a signatory to this treaty, to follow its spirit. Moreover, although the justifications for parental medical decision-making power may be appropriate for young children, it is unclear that they are as relevant for adolescents in genomic research. Studies indicate that adolescents' (greater than thirteen years old) medical decision-making capacity is comparable to adults' (Weithorn and Campbell 1982; Santelli et al. 2003) and that their genomic literacy is at least as good as adults' (Rew, Mackert, and Bonevac 2010; Sabatello et al. 2019). And, while adults, including health care providers, have a hard time keeping up with the pace of genetic tests and genomic knowledge (Secretary's Advisory Committee on Genetics, Health, and Society 2011; Genomic Literacy, Education, and Engagement 2017), adolescents may be particularly equipped for the role of informed decision-makers. They are more likely than any other age group to be exposed to genomic data in school (McQueen, Wright, and Fox 2012), online

(Borzekowski and Rickert 2001), and through regular use of mobile devices that offer genomic apps (Sabatello and Appelbaum 2016). As the ethical underpinning of consent and ambiguity of assent are increasingly being questioned (Wetheimer 2014; Wilfond and Diekema 2012; Alderson 2007), it will be key for researchers and policy makers to consider what role adolescents should have in genomic research.

A further complicating factor is that genomic research programs increasingly offer return of individualized results. This possibility opens the door for the disclosure of extensive information about children's genomic makeup, including immediately relevant medical information to findings about children's carrier status (e.g., cystic fibrosis), data about preventable adult onset genomic predispositions (e.g., BRCA 1/2), genomic findings about adult onset untreatable conditions (e.g., Huntington's disease), as well as (in the future) personal behavioral and other traits. Whether and which results from pediatric genomic research should be returned to parents and children has been the focus of heated debates (e.g., Abdul-Karim et al. 2013; Hens, Levesque, and Dierickx 2011; Hens et al. 2009). Studies indicate that parents and health care professionals often disagree about this question, especially, when there is no near-future urgency in knowledge of these data. Parents tend to view access to their children's genomic data as part of their parental responsibility to care for them (Rew, Mackert, and Bonevac 2010; Levenseller et al. 2014; Kaufman et al. 2008; Sapp et al. 2014), whereas health care professionals worry that overdisclosure of children's genomics data would violate children's "right to an open future," that is, the power to decide whether and when they want to know about their genetic makeup (Strong et al. 2014; Appelbaum et al. 2014). Regardless, one consequence of the possibility of return of results from pediatric genomic research is that it brings us closer to clinical settings (Berkman and Hull 2014), where the parental prerogative of providing consent has been largely solid.

Nonetheless, there are several reasons increasing children's, especially adolescents', involvement in genomic decisions is important. First, pediatric engagement in genomic decisions has a legal and philosophical grounding. Although countries and cultures vary in the way they construct childhood and adulthood (Helman 2000), there is a general agreement that a minor's age and maturity are important factors (Levenseller et al. 2014). It is explicitly recognized in Articles 5 and 12 of the Convention on the Rights of the Child and a recommended practice in clinical genomics settings (Holm et al. 2014). A categorical exclusion of children and adolescents from genomic conversations thus not only disregards minors' competence (Borry et al. 2009) but also treats them as a group, rather than as subjects of the law as envisioned in international human rights law.

Second, the goals of the genomic revolution are unlikely to succeed without active engagement of pediatric research participants in the discussion. Although the clinical aspects of genomic data, that is, genomic-based individualized treatment for rare conditions, often receive the spotlight, the deeper promise for genomic research lies in the goal of prevention. The idea that health predictions based on genetic data would allow developing tailored, genomic-based risk-reducing interventions for healthy populations (Meagher et al. 2017). To date, the rhetoric of "precision prevention" (Meagher et al. 2017) has focused primarily on empowering adult patients and research participants to mitigate their health risks through knowledge of their genetic predispositions. However, disregard for the empowerment of healthy, pre- and asymptomatic children and adolescents is counterintuitive to achieving the desired outcome. Many common disorders have pediatric and juvenile onset (e.g., obesity, depression, and schizophrenia) (Katzmarzyk et al. 2014; Salagre et al. 2018; Wilde et al. 2011) but may be averted or mitigated through early preventive intervention, including by increased knowledge of genetic risks and provision of appropriate supports (Rew, Mackert, and Bonevac 2010; Ryan, Virani, and Austin 2015).

Moreover, although studies have shown that genetic information alone has had no impact on risk-reducing health behaviors among adults (Austin 2015; Hollands et al. 2016), childhood, especially adolescence, offers a unique window of opportunity to develop long-term health behaviors that take account of individualized genomic risks. Because adolescents are less ambiguity averse than adults (Blankenstein et al. 2016), they may be better positioned than adults to receive genomic results indicating an increased risk for a condition (rather than a diagnostic value), without this information leading to anxiety, which is a common concern raised in studies with adults (Hollands et al. 2016; Wilhelm et al. 2009; Semaka, Balneaves, and Hayden 2013). Adolescents may also be more amenable to changes in health practices than adults, who need to alter long-standing behaviors (Sabatello and Appelbaum 2016). Indeed, studies of healthy adolescents found that many are willing to make behavioral changes in light of genetic data indicating increased risk for breast cancer, heart disease, hypercholesterolemia, and psychiatric conditions (Harel, Abuelo, and Kazura 2003; Bradbury et al. 2009; Ryan, Virani, and Austin 2015; Sabatello et al. forthcoming A).

Whether the "precision prevention" goal of the genomic revolution can materialize will thus largely depend on the extent to which *healthy* children and adolescents are empowered to be involved in genomic decisions. However, providing genetic counseling and appropriate social supports to children and adolescents raises unique challenges that mirror and are connected with the traditional focus on adults. Studies indicate that parents and teachers play an instrumental role in developing children's and adolescents' sense of empowerment in health-related decisions (Simonsen et al. 2018) but also that parents may be reluctant or not know how to discuss such information with their children (Levenseller et al. 2014; Bernhardt et al. 2003; Metcalfe et al. 2008) and that the genomic knowledge of both parents and teachers may be limited (Johnson et al. 2019; Dougherty 2009). Health care professionals may equally have difficulty empowering children in genomic conversations. Not only that mitigating the parent–child relationship may be challenging (Levenseller et al. 2014; Townsend et al. 2012), but studies also indicate that health care professionals, including genetic counselors, are insufficiently trained in adolescent medicine (Duncan and Young 2013). Finally, it is unclear how inclusive pediatric empowerment will be in a society that is marked by increasing health disparities, including lack of consistent access to health care providers, socioeconomic deprivation that is concentered in racial/ethnic minorities (Bentley, Callier, and Rotimi 2017; Sabatello 2017), and human biorepositories that are overwhelmingly composed of European-ancestry samples and thus are inappropriate for accurate, race-sensitive genomic risks assessment to occur (Popejoy and Fullerton 2016; Palk et al. 2019). Larger systematic changes are urgently needed for the genomic revolution to be implemented for all children.

PRECISION EDUCATION

Another nonclinical setting on the horizon for children's genomic makeup to play a role is education. Of course, there is a long (ugly) history to this development. Genetic research relating to IQ and the idea that educational attainment (and other social success) is only the outcome of "inborn ability" have served to justify eugenic practices and racial/ethnic segregation policies in the twentieth century (King 1992; Martschenko, Trejo, and Domingue 2019). Yet genomics is increasingly making its way back into schools.

Since the 1970s, genetic screening programs have begun to spread. Emerging, initially, among Jewish Orthodox communities in Canada to inform future reproductive decisions by identifying carrier status of Tay-Sachs disease (Gason 2006), such programs have expanded over time to other countries and encompass a growing number of genetic conditions for which students are tested (e.g., cystic fibrosis) (Ross 2006). In line with the agenda of precision prevention (see above), more recent efforts have further shifted to focus on genetic *susceptibility* testing of high school students for hereditary hemochromatosis, a preventable and treatable adult onset disorder (Delatycki et al. 2010). Concurrently, ongoing research is conducted to identify the complex genetic underpinning of a variety of conditions associated with educational attainment, from dyslexia and attention deficit hyperactivity disorder (ADHD) to autism, intelligence, learning disabilities, and behavioral and personality traits, with some researchers explicitly calling for incorporating these data, at some point, into the classroom (Bouregy et al. 2017).

The rationales for the use of genetic data in schools vary. Insofar as genomic screening programs are viewed as promoting public health, school settings are ideal. From a practical perspective, schools provide an opportunity to reach out to a large number of children who are clearly connected with adults' communities (parents, teachers, and the larger community) in ways that can promote awareness and preventive efforts (Gason et al. 2006). The introduction of a diagnostic genomic test in schools may also support a claim for eligibility and facilitate access of children with disabilities for special services, a process that is often contested, time consuming, and cumbersome on parents (Borgelt et al. 2014). Others argue that genomic data may allow for better tailoring of educational interventions to the needs of children with disabilities (e.g., instructing teachers to respond to students with Fragile X in ways that take into account the possible heightened anxiety among such students) (Reilly 2012).

More generally, proponents of precision education suggest that understanding the genetic bases of abilities and behaviors that impact learning-related processes will enable identification of environmental and pharmacological interventions that may enhance students' educational attainment (e.g., Grigorenko 2007; Reilly, Senior, and Murtagh 2015). Thus, although the notion of precision education emerged in the context of children with disabilities, some proponents further suggest that precision education could benefit *all* students (Plomin and Ashbury 2014); indeed, that a genomically tailored approach to education would reflect an up-to-date concept of equality (Rothstein 2007).

Although proponents of precision education have cushioned the issue in concepts of the child's best interests, there are several issues that merit attention. First, who should decide about children's genetic testing in schools? Current approaches to children's genetic testing in connection with schools have generally relied on parental consent, even as there have been concerns about the possible peer pressure for testing in this environment (Gason et al. 2006; Frumkin and Zlotogora 2008). However, this was not always the case. For example, in the early 1970s, twelve states in the United States enacted laws mandating African Americans to undergo genetic screening for sickle cell disease, and untested children were denied access to school (Reilly 2000). Although these laws were repealed in 1972 and it is now well accepted that these laws were mobilized by genetic misperceptions, genetic discrimination, and genetic racism (Fulda and Lykens 2006; King 1992), it is unclear that mandatory screening of *all* students would have a similar fate.

Indeed, with the Child Find Mandate requiring schools to identify, locate, and evaluate *all* children who are eligible for special services, regardless of the severity of their disabilities (IDEA 2004), it seems plausible that increased genomic knowledge about conditions associated with educational outcomes will translate into efforts—even a requirement—that students will be tested or that their genomic data be provided in schools. And while a study of a nationally representative sample of parents in the United States found disapproval of mandatory genetic testing by school authorities (Sabatello et al. forthcoming C), the expansion of newborn screening using next-generation sequencing (Knoppers et al. 2014), along with stakeholders' attitudes that espouse the use of genomic data in a variety of settings (Collins 2014), are indicative of what the future may hold.

For instance, studies found that teachers support knowing of, and adjusting their educational styles to, students' genetic-influenced learning difficulties (Walker and Plomin 2005; Gason et al. 2005). Studies of parents and potential parents indicate high interest in genetic testing of their children for conditions that are associated with educational attainment, such as ADHD (Sabatello et al. forthcoming C), and use of such data to support a claim for their child's eligibility for special services (Borgelt et al. 2014), as well as support for preventive behavioral, environmental, and therapeutic interventions on the basis of children's genetic susceptibility for such disorders (Wilde et al. 2011; May, Brandt, and Bohannan 2012). And, as the scientific community marches ahead with expanding the knowledge of the impact of children's genomic makeup on their educational achievements (Bouregy et al. 2017), there are concurrent efforts to incorporate genetic experts in education-related decisions (Grigorenko 2007), along with calls to enhance the involvement of educational psychologists in deciding how genomic knowledge can inform educational interventions in the classroom (Haworth and Plomin 2012).

Children's voices have been largely absent from these discussions. On the one hand, the seemingly high uptake of genetic testing in schools for carrier status and susceptibility screening may suggest high interest among teenagers. In the aforementioned study of high school students and their parents about genetic susceptibility testing for hereditary hemochromatosis, the researchers found that students' positive views about such screening even exceeded those of parents (Gason et al. 2005; Delatycki et al. 2010). On the other hand, no study to date has explored whether children and teenagers would support testing in schools for learning and behavioral-related genetic conditions. The latter conditions are more genomically complex (as explained above) and have fewer well-established interventions than other medical and physical conditions (e.g., preimplantation genetic testing to avoid conception of a child with Tay-Sachs). Nor is it clear that children and adolescents would support the use of such data by nonmedical professionals, such as educators and educational staff. Learning and especially behavioral and psychiatric conditions are highly stigmatized in society (Mueller et al. 2012; O'Driscoll et al. 2012; Kinnear et al. 2016) and given conventional misperceptions about genomic determinism—the idea that there is an unbreakable, causative one-sided relationship between genes and behavioral outcomes (Wachbroit 2000)—there is a risk that sharing of such data will lead to biases in assessment of a student's educational capabilities and in decisions about educational placement (Sabatello 2017).

The possible testing and use of children's genetic data in school further raises unique privacy concerns. Teachers' knowledge of students' genetic makeup raises the possibility of their (at least perceived) knowledge of the genetics of the student's family members, thus extending the potential bias to a student's siblings and other relatives (Sabatello 2017). Privacy issues also arise in the relationship between children and their parents, especially with regard to behavioral traits. Even if parents' knowledge of their children's behavioral disorders is acceptable, it is unclear that parents' knowledge of their children's behavioral genetic *predispositions* fit the criteria of "best interests" nor which predispositions parents should know about (consider, e.g., athletic and musical talent versus risk for schizophrenia). Indeed, as a Belgian study of children ages fifteen to nineteen found, although they approve of sharing "medically important information" with parents, they are more reluctant to share data about behavioral predispositions (e.g., alcoholism) when no medical necessity exists (Hens et al. 2011).

These concerns are all the more acute give the limitations of the Genetic Information Non-Discrimination Act (GINA). This law prohibits the use of genetics in determining health insurance eligibility and employment decisions but does not extend to school settings or to situations in which individuals voluntarily shared their genomic data (e.g., posted it online). Insofar as teachers and parents may disclose students' genomic information, the protections afforded by GINA will be lost. Before moving ahead with precision education, there is a need to think about how to balance children's legitimate genomic privacy concerns, as well as adults' (i.e., parents, teachers, and scientists) responsibilities in protecting children's interests in both better educational achievements and other important goals.

CHILDREN'S GENETIC MAKEUP IN JUDICIAL PROCEEDINGS

Although children cannot generally file an independent claim in courts, children's genetic makeup is increasingly introduced in judicial proceedings. Historically, children's genetic testing was sought predominantly in paternity cases, where a litigant (the mother and a putative father) aimed to establish whether an individual was the biological parent of a child (Uniform Parentage Act 2002). Genetic testing for identification purposes has obtained a high level of accuracy—it can confirm father–child genetic relationships with 99.9 percent probability—and has been initially viewed as divulging important data to improve the child's financial and emotional future.

In past decades, however, children's genetic data have been entering into other judicial proceedings and they are entering with a twist. Rather than testing children for identification purposes, genetic tests are increasingly aimed to determine health status. So far, children's genetic data have been used particularly to rebut causation of injury in medical malpractice and toxic tort litigation, where genetic evidence may elucidate whether a child's medical condition is due to genetic causes or medical malpractice (e.g., Marchant and Robert 2009; Brice and Christian 2017). There is yet indication that such data are likely to enter other judicial proceedings as well. First, studies have found that judges are receptive to genetic data and that they are willing not only to admit such evidence but also to compel testing (Hoffmann and Rothenberg 2007). This receptiveness may fit with common views of genomics as "hard evidence" (John 2015), even as genomics—especially in the context of complex conditions— are often far from being deterministic. Second, the blooming market of DTC genetic testing companies further facilitates (and will likely continue to facilitate) the introduction and use of children's genomic data in courts. Such companies have not only adjusted their genomic services to assure that, for example, their paternity tests can meet judicial admissibility criteria (for additional costs), but also their home kits have enabled and are likely to continue to enable an easy process for adults to test their children for a growing number of conditions (Phillips 2016) and genomic predispositions that, notwithstanding the testing's questionable scientific value (Evans 2008), may impact litigants in judicial proceedings.

Finally, it is likely that information about *adults'* genetic predisposition that began entering courts will, in the future, expand to children who are embroiled in judicial proceedings. For instance, a few defendants in criminal courts have already requested to be tested or to have admitted their genetic test results showing low activity of the MAOA gene to mitigate judicial decisions of culpability and punishment (Denno 2009; Denno 2011; McSwiggan, Elger, and Appelbaum 2017). The MAOA gene has been associated with impulsive behavior among individuals who experienced childhood adversity, and its introduction in juvenile criminal proceedings may gain a similar traction, especially because some scholars advocate for early testing of children for this gene (Marchant 2012). Indeed, the use of genomic data in criminal proceedings may further extend in the future to other behavioral traits or conditions that have juvenile onset, such as opioid addiction (Eitan et al. 2017). With a growing number of studies to identify genetic markers associated with a propensity to addiction (Randesi et al. 2019; Crist, Reiner, and Berrettini 2019) and developing pharmacogenomic treatment options to improve clinical outcomes, the introduction of such data may have significant impact on judicial determination of responsibility and rehabilitation options.

Similarly, information about children's behavioral and psychiatric genetic makeup will likely make its way to child custody proceedings. Such proceedings—including termination of parental rights, adoption, and determination of primary custody of children—revolve around future predictions of both parents' fitness and children's psychosocial adjustment. In the absence of genetic tests to diagnose or confirm common psychiatric conditions (e.g., depression), existing court cases have largely been made on the basis of family history or in the abstract. For example, in *William S. v. State, Dept. of Health & Social Services* (2014; WL 199882, Supreme Court of Alaska), parents appealed a decision to terminate their parental rights, claiming that their child's psychiatric conditions (including depression, ADHD, and oppositional defiant behavior) were the result of his genetics rather than their neglect and family home environment as determined by the court. Yet, as knowledge of psychiatric genetics and advanced sequencing technologies continues to emerge, it is likely that, once available, genetic tests showing children's predispositions for behavioral and psychiatric conditions will be used in family courts.

Whether the use of children's genomic data in courts will positively facilitate judicial resolution is open for debate (Sabatello and Appelbaum 2016; Sabatello and Appelbaum, 2017). Insofar as genomic data will provide a more accurate prediction about the child's future well-being, judicial actors may find them useful. Conversely, there is a concern that genomic data may introduce biases into the decision-making process. Studies indicate that the general public has only limited understanding of how genetic risk factors affect multifactorial diseases (Etchegary 2014) and tends to view genetics through essentializing frames and as immutable characteristics (Heine et al. 2017). Although no study has explored judicial genomic literacy, it is likely that judges and other judicial actors are prone to similar conceptualizations of genomics. Even as the public's endorsement of genomic determinism may be overrated (Condit 2011), a study of the use of psychiatric genetic evidence in child custody proceedings found that the general public often conflates psychiatric genetic predisposition and the presence of symptoms (Sabatello et al. forthcoming B). The introduction of children's genomic data in court may thus lead to increased medicalization of children who are involved in judicial proceedings, also in the absence of symptoms. Concurrently, studies indicate that the public's understanding of genomic data is often strategic (Condit 2019). That is, people interpret genomic data in light of other social constructs that they hold and which they use as they find fit to advance their interests. When considered in light of the heightened racism, sexism, ableism, and other social ills that differentiate groups, rather than unite them, this finding of biased interpretation should be a cause for concern, all the more so when they may negatively impact the administration of justice.

CONCLUSION

The genomic train has left the station and children are increasingly taking the ride. Whether they should be tested, for what conditions or predispositions, who is to determine, and how their data should be used in nonclinical settings are issues that we should all consider—and be aware of the risks.

Whether the historical justifications for children's relative passive involvement in medical settings are still applicable to genomic research and other geneticized settings such as schools and courts is open for debate. The possible costs of such uses are not negligent. They involve core values in American society, including autonomy, capacity, and privacy, as well as key challenges within it, namely, stigma against racial/ethnic minorities and bias against other historically marginalized groups (e.g., people with behavioral and psychiatric conditions). Ultimately, however, all these issues touch upon social, political, and judicial justice and thus require ongoing engagement and regulations to ensure that everyone indeed can enjoy the benefits of scientific progress.

The questions above are all the more pivotal for adolescents—an age group that is uniquely positioned in the genomic era but often remains in the shadow. Their exposure to genomic data and expertise in technology not only surpasses that of adults but may have significant impacts on both their and society's health. Further research with this population is needed. and we shouldn't miss the opportunity for engaging this population in genomic conversations.

ACKNOWLEDGMENT

This work was supported by grant funding from the National Institute of Health (NIH), K01HG008653 and RM1HG007257.

REFERENCES

Abdul-Karim, R., et al. 2013. "Disclosure of Incidental Findings from Next-Generation Sequencing in Pediatric Genomic Research." *Pediatrics* 131, no. 3: 564–71.

Alderson P. 2007. "Competent Children? Minors' Consent to Health Care Treatment and Research. *Social Science & Medicine* 65: 2272–83.

American Academy of Pediatrics. 2013. "Ethical and Policy Issues in Genetic Testing and Screening of Children." *Pediatrics* 131, no. 3: 620–22.

Appelbaum, P. S., et al. 2014. "Researchers' Views on Informed Consent for Return of Secondary Results in Genomic Research." *Genetics in Medicine* 17, no. 8: 644–50.

Austin, J. 2015. "The Effect of Genetic Test-Based Risk Information on Behavioral Outcomes: A Critical Examination of Failed Trials and a Call to Action." *American Journal of Medical Genetics Part A* 167a: 2913–15.

Bentley, A. R., S. Callier, and C. N. Rotimi. 2017. "Diversity and Inclusion in Genomic Research: Why the Uneven Progress?" *Journal of Community Genetics* 8, no. 4: 255–66.

Berkman, B. E., and S. C. Hull. 2014. The "Right Not to Know" in the Genomic Era: Time to Break from Tradition? *American Journal of Bioethics* 14, no. 3: 28–31.

Bernhardt, B. A., et al. 2003. "Parents' and Children's Attitudes toward the Enrollment of Minors in Genetic Susceptibility Research: Implications for Informed Consent." *American Journal of Medical Genetics Part A* 116a, no. 4: 315–23.

Blankenstein, N. E., E. A. Crone, W. van den Bos, and A. C. van Duijvenvoorde. 2016. "Dealing with Uncertainty: Testing Risk- and Ambiguity-Attitude across Adolescence." *Developmental Neuropsychology* 41: 77–92.

Blum, K., L. Lott, D. Siwicki, L. Fried, and M. Hauser. 2018. "Genetic Addiction Risk Score (GARS™) as a Predictor of Substance Use Disorder: Identifying Predisposition Not Diagnosis." *Current Trends in Medical Diagnostic Methods* CTMDM-101.

Borgelt, E. L., D. Z. Buchman, M. Weiss, and J. Illes. 2014. "In Search of 'Anything That Would Help': Parent Perspectives on Emerging Neurotechnologies." *Journal of Attention Disorders* 18: 395–401.

Borry, P., et al. 2009. "Genetic Testing in Asymptomatic Minors: Background Considerations towards ESHG Recommendations." *European Journal of Human Genetics* 17, no. 6: 711–19.

———. 2010. "Health-Related Direct-to-Consumer Genetic Testing: A Review of Companies' Policies with Regard to Genetic Testing in Minors." *Familial Cancer* 9: 51–59.

Borzekowski, D. G., and V. I. Rickert. 2001. "Adolescent Cybersurfing for Health Information: A New Resource That Crosses Barriers." *Archives of Pediatrics & Adolescent Medicine* 155, no. 7: 813–17.

Bouregy, S., E. Grigorenko, M. Tan, and S. Latham, eds. 2017. *Genetics, Ethics and Education*. Cambridge: Cambridge University Press.

Bradbury, A. R., et al. 2009. "Learning of Your Parent's BRCA Mutation during Adolescence or Early Adulthood: A Study of Offspring Experiences." *Psycho-Oncology* 18, no. 2: 200–208.

Brice, S. E., and W. V. Christian. 2017. "The Use of Genetic Evidence to Defend against Toxic Tort Claims." *Intellectual Property & Technology Law Journal* 29, no. 3: Parts I & II. https://www.bclplaw.com/images/content/9/6/v2/96913/genetic-evidence-defend-against-toxic-tort-parts1and2.pdf.

Capron, A. M. 1982. "The Authority of Others to Decide about Biomedical Intervention with Incompetent." In *Who Speaks for the Child?: The Problems of Proxy Consent*, edited by Willard Gaylin and Ruth Macklin, 115–52. New York: Plenum Press.

Caulfield, T., et al. 2015. "Marginally Scientific?: Genetic Testing of Children and Adolescents for Lifestyle and Health Promotion." *Journal of Law and Bioscience* 2, no. 3: 627–44.

Clayton, E. W. 2015. "How Much Control Do Children and Adolescents Have over Genomic Testing, Parental Access to Their Results, and Parental Communication of Those Results to Others? *Journal of Law, Medicine & Ethics* 43, no. 3: 538–44.

Collins, F. S. 2014. "Francis Collins Says Medicine in the Future Will Be Tailored to Your Genes." *Wall Street Journal*, July 7, 2014. https://www.wsj.com/articles/francis-collins-says-medicine-in-the-future-will-be-tailored-to-your-genes-1404763139.

Condit, C. M. 2011. "When Do People Deploy Genetic Determinism?: A Review Pointing to the Need for Multi-Factorial Theories of Public Utilization of Scientific Discourses." *Sociology Compass* 5, no. 7: 618–35.

———. 2019. "Laypeople Are Strategic Essentialists, Not Genetic Essentialists." *Hastings Center Report* 49, no. S1: S27–S37.

Crist, R. C., B. C. Reiner, and W. H. Berrettini. 2019. "A Review of Opioid Addiction Genetics." *Current Opinion in Psychology* 27: 31–35.

Delatycki, M. B., et al. 2010. "Implementation of IronXS: A Study of the Acceptability and Feasibility of Genetic Screening for Hereditary Hemochromatosis in High Schools." *Clinical Genetics* 77, no. 3: 241–48.

Denno, D. W. 2009. "Behavioral Genetics Evidence in Criminal Cases: 1994–2007." In *The Impact of Behavioral Sciences on Criminal Law*, edited by N. A. Farahany. New York: Oxford University Press, 317–54, 465–98.

———. 2011. "Courts' Increasing Consideration of Behavioral Genetics Evidence in Criminal Cases: Results of a Longtitudinal Study." *Michigan State Law Review* 2011: 967–1047.

Dougherty, M. J. 2009. "Closing the Gap: Inverting the Genetics Curriculum to Ensure an Informed Public." *American Journal of Human Genetics* 85, no. 1: 6–12.

Duncan, R. E., and M.-A. Young. 2013. "Tricky Teens: Are They Really Tricky or Do Genetic Health Professionals Simply Require More Training in Adolescent Health?" *Personalized Medicine* 10, no. 6: 589–600.

Eitan, S., M. A. Emery, M. S. Bates, and C. Horrax. 2017. "Opioid Addiction: Who Are Your Real Friends?" *Neuroscience & Biobehavioral Reviews* 83: 697–712.

Etchegary H. 2014. "Public Attitudes toward Genetic Risk Testing and Its Role in Healthcare." *Personalized Medicine* 11, no. 5: 509–22.

Evans, J. P. 2008. "Recreational Genomics; What's in It for You?" *Genetics in Medicine* 10, no. 10: 709–10.

Frumkin, A., and J. Zlotogora. "Genetic Screening for Reproductive Purposes at School: Is It a Good Strategy?" *American Journal of Medical Genetics Part A* 146a, no 2 (2008): 264–69.

Fulda, K. G., and K. Lykens. 2006. "Ethical Issues in Predictive Genetic Testing: A Public Health Perspective." *Journal of Medical Ethics* 32: 143–47.

Gason, A. A., et al. 2005. "Genetic Susceptibility Screening in Schools: Attitudes of the School Community towards Hereditary Haemochromatosis." *Clinical Genetics* 67, no. 2: 166–74.

———. 2006. "It's 'Back to School' for Genetic Screening." *European Journal of Human Genetics* 14, no. 4: 384–89.

Genomic Literacy, Education, and Engagement (GLEE) Initiative. 2017. "Community-Public Working Group." March 2017. https://www.genome.gov/Pages/About/OD/ECIB/GLEE/GLEE_white_paper_CmtyPublic_WG.pdf.

Grand View Research. 2019. "Predictive Genetic Testing & Consumer/Wellness Genomics Market Size, Share & Trends Analysis Report By Test Type (Population Screening, Susceptibility), by Application, by Setting Type, and Segment Forecasts, 2019–2025." Published June 2019. https://www.grandviewresearch.com/industry-analysis/predictive-genetic-testing-consumer-wellness-genomics-market.

Grigorenko, E. L. 2007. "How Can Genomics Inform Education?" *Mind, Brain and Education* 1, no. 1: 20–27.

Harel, A., D. Abuelo, and A. Kazura. 2003. "Adolescents and Genetic Testing: What Do They Think About It?" *Journal of Adolescent Health* 33, no. 6: 489–94.

Haworth, C. M. A., and R. Plomin. 2012. "Genetics and Education: Toward a Genetically Sensitive Classroom." In *APA Educational Psychology Handbook*, edited by K. R. Harris et al., 529–59. American Psychological Association.

Heine, S. J., et al. 2017. "Essentially Biased: Why People Are Fatalistic about Genes." In *Advances in Experimental Social Psychology*, edited by J. M. Olson, 137–92. Cambridge, MA: Academic Press.

Helman, Cecil G. 2000. *Culture, Health and Illness.* Oxford: Butterworth.

Henderson, G. E., et al. 2013. "Characterizing Biobank Organizations in the U.S.: Results from a National Survey." *Genome Medicine* 5, no. 1: 1–12.

Hens, K., et al. 2009. "Genetic Research on Stored Tissue Samples from Minors: A Systematic Review of the Ethical Literature." *American Journal of Medical Genetics A* 149a, no. 10: 2346–58.

———. 2011. "The Storage and Use of Biological Tissue Samples from Minors for Research: A Focus Group Study." *Public Health Genomics* 14, no. 2: 68–76.

Hens, K., E. Levesque, and K. Dierickx. 2011. "Children and Biobanks: A Review of the Ethical and Legal Discussion." *Human Genetics* 130, no. 3: 403–13.

Hoffmann, D. E., and K. H. Rothenberg. 2007. "Judging Genes: Implications of the Second Generation of Genetic Tests in the Courtroom." *Maryland Law Review* 66: 858–922.

Hollands, G. J., D. P. French, S. J. Griffin, et al. 2016. "The Impact of Communicating Genetic Risks of Disease on Risk-Reducing Health Behaviour: Systematic Review with Meta-Analysis." *BMJ* 352: i1102.

Holm, I. A., et al. 2014. "Guidelines for Return of Research Results from Pediatric Genomic Studies: Deliberations of the Boston Children's Hospital Gene Partnership Informed Cohort Oversight Board." *Genetics in Medicine* 16, no. 7: 547–52.

John, P. 2015. "When Neurogenetics Hurts: Examining the Use of Neuroscience and Genetic Evidence in Sentencing Decisions through Implicit Bias." *California Law Review* 103: 1019–45.

Johnson, L. M., et al. 2019. "Speaking Genomics to Parents Offered Germline Testing for Cancer Predisposition: Use of a 2-Visit Consent Model." *Cancer* 125, no. 14: 2455–64.

Jones, S., and S. Fox. 2009. "Generations Online in 2009." Pew Research Center. Published January 28, 2009. http://www.pewinternet.org/2009/01/28/generations-online-in-2009/.

Katzmarzyk, P. T., S. Barlow, C. Bouchard, et al. 2014. "An Evolving Scientific Basis for the Prevention and Treatment of Pediatric Obesity. *International Journal of Obesity (London)* 38: 887–905.

Kaufman, D., et al. 2008. "Ethical Implications of Including Children in a Large Biobank for Genetic-Epidemiologic Research: A Qualitative Study of Public Opinion." *American Journal of Medical Genetics Part C* 148c, no. 1: 31–39.

King, Patricia A. 1992. "The Past as Prologue: Race, Class, and Gene Discrimination." in *Gene Mapping: Using Law and Ethics as Guides*, edited by G. Annas and S. Elias, 94–111. New York: Oxford University Press.

———. 1984–1985. "Treatment and Minors: Issues Not Involving Lifesaving Treatment." *Journal of Family Law* 23: 241–65.

Kinnear, S. H., et al. 2016. "Understanding the Experience of Stigma for Parents of Children with Autism Spectrum Disorder and the Role Stigma Plays in Families' Lives." *Journal of Autism and Developmental Disorders* 46, no. 3: 942–53.

Knoppers, B. M., et al. 2014. "Whole-Genome Sequencing in Newborn Screening Programs." *Science Translational Medicine* 6, no. 229: 229cm222.

Lazaro-Munoz, G., et al. 2015. "Looking for Trouble: Preventive Genomic Sequencing in the General Population and the Role of Patient Choice." *American Journal of Bioethics* 15, no. 7: 3–14.

Lee, Soo-Jin S., and L. Crawley. 2009. "Research 2.0: Social Networking and Direct-to-Consumer (DTC) Genomics." *American Journal of Bioethics* 9, no. 6-7: 35–44.

Levenseller, B. L., et al. 2014. "Stakeholders' Opinions on the Implementation of Pediatric Whole Exome Sequencing: Implications for Informed Consent." *Journal of Genetic Counseling* 23, no. 4: 552–65.

Marchant, Gary. 2012. "Should We Screen Kids' Brains and Genes to ID Future Criminals?" *Slate*. Published October 17, 2012. https://slate.com/technology/2012/10/should-kids-brains-and-genes-be-screened-to-detect-future-criminals.html.

Marchant, G., and J. Robert. 2009. "Genetic Testing for Autism Predisposition: Ethical, Legal and Social Challenges." *Houston Journal of Health Law and Policy* 9: 203–35.

Martschenko, D., S. Trejo, and B. W. Domingue. "Genetics and Education: Recent Developments in the Context of an Ugly History and an Uncertain Future." *AERA Open* 5, no. 1 (2019): 2332858418810516.

May, M. E., R. C. Brandt, and J. K. Bohannan. 2012. "Moderating Effects of Autism on Parent Views of Genetic Screening for Aggression." *Intellectual and Developmental Disabilities* 50, no. 5: 415–25.

McCabe, E., and L. McCabe. 2007. "Genomic Medicine: A Future Flooded with Risk Information." *Minnesota Journal of Law, Science and Technology* 8, no. 2: 429–39.

McQueen, J., J. Wright, and J. A. Fox. 2012. "Design and Implementation of a Genomics Field Trip Program Aimed at Secondary School Students." *PLoS Computational Biology* 8, no. 8: e1002636.

McSwiggan, S., B. Elger, and P. S. Appelbaum. 2017. "The Forensic Use of Behavioral Genetics in Criminal Proceedings: Case of the MAOA-L Genotype." *International Journal of Law and Psychiatry* 50: 17–23.

Meagher, K. M., et al. 2017. "Precisely Where Are We Going? Charting the New Terrain of Precision Prevention." *Annual Review of Genomics and Human Genetics* 18: 369–87.

Metcalfe, A., et al. 2008. "Family Communication between Children and Their Parents about Inherited Genetic Conditions: A Meta-Synthesis of the Research." *European Journal of Human Genetics* 16, no. 10: 1193–2000.

Mueller, A. K., et al. 2012. "Stigma in Attention Deficit Hyperactivity Disorder." *Attention Deficit Hyperactivity Disorder* 4, no. 3: 101–14.

Nelkin, D., "Molecular Metaphors: The Gene in Popular Discourse." Nature Reviews Genetics, 2 no. 7 (2001): 555–9.

Nordgren, A., and E. T. Juengst. 2009. "Can Genomics Tell Me Who I Am? Essentialistic Rhetoric in Direct-to-Consumer DNA Testing." *New Genetics and Society* 28, no. 2: 157–72.

O'Driscoll, C., et al. 2012. "Explicit and Implicit Stigma towards Peers with Mental Health Problems in Childhood and Adolescence." *Journal of Child Psychology and Psychiatry* 53, no. 10: 1054–62.

Palk, A. C., et al. 2019. "Potential Use of Clinical Polygenic Risk Scores in Psychiatry: Ethical Implications and Communicating High Polygenic Risk." *Philosophy, Ethics, and Humanities in Medicine* 14, no. 1: 4.

Phillips, A. M. 2016. "Only a Click Away: DTC Genetics for Ancestry, Health, Love . . . and More: A View of the Business and Regulatory Landscape." *Applied & Translational Genomics* 8: 16–22.

Plomin, R., and K. Ashbury. 2014. *G is for Genes: The Impact of Genetics on Education and Achievement.* Chichester, UK: Wiley Blackwell.

Popejoy, A. B., and S. M. Fullerton. 2016. "Genomics Is Failing on Diversity." *Nature* 538, no. 7624: 161–64.

Randesi, M., W. van den Brink, O. Levran, P. Blanken, J. M. van Ree, et al. 2019. "VMAT2 Gene (SLC18A2) Variants Associated with a Greater Risk for Developing Opioid Dependence." *Pharmacogenomics* 20, no. 5: 331–41.

Reilly, C. 2012. "Behavioural Phenotypes and Special Educational Needs: Is Aetiology Important in the Classroom?" *Journal of Intellectual Disability Research* 56, no. 10: 929–46.

Reilly, C., J. Senior, and L. A. Murtagh. 2015. "A Comparative Study of Educational Provision for Children with Neurogenetic Syndromes: Parent and Teacher Survey." *Journal of Intellectual Disability Research* 59, no. 12: 1094–107.

Reilly, P. R. 2000. "Ethical and Legal Issues in Genetic Testing to Predict Risk of Heart Disease." *American Heart Journal* 140, no. 4: S6–S10.

Rew, L., M. Mackert, and D. Bonevac. 2010. "Cool, But Is It Credible? Adolescents' and Parents' Approaches to Genetic Testing." *Western Journal of Nursing Research* 32: 610–27.

Ross, L. F. 2006. "Heterozygote Carrier Testing in High Schools Abroad: What Are the Lessons for the U.S.?" *Journal of Law, Medicine and Ethics* 34, no. 4: 753–64.

Rothstein, M. 2007. "Legal Conceptions of Equality in the Genomic Age." *Law and Inequality* 25: 429–71.

Ryan, J., A. Virani, and J. C. Austin. 2015. "Ethical Issues Associated with Genetic Counseling in the Context of Adolescent Psychiatry." *Applied & Translational Genomics* 5: 23–29.

Sabatello, M. 2018. "A Genomically Informed Education System? Challenges for Behavioral Genetics." *Journal of Law, Medicine and Ethics* 46, no. 1: 130–44.

Sabatello, M. 2017. "Psychiatric Genomics and Public Mental Health in the Young Mind." *American Journal of Bioethics* 17, no. 4: 27–29.

Sabatello, M., and P. S. Appelbaum. 2016. "Psychiatric Genetics in Child Custody Proceedings: Ethical, Legal, and Social Issues." *Current Genetic Medicine Reports* 4, no. 3: 98–106.

———. 2017. "Behavioral Genetics in Criminal and Civil Courts." *Harvard Review of Psychiatry* 25, no. 6: 289–301.

Sabatello, M., Y. Chen, J. Austin, C. F. Herrere, E. Brockhoff, and P. S. Appelbaum. Forthcoming. "Teenagers, Precision Psychiatry and Translational Genomics: A Window of Opportunity."

Sabatello, M., Y. Chen, S. C. Sanderson, W. K. Chung, and P. S. Appelbaum. 2019. "Increasing Genomic Literacy among Adolescents." *Genetics in Medicine* 21, no. 4: 994–1000.

Sabatello, M., B. Insel, J. Phelan, B. Link, and P. S. Appelbaum. Forthcoming B. "The Double Helix in Schools: Behavioral Genetics, Disability, and Precision Education."

———. Forthcoming C. "Children's Psychiatric Genetic Data in Judicial Proceedings to Terminate Parental Rights."

Salagre, E., S. Dodd, A. Aedo, et al. 2018. "Toward Precision Psychiatry in Bipolar Disorder: Staging 2.0." *Frontiers in Psychiatry* 29, no. 9: 641.

Santelli, J. S., et al. 2003. "Guidelines for Adolescent Health Research: A Position Paper of the Society for Adolescent Medicine." *Journal of Adolescent Health* 33, no. 5: 396–409.

Sapp, J. C., et al. 2014. "Parental Attitudes, Values, and Beliefs toward the Return of Results from Exome Sequencing in Children." *Clinical Genetics* 85, no. 2: 120–26.

Secretary's Advisory Committee on Genetics, Health, and Society. 2011. "Genetics Education and Training: Report of the Secretary's Advisory Committee on Genetics, Health, and Society." Genetics Education and Training. February 2011. https://www.genome.gov/Pages/Careers/HealthProfessional Education/SACGHS-EducationReport2011.pdf.

Semaka, A., L. G. Balneaves, and M. R. Hayden. 2013. "'Grasping the Grey': Patient Understanding and Interpretation of an Intermediate Allele Predictive Test Result for Huntington Disease. *Journal of Genetic Counseling* 22: 200–217.

Simonsen, N., A. Lahti, S. Suominen, et al. 2018. "Empowerment-Enabling Home and School Environments and Self-Rated Health among Finnish Adolescents." *Health Promotion International*. Published December 24, 2018.

Strong, K. A., et al. 2014. "Views of Primary Care Providers Regarding the Return of Genome Sequencing Incidental Findings." *Clinical Genetics* 86, no. 5: 461–68.

Townsend, A., et al. 2012. "'I Want to Know What's in Pandora's Box': Comparing Stakeholder Perspectives on Incidental Findings in Clinical Whole Genomic Sequencing." *American Journal of Medical Genetics A* 158a, no. 10: 2519–25.

Uniform Parentage Act (amended 2002), 9B U.L.A. 4, 2002.

Wachbroit, R. 2000. "Genetic Determinism, Genetic Reductionism, and Genetic Essentialism." In *The Encyclopedia of Ethical, Legal and Policy Issues in Biotechnology*, Vol. 1, edited by T. H. Murray and M. J. Mehlman, 352–56. Hoboken, NJ: Wiley-Interscience.

Walker, S. O., and R. Plomin. 2005. "The Nature–Nurture Question: Teachers' Perceptions of How Genes and the Environment Influence Educationally Relevant Behavior." *Educational Psychology* 25: 509–16.

Weithorn, L. A., and S. B. Campbell. 1982. "The Competency of Children and Adolescents to Make Informed Treatment Decisions." *Child Development* 53, no. 6: 1589–98.

Wilde, A., et al. 2011. "Community Attitudes to Genetic Susceptibility-Based Mental Health Interventions for Healthy People in a Large National Sample." *Journal of Affective Disorders* 134, no. 1–3: 280–87.

Wilde, A., P. B. Mitchell, B. Meiser, P. R. Schofield. 2013. "Implications of the Use of Genetic Tests in Psychiatry, with a Focus on Major Depressive Disorder: A Review." *Depression and Anxiety* 30: 267–75.

Wilfond, B. S., and D. S. Diekema. 2012. "Engaging Children in Genomics Research: Decoding the Meaning of Assent in Research." *Genetics in Medicine* 14: 437–43.

Wilhelm, K., B. Meiser, P. B. Mitchell, et al. 2009. "Issues Concerning Feedback about Genetic Testing and Risk of Depression." *British Journal of Psychiatry* 194: 404–10.

2

The Abortion Debate in the Twenty-First Century

Michael Boylan

ABSTRACT

This essay seeks to formulate a structure by which people might more profitably discuss abortion. This structure is tied to a conception of both personal worldview and a practical linking principle connected with the vocabulary of maternal threat versus fetal respect. This structure does not create a firm line to cross but instead suggests a continuum by which various arguments can be made that differ only through their various emphases.

INTRODUCTION

There are very few conversations in the public square that have had such a long life with so little agreement to show for it as the abortion debate. This essay does not intend to "settle" the issue in a manner that everyone will accept but instead aspires to outline a way to view the problem so that each person may decide how a universal moral theory along with a "linking principle" can resolve this problem.[1] It is suggested that the means for doing so will lie in the personal worldview imperative: "All people must develop a single comprehensive and internally coherent worldview that is good and that we strive to act out in our daily lives."[2]

To this end I will present my argument in the following way. First, I will review some of the history of the debate. Second, I will critically examine the key premises in a version of the arguments from each side. Finally, I will suggest a way of thinking about the problem that does not force a single solution upon the reader but rather suggests a way to frame the problem so that each reader might legislate his or her own "universal maxim."

THE HISTORY OF THE DEBATE

One can summarize the debate over abortion as being between two camps:

A. The Pro-Abortion Position[3]
   1. A woman's body is her own—Assertion
   2. Whatever is one's own is under her discretion to dispose of at will—Fact

190

3. A woman's body is under her discretion to dispose of at will—1, 2
4. The fetus is wholly dependent upon the woman's body (at least through most of the first two trimesters of pregnancy)—Fact
5. That which is wholly dependent upon one's body is (barring any other intervening duties) wholly under one's discretion to dispose of at will—Assertion
6. The fetus inside a woman is hers to dispose of at will—3–5
7. To "abort" a fetus is to remove it from one's body—Fact
8. Removing a fetus from a mother's body will, in most cases, cause it to be biologically nonfunctional—Fact
9. To abort a fetus is to cause it to be biologically nonfunctional—7, 8
10. Removing something from one's body (which is at one's disposal, at will) is permissible—2, 3
11. Removing the fetus from a woman's body is permissible even if such removal renders the fetus biologically nonfunctional—6, 9, 10

B. The Anti-Abortion Position
1. From the moment of conception there is a person—Assertion
2. All persons should be accorded full human rights—Fact
3. To kill an innocent human agent, at will, is impermissible—Fact (generally accepted by most moral theories)
4. A fetus is an innocent human agent—Assertion
5. To kill a fetus is impermissible—1–4
6. All morally impermissible acts should be sanctioned by society as impermissible—Fact
7. Abortion kills the fetus—Fact
8. Abortion is impermissible and should be sanctioned by society as impermissible—5–7

Obviously, there is a tremendous gap between these two arguments. Let's examine some aspects of the worldviews that drive each side and then turn to key premises in the above arguments, as well as other classic renditions of the argument.

To make the worldview of each group seem understandable and sympathetic, I will adopt the persona of an advocate of each as I encourage each of you to explore these worldviews to evaluate what positive and negative points they have to offer.

The Worldviews of Position A. To properly review an ethical argument, it is my opinion that one must assess the worldview(s) of those who make such arguments. I believe that much of the power of *Position A*'s argument is tied to (1) the unequal consequences that women face in sexual relations, (2) the issue of personal autonomy, and (3) the general societal repression of women. Let's examine these in order.

1. The consequences of a woman engaging in sexual intercourse are (among other things) the possibility of a pregnancy. A man can engage in intercourse as often as he chooses, and he will never become pregnant. He can (if he is a purely egoistic sort of fellow) walk away when his sexual partner becomes pregnant. Though the consequence of their actions is just as much *his* fault as it is *hers*, still, only she will have to bear the physical debt of their joint behavior. This is unfair. If both the man and woman *jointly* engaged in an action, then they should jointly have to bear the consequences. But history has shown that this has never been the case. In fact, some have speculated that the entire institution of marriage evolved solely to protect the woman from this brute inequality.

Why should men get off without consequence? The large number of single mothers who must raise families around the world is a testament to the brute inequality of the biological scenario that some sociobiologists have termed "a battle of genetic strategies." Under this account all organisms have a single biological imperative: to send their genes into future filial generations. The best strategy for a man is to inseminate as many women as possible—hoping that some of these forays may result in pregnancies and thus fulfill his biological imperative.

The best strategy for a woman is to be very selective and try to get a commitment from the biological father to assist in raising their child. This is because a woman when pregnant loses a proverbial "a step or two" in her ability to compete for food and shelter. Also, when the child is born, the woman needs to nurse it for at least six months and needs some protection. (Some have also theorized that this protection can come from a grandmother—hence, the notion that menopause may also be biologically adaptive.)

If this scenario has any truth to it, the brute biological reproductive strategies of men and women differ. For thousands of years, a mistake on the part of women in the execution of their strategy has had far more deleterious consequences than any failures on the part of men.

It is often seen as a curiosity among many women that some of the most vocal critics of women and their reproductive decisions are men (who bear no brute biological consequences for their actions, i.e., "it's easy for *you* to say . . . ").

Thus, I believe that is fairly clear why women would aspire to have the *option* for their gender to be able to walk away from an unfortunate sexual relationship in the same way that men always have.

Some critics say that men as well as women ought to face equal consequences. This is a rejoinder that meets this argument at its essence. However, how are such consequences to be enforced? Even in the United States (which aspires to be a nation under law), we cannot make divorced fathers and those who abandon their reproductive partner pay legally sanctioned child support. How can we ever realistically aspire to make men pay the same price that women pay for the consequences of sexual intercourse?

2. The issue of autonomy relates to the ownership of one's own body. All things equal, it is difficult to know who would own your body except yourself.[4] This means that whatever you own is yours (unless some intervening duty can be proven). If you want to tattoo yourself, put pierced rings in various places, or cut off a limb, it is your privilege because whatever is entirely yours is at your disposal. Thus, if you don't choose to use your body as a "growth chamber" for an embryo, you needn't. It is your body to do with as you wish.

3. The general station of women in this society, as well as most societies in history, has been as a repressed and enslaved group. This is a broad, sociological statement. This does not mean that there are not individual men who are sensitive and nurturing of their spouses, daughters, and women in general. But one need only engage in some volunteer work with women's shelters and other facilities that deal with those in need to know the truth of this generalization. Despite all our laws and aspirations as a society, women are treated differently than men. And this difference *is* an added hurdle that women must overcome and that is not present for men.

To make the point rather sharper, women are the oppressed gender. For men to say to them that they must abide by laws enacted by men that constrict their reproductive freedom (so that they might not be as free as men) is an act of political enslavement. In this way, it is the *freedom of choice* that is essential—not the actual execution of an act of abortion. Most women will never have an abortion. Most women would never want to have an abortion. Many women will carry an impaired infant to term rather than abort it. Nonetheless, despite the fact that most women will never avail themselves of the political right of abortion (within the United States and a number of other countries), still, it is important to maintain the freedom of choice.

This is because this freedom of choice is a cornerstone in the edifice that stands against gender enslavement. The struggle of oppressed women demands that they not be subjected to the brute will of men on something so close to their biological nature, viz., their reproductive equality. The *choice* for pregnancy termination is merely one part of a very large structure. However, it is symbolically a very important part. It was not very long ago that women who had to pay for the outcomes of their loving relationships were relegated to disbarred physicians who used dirty tools and whose rate of sepsis was exceeded only by their blood-alcohol ratio.[5]

This image of a woman alone, abandoned by her partner and abandoned by society, is one that resonates with most women (even if they feel that such a situation will never happen to them). It is a sort of "but for the grace of God, go I" scenario. For this reason, most women feel solidarity for their sisters in need and strive to protect them from a solitary journey into hell.

The freedom of choice is importantly symbolic as a balance against gender oppression.

The Worldviews of Position B. The second group views reality in a much different fashion. To begin with, there is a very strong belief in relatively unencumbered free will. Each person can act as she pleases without much real perturbation. The perception of one gender being oppressed is viewed in several ways by different sides as follows: (1) This is just a lot of belly-aching by a sex that is already protected and is given more than ample opportunities. "Why, a woman today has it so much easier than a man because all she has to do is to be 'near' a man in skill and she will be automatically hired." (2) Sexual intercourse is an activity given by God for the creation of children. When people go against the laws of God, then they must be prepared to "face the music." Abortion is the "easy way out." "Living with a few more unfortunate consequences in life would be good for most of these unregulated young people, anyway."

A third perspective is more profound. It asserts that human life is precious. We should do everything in our power to preserve the life of someone unable to protect him/herself, viz., the unborn. We have so much empathy in society for the handicapped—and rightly so. What is the basis of this empathy? It is because they need the protection and support of others.

When someone is impaired, s/he needs the protection and support of others. A fetus is in a similar position as one impaired. This impairment is not due to a defect in the genotype or in development but is a natural consequence of the biological stage this individual is in his/her point of life. All other things being equal, this embryo will become a human agent capable of reason and action.

According to the doctrine of "*novus actus interveniens*," the normal process of nature is taken to be the standard. This doctrine is well entrenched in the law.[6] The idea is this. If you interfere with the normal operation of nature as a new intervening action, then you are responsible for all the ensuing consequences. For example, John is robbing a bank and says to the teller, "If you move, I'll shoot," and the teller moves slightly as she presses the alarm button with her foot. The bank robber shoots, and his bullet ricochets off one of the iron bars of the teller's cage and lodges in the neck of a person standing in line behind the gunman.

Now, who "caused" the person to be shot? If one takes an "inciting incident" theory of causation (which is often taken as definitive in the philosophy of science), then the teller is to blame. But this is ridiculous. The teller was put into an abnormal situation by the gunman. The natural order had been changed by the gunman with his gun and his demands. Thus, according to the doctrine of *novus actus interveniens*, it is the gunman who is at fault for the bullet in the customer's neck and not the teller. This is because the gunman changed the natural order, and thus all ensuing events (in an appropriately fashioned action description) can be attributed to him.

How does this apply to abortion? The natural order would have the fetus grow and develop as it normally would. Any event that intervened to stop this process would be considered to be the causally responsible party for the fetus's demise. If the fetus is a person, then the intervening party is a murderer.

Thus, abortion is murder. Now, if you were a part of a society that institutionalized murder and you did nothing about it, then you would be some sort of accessory to the murder. Thus, to live in a society that permits abortion and to do nothing about it would be tantamount to someone who turned a blind eye to Hitler, Stalin, or Pol Pot (if you lived in their societies or in the world at large and could have reacted in some meaningful way). Despite societal acceptance, you must do everything you can to stop it.

We have created a society that legalizes the continual killing of thousands of fetuses every year. If these fetuses are children, then aren't we guilty of mass murder? Aren't we to be compared to the great murdering societies of history? Isn't this cause enough to prohibit abortion now?

A CRITICAL EXAMINATION OF THE PREMISES OF EACH SIDE

The last section dealt with a version of the pro and con arguments, per se, and explored in brief the worldviews of each side. Let us begin with defining what I mean by "abortion." Abortion is the removal of the fetus from the female by natural or artificial means. The "natural" abortion is called "spontaneous abortion" and occurs in 20 to 25 percent of all pregnancies (depending on how one frames the data). Most spontaneous abortions occur during the first trimester of pregnancy. They are called miscarriages. Miscarriages generally occur because the developing embryo is malformed. It is nature's way of ensuring that potential children with no real chance of survival are given an exit at the beginning of life's journey.

Artificial abortion is the removal by medical means of a fetus from the female. Abortion is *not* the killing of that fetus. As a matter of fact, many embryos removed from the female do die. They don't die because they are removed from the mother, as such. For example, one might imagine a time in which there might be an artificial womb in the laboratory. In this case, an embryo might be removed from a woman at any time, and it would not necessarily result in its death. All this is to say that, if there is a right to abortion, it is a right to remove the fetus from your body. This is not a right to kill the fetus.

If the fetus, for example, were able to be preserved, then it would be a separate question of what to do with that fetus.[7] The right to abortion, *simpliciter*, is a right to remove a fetus from one's body. This follows from the sample argument and the worldview enhancement of the same. Therefore, the abortion question changes drastically after the point of viability. In principle, one might be able to remove the fetus from the female and raise it separately in some sort of nursery. In these cases, removing a fetus would not be tantamount to causing it to die. One could remove the fetus and allow it to develop without any further contact with its biological mother.

Having clarified this, let's turn to a few key premises in the arguments on each side. First, let's examine the pro-abortion position as represented by the generic argument as I presented it. The argument given the worldview background to the argument is very persuasive. Detractors are likely to focus on premise 5: That which is wholly dependent on one's body is (barring any other intervening duties) wholly under one's discretion to dispose of at will—Assertion.

The move is from autonomy over one's own body parts to sovereignty over entities dependent on one's body. This is an argument that Judith Jarvis Thomson elaborates in her famous article.[8] Deontologists might object to a blanket endorsement of this position. It seems to violate the "duty to rescue." This duty is a moral obligation that is supported by Kant, Gewirth, and Donagan.[9] In the duty to rescue, one is obliged to aid another whenever that other person's basic goods of agency are threatened so long as doing so does not entail that one risks his or her own basic goods of agency.[10] For example, in the case of Kitty Genovese (which Thomson cites), the apartment dwellers could have screamed from their window at the attacker or called the police or both. I can attest from personal experience that this is an effective way to thwart a criminal in the inner city. Thus, if one can aid another whose basic goods of agency are being threatened without risking one's own basic goods of agency, then one is obliged to do so. This is a little different than the depiction given by Thomson. She says we are not obliged to go out and confront the mugger ourselves and that one who does so is a Good Samaritan.

But this implies that there are only two sorts of response to the Kitty Genovese case—either fight or flight. But this is too simple. Surely, everyone is obliged to aid another when it does not risk one's own basic goods of agency. But what of abortion?

Is abortion properly analogous to one of these options (in the above example): (a) calling the police and yelling outside one's window or (b) leaving the apartment complex to do physical battle with the assailant? In the first case one is merely fulfilling a moral duty. This does not deserve praise but a mere statement of gratitude. In the second case, one has risked his or her basic goods of agency. He or she might also might have been killed. This person is a hero.

Is the woman who chooses to carry a fetus to term more like the person doing her duty or the hero? This can be an important component in evaluating this argument.

Returning to premise 5, we can also note that there is a difference between what one does to one's own body and to other entities that are not of one's body. In the case of bacteria, viruses, cysts, and growths, we pay no mind to eliminating them. They are not of our body, and they have no intrinsic worth—nor would a reasonable interpretation of precautionary reasoning dictate that they have any worth.[11]

But a fetus is certainly different. A fetus will, all things being equal, develop into a moral agent who has absolute rights to freedom and well-being. Thus, the argument for potentiality is not wholly without merit. Though the fetus is not *actually* a person in the strong sense of the word, it is still a *potential* person. This potentiality of personhood is not trivial and cannot be dismissed.

Next, let's examine the anti-abortion position as represented by the generic argument as I presented it. The argument given the worldview background to the argument is very persuasive. Detractors are likely to focus on premise 3: To kill an innocent human agent, at will, is impermissible—Fact (generally accepted by most moral theories). Now, some would want to discuss the nature of "innocent." Is the word meant to be some sort of absolute term (i.e., "in no way deserves to die") or relative to the action description at hand (i.e., "is in no way threatening the life of any other agent [knowingly or unknowingly]").[12] The first sense is rather silly as depicted because it presupposes so many unstated propositions that need to be argued and defended.

The second, on the other hand, has merit. "Innocent" on this reading implies that one is not materially involved in the loss of fundamental rights of agency for another (intended or otherwise). For example, take the example of the deer hunter who begins firing at another person thinking s/he is a deer. That other person could justifiably kill the one firing at him or her. (We assume that the person firing thinks s/he is firing at a deer. We also assume that the only way to stop the gunman is to use lethal force.)[13] Under this reading, the unwitting gunman is not innocent. S/he is materially guilty because s/he jeopardizes the life of another.

Under this definition, a person may be innocent only if s/he is not materially threatening the life of another.[14] Thus, a fetus who threatens the life of a mother and is killed as a result is not a case of killing an "innocent."

But let's explore further the sense of "threatens." There are certainly many senses of this word. The most severe sense is to kill the mother. A fetus (without motive) may be the cause of a mother's death. There are other senses of "threatens."

One of these senses identifies "threatens" as ripping apart the worldview in which the pregnant woman lives. This threatens her because it challenges everything that she holds as precious in her life plan (stated or only imagined). This is not trivial. People kill themselves for as much. Where does one draw the line at delineating harm?

Is this a question of balancing?

It is always a question of balancing. The difference between theories that explicitly balance— such as utilitarianism, intuitionism, and virtue ethics—is that they balance on the "back end." They balance at the moment of decision.

Deontological theories balance, too. But they aspire to balance at the front end (i.e., in the depiction of the act to be judged). One balances in judging what *sort* of action is being depicted. The operation of forming an action description is not value neutral. It involves balancing competing understandings of what is happening (i.e., what is relevant). Thus, there is always balancing. The question is what drives the decision. In this case, I am suggesting that it ought to be the personal worldview imperative. The "consistency" portion of this imperative requires that one treat all cases alike and create rules (whatever they are) that fulfill the aspirations of that moral theory and do not contradict each other.

Thus, there have to be some boundaries as to what should be regarded as "threatening" to one's worldview. For example, when I used to be a track runner, we had a very talented runner on our club who had the potential to be an Olympic runner. He had joined the club because we had four other runners who were favorites to make the 1976 Olympic team. The only problem was that this runner never finished a race in the four years I ran with the club. Something would always get in the way. Either his splits were not exactly as he had wanted them to be, or a black bird flew over the track (he hated black birds), or he thought he heard someone yelling something at him, or the humidity suddenly changed, *et aliud*. Surely, these distractions, while real and important to him, would be viewed by the rest of us as ultimately trivial. So it is with some senses of "threaten." What should count as a legitimate sense of the word? To make this point more starkly, let me contrast seven motivations for an abortion that women might bring forward as instances of being threatened.[15]

A. Ms. A is pregnant, and it has been determined that, if she were to bring this fetus to term, she would die. Ms. A feels threatened because her life is in danger.

B. Ms. B is pregnant. She is a married mother of five other children and of very modest financial means. If she carries this fetus to term, her other five children will be pushed over the edge of starvation. There are not enough resources for six children. Ms. B feels threatened because the lives of her other children are at stake.

C. Ms. C is pregnant. She is married, and her obstetrician has told her that the baby she is carrying has a fatal disease that will kill the child at the age of six. It will be a painful death. Maybe medical science will find a cure for this disease, but probably this will not occur. Ms. C feels threatened on behalf of her unborn child.

D. Ms. D is pregnant. She is a thirty-something single and in a career that is just about to "take off." Her profession is so competitive and limited in size that it is reasonable to assume that if she muffs this opportunity, she will never have another chance. Ms. D feels threatened because her career and personal life plan are at stake.

E. Ms. E is pregnant. She is a high school senior who has been admitted to a very selective college. Her parents would be furious if they knew she was pregnant. Her college admission might not be renewable if she does not attend this fall. Her whole future is in front of her. This plan did not include a pregnancy. There is no way that she could be a good mother at this point in her life. It wasn't supposed to work out this way. Ms. E feels threatened because her future and her reputation are at stake.

F. Ms. F is pregnant. She is married and has decided that she would like to have a boy and a girl. They already have the girl and amniocentesis has indicated that the fetus within her will be a girl, too. They do not want to have more than two children because it is not part of the plan that they have created for themselves. Ms. F feels threatened because she has a girl within her when she wanted a boy.

G. Ms. G is pregnant. She is married and has decided that she would like a male child who is very intelligent and fits the profile of physical features that she feels represents the perfect child: blonde hair, blue eyes, six feet tall, 1,500+ on the SATs. Assume that there is some battery of tests that pretends to predict a genotype that is most compatible with the desired phenotype/developmental end product. Ms. G's test results indicate that her fetus is deficient in several areas: (a) not perfectly blonde hair—several color shades of brown seem more likely, (b) five feet eleven inches tall is the prognosis, and (c) probable SAT score of only 1200. Ms. G feels threatened because she has a fetus that will not meet her standard for the child she really wants.

Each of these scenarios illustrates on a sliding scale of relative senses of being threatened. If one is entitled to kill an otherwise innocent agent who is materially guilty because s/he threatens you, then it is important to create a "floor" that demarcates what is a suitable ground of threat.

In case A, we have a pure sense of self-defense. In B, one may be said to be acting in self-defense on behalf of another (in this case the children)—though the case is rather more difficult because there are more contingencies. In C, the question transforms into a structure that is similar to those found in active euthanasia. One is paternalistically acting on behalf of another's best interest. The mother thinks, "I know that this child will not want to die so early and with so much suffering." She may also think, "I cannot face the trial of caring for another knowing that the future is both fixed and fatal."

Cases D and E are similar except for the age of the parties. The age issue can work both ways. One might give greater latitude to the younger person because she is not fully mature and responsible for her actions. Or one might give greater latitude to the older person because, as one ages, doors of opportunity close. The consequences to the older woman are probably more severe than to the younger. In each case we have "threaten" in the context of "very disruptive to my life plan."

Cases F and G are also similar because they indicate a sense of eugenics. It is a fact that a great number of abortions that are performed in the world revolve around the sex of the fetus. Thousands of female fetuses have been aborted because the mother desired a son. In case G, we have a science fiction scenario in which people desire to have "designer babies." To some, this is a desirable future. To others it is a nightmare.

More will be said about these senses of "threaten" in the last section of this essay.

The other aspect of premise 3 concerns the definition of an agent. This issue has been much discussed in the literature with little to show for it.[16] I would like to preface my remarks by referring to Deryck Beyleveld's essay on precautionary reasoning.[17] Beyleveld makes the point that *full human rights*, viz., those that confer absolute respect for freedom and well-being, become operative only when there is an agent who clearly meets the criteria of being a prospective, purposive agent.

In a strong sense, this would not be evident without objection until some time in the child's second year of life.[18] If we grant this, then everyone under the age of thirty months or so has no dialectically necessary claim to agency. Then, *quod erat demonstrandum*, s/he has no dialectically necessary claim to life (one of the goods of well-being).

This is certainly a very high standard. Does this mean that we are entitled to kill at will all those under the age of thirty months? Surely not. Precautionary reasoning indicates that various actions, such as walking and feeding oneself, indicate that the infant may be more cognizant than we can scientifically document. In these cases, the infant is doing no more than what many other animals also do[19]—yet we do not ascribe to them the sorts of rights afforded to human agents. Why? To answer this we need to turn back to the personal worldview imperative.

THE PERSONAL WORLDVIEW IMPERATIVE AND ABORTION

The personal worldview imperative says: "All people must develop a single comprehensive and internally coherent worldview that is good and that we strive to act out in our daily lives." The personal worldview imperative enjoins each of us to create both a comprehensive and an internally coherent vision of life. One aspect of this is to be able to will oneself to have an action performed upon him/herself without violating the laws of nature as the s/he understands them.[20] This is similar to the Kantian notion of imperfect duties.

In the case of a fetus, no one could will his/her own demise (i.e., being aborted) without contradicting the natural law that says that, *ceteris paribus*, we all act for our preservation and happiness.

But what if we could not will? Certainly, this situation may exist when we are at the beginning of life. In these cases, the fetus does not act and, since "willing" is a precondition to action, the fetus does not will. This would seem to be an exception to the Kantian interpretation of the personal worldview imperative above. However, some might claim that such situations should be judged like we would assess a person who is asleep (to use Aristotle's example) (i.e., the fetus is not willing *now* but will be in the position to will in the near future). Such an argument is a form of precautionary reasoning.

The essence of this doctrine (as I choose to use it) is to make precautionary reasoning a form of Aristotelian potentiality that holds open the possibility that the individual in question may be more empowered than we can scientifically determine. At some point, we must "draw a line" and say that past that point it is impossible (from the worldview perspective of the speaker) that the individual in question should be afforded the moral rights of agency—even using precautionary reasoning.

Does this mean that, past the point of affording the fetus proportional rights[21] through precautionary reasoning, we are entitled to give the fetus no consideration at all and thus be entitled to kill it "at will"? No. This is because I have linked "precaution" with a sense of Aristotelian potentiality. Under this interpretation of cautionary reasoning, one will give some level of respect to any fetus no matter how immature. On the principle of proportionality I have been exposing, one would give more respect to a thirteen-week fetus than to a four-week fetus. This is because the thirteen-week fetus is closer to enjoying precautionary reasoning than a four-week fetus is. Just how much respect, vis-à-vis various threats that face the mother, must be determined by the agent.

The process goes like this. First, one must establish for him/herself the floor of precautionary reason. This requires judgment. Personally, I would put the floor at the end of the first trimester of pregnancy (thirteen weeks). Before this point, the brain and spinal cord are not connected; therefore, according to my own best understanding, it would be impossible for the fetus to deliberate, plan, and act. Others may disagree with me moving in either direction (i.e., earlier or later in pregnancy).

Second, one must determine the limit of respect one will accord to a fetus who is not (a) an actual agent nor (b) a possible agent (even under a liberal sense of precautionary reasoning). The agent in question is *potentially* a *possible* agent. As a potentially possible agent, the fetus has some respect accorded to it because, barring intervention, it will become a possible agent (protected by precautionary reason) and eventually a full-blown agent (protected by most theories of morality).

This interpretation would invalidate the given form of the pro-abortion argument because it would suggest that the "at will" provision is incorrect. One may eliminate some entity "at will" only when there is no justifiable respect owed to it. Under the interpretation outlined above, there is always some level of respect due to potentiality tied to precautionary reasoning. It is up to the agent involved to determine the *level of respect*. This is a personal assessment. But to say so does not imply relativism. Rather, it is the proper expression of the personal worldview imperative in which one legislates a universal interpretation of reality (which would include valuing this level of respect).

I do not feel one may abort a fetus at will. One must have a threat that supersedes the level of respect one has assigned to the fetus. In the above examples, I would say that the sort of threat represented by F and G does not meet this standard. Thus, abortion for the sake of the baby's sex or due to some eugenics desire would be impermissible at any stage of pregnancy. The level of respect due to the fetus as a mere potential possible agent is greater than that level of maternal threat.

I would assess cases A–E as meeting this standard of threat during the first trimester of pregnancy. Others might demur because they would quarrel with me about balancing of threats.

I would always view case A as meeting a sufficient standard of threat throughout the pregnancy.[22] However, in third-trimester abortions, there may be opportunity to remove the fetus without destroying it. The right to an abortion is not a right to have the embryo destroyed but merely a right to have it removed from one's body.

Cases B and C and D and E both form units that revolve around similar themes (self-defense for the sake of another and severe disruption to one's personal life plan, respectively). Since averting death is more disastrous to agency than mere roadblocks (no matter how disruptive), I would assess B and C as being a higher-order threat than D and E. This differentiation must make itself felt in different stages of pregnancy in which an abortion may be permissible. For example, I would lean toward D and E as being permissible during the first trimester and B and C as being permissible during the first two trimesters.

The general principle in operation is how to weigh "threat" and "response." In the latter case, the nature of the response changes as the fetus develops. Thus, a response to a fetus in the first trimester is different from a response in the second trimester, is different from a response in the third trimester. This is because, in the first trimester, one has merely the principle of potentiality by which to refer.

After the first trimester, I believe the principle of precautionary reason kicks in and becomes proportionally more relevant until the minimal stages of operationally verifiable agency are evidenced (thirty months after birth—or less). After thirty months (or whatever time frame is chosen), it would be absolutely impermissible to kill the entity unless it was materially threatening the life of the mother.[23]

CONCLUSION

This essay has aspired to be suggestive rather than definitive on the question of abortion. To this end, I have suggested criteria that can be used by different people to set the universal limits of permissibility and impermissibility. This variation is due to the variation in personal worldviews in which one may weigh maternal threats and fetal respect differently. Instead of focusing on the definition of personhood or the expression of autonomy, I would suggest that it is more productive to focus on maternal threats versus fetal respect.

This approach suggests that three levels exist that should be considered when evaluating how much respect anyone deserves. A. Full personhood (at some time in the first few years of development). B. Possible personhood (protected by precautionary reason from some base level to personhood—I would put this moment at the end of the first trimester of pregnancy). C. Potential possible personhood (from the moment of conception to possible personhood).

Full moral rights obtain necessarily to those enjoying full personhood (since they are actual deliberating agents). Something proportionally approaching full moral rights may be claimed for the possible agent. And some proportionally lesser level of respect (with its associated rights) should be granted to those on the lowest level.

Contra the traditional anti-abortionists who generally argue for full moral rights for the fetus from conception, this theory creates three levels of respect that move well past birth in order to be complete. Contra the traditional pro-abortionists, who generally argue for the right of abortion at will, this theory denies abortions at will. What is requisite is demonstrating a level of maternal threat that is greater than the level of respect we ought to give the developing (though not yet actual) person.

The levels that one sets for threats versus respect will follow from one's complex web of values that I call the worldview. Through a dialectical interaction between the question at hand and these values emerges personal ownership of a universal theory dealing with "if, when, and under what conditions" an embryo may be separated from its biological mother.

The question of abortion has stayed with us so long in the public square because it addresses so many key issues about the rights of others versus our own individual expressions of autonomy. I believe that total consensus on this issue will never occur in the present framework because consensus is a derivative property of one's worldview. And since worldviews differ, so will the imperatives they endorse. This is not a statement of relativism, but a factual description of various people working on a common problem (each thinking s/he has *the* correct answer).

However, on the optimistic side, I believe that, if the abortion question is viewed from the personal worldview imperative, at least there will be more understanding of (a) where the other side is "coming from" and (b) a vocabulary that is structured so that it does not prejudge the issue (viz., the vocabulary of maternal threat vs. fetal respect). These sorts of understanding will be essential if there is to be any real progress in the public debate on abortion.

NOTES

1. I define a linking principle as one that follows from a moral theory but that is "action guiding" in its application. One example of a linking principle is Deryck Beyleveld's "cautionary reasoning." See Deryck Beyleveld and Shaun Pattinson, "Precautionary Reason as a Link to Moral Action," in *Medical Ethics*, ed. Michael Boylan (Upper Saddle River, NJ: Prentice Hall, 2000).

2. An argument for the personal worldview imperative is given in my book *Basic Ethics* (Upper Saddle River, NJ: Prentice Hall, 2000). See especially the introduction.

3. There is obviously not a single argument that represents either position entirely. There are, in fact, many distinct arguments meant to argue for the conclusion that abortion is or is not permissible. My reconstructions here are meant to represent my opinion about the strongest version of each argument in a simple, generic form.

4. There are at least two objectors to this position: (a) To say that one "owns" one's body splits the person in two. There is no proper distinction between one's self and one's body. They are one and the same. Thus, all metaphors of "ownership" are faulty and do not fit legal notions of ownership. For a statement of this position, see Hugh V. McLachlan, "Bodies, Rights and Abortion," *Journal of Medical Ethics* 23, no. 3 (1997): 176–80. (b) Of course, those who accept a theology that posits an all-powerful creator God—such as Judaism, Christianity, and Islam (a sizable portion of the world's population)—will demur on this point since it is dogma that God created everything and therefore "owns" what s/he/it has created. In this case one's body is not one's own but God's. This tenet can have an effect upon the argument.

5. For a description of these times, see Leslie J. Reagan, *When Abortion Was a Crime: Women, Medicine, and Law in the United States, 1867–1973* (Berkeley, CA: University of California Press, 1997).

6. H. L. A. Hart and A. M. Honoré, *Causation in the Law* (Oxford: Clarendon Press, 1959), 129 ff., cf. 127, 292–96.

7. In this case, the state would enter the equation as an interested party in order to govern the interests of the newly born, premature infant.

8. Judith Jarvis Thomson, "A Defense of Abortion," *Philosophy and Public Affairs* 1 (1971): 47–66. The responses to this article have been enormous. Some of the most interesting of these include Robert N. Wennberg, *Life in the Balance: Exploring the Abortion Controversy* (Grand Rapids, MI: Eerdmans, 1985); John T. Wilcox, "Nature as Demonic in Thomson's Defense of Abortion," in *The Ethics of Abortion: Pro-Life vs. Pro-Choice*, rev. ed., ed. Robert M. Baird and Stuart E. Rosenbaum (Buffalo, NY: Prometheus, 1993), 212–25; Mary Anne Warren, "On the Moral and Legal Status of Abortion," in *Arguing about Abortion*, ed. Lewis M. Schwartz (Belmont, MA: Wadsworth, 1993), 227–24; Keith J. Pavlischek, "Abortion Logic and Paternal Responsibility: One More Look at Judith Thomson's 'A Defense of Abortion,'" *Public Affairs Quarterly* 7 (1993): 341–61; and David Boonin-Vail, "A Defense of 'A Defense of Abortion': On the Responsibility Objection to Thomson's Argument," *Ethics* 107 (1997): 286–313.

9. Immanuel Kant, *Grundlegung zur Metaphysik der sitten*, 1st ed., 1785; 2nd ed., 1786, Prussian Academy edition, vol. 4 (Berlin: G. Reimer, 1902–1942), 421; Alan Gewirth, "Replies to My Critics," in *Gewirth's Ethical Rationalism: Critical Essays with a Reply by Alan Gewirth*, ed. Edward Regis, Jr. (Chicago: University of Chicago Press, 1984), 228–29; Alan Donagan, *The Theory of Morality* (Chicago: University of Chicago Press, 1977), 154 ff.

10. The reason for this caveat is that one is not *obliged* ever to risk his or her own basic goods of agency for the sake of another. To do so would be to admit that the other person had more of a right to the basic goods of agency more than I do. This would entail that the other person is better qua being an agent than I am. There is no support for such an assertion under the deontological theories I am citing since all agents are equally entitled to the basic goods of agency simply by being human beings alive on this earth. Those who choose to risk their own basic goods of agency for the sake of others go "above and beyond" their moral duty (i.e., they are heroes). But one who fulfills his or her duty to save another only when his or her basic goods of agency are not at risk is only an ordinary person doing his or her duty.

11. Beyleveld and Pattinson, "Precautionary Reason as a Link to Moral Action."

12. I discuss what I mean by "action description" in the introduction to *Basic Ethics*.

13. The proportionality of "threat" to "minimal response necessary to alleviate the threat" is very important in cases of self-defense. However, in the instance of abortion, the response (abortion) will have a fixed effect (the death of the fetus) until near the end of the second trimester. In this case the only variable is the level of threat. After viability, of course, the situation changes if there is a policy to use an abortion procedure that seeks to preserve the fetus's life.

14. Donagan makes a similar distinction; see *The Theory of Morality*, 87 ff.

15. These cases are not meant to be comprehensive but merely suggestive of certain levels of threat. They deal with only those who have engaged in sexual intercourse willingly and are faced with the resulting pregnancy. I would characterize all nonvoluntary acts of sexual intercourse (such as rape or incest) as creating a very high sense of threat for the woman, which might be characterized as being between A and B. In this case, the carrying of the fetus (as innocent as s/he may be) constantly reinforces the horror and degradation of the initial act. This humiliation is a primary threat to human action and well-being so that the woman would be fully within her rights to remove the fetus from her body at any time.

16. For a discussion of this literature, see Bonnie Steinbock, *Life before Birth: The Moral and Legal Status of Embryos and Fetuses* (Oxford: Oxford University Press, 1992).

17. Beyleveld and Pattinson, "Precautionary Reason as a Link to Moral Action."

18. This is a troubling point because it invokes both methodologies and measurements. Some may want to push the point back a bit, but the ultimate measure in this case is whether the child has shown that s/he has a sense of self and that the sense of self deliberates and carries out action. Thus, walking might count or beginning to speak. *Wherever* one wishes to set this point, it will be well past birth.

19. In most cases, human infants go through many developmental stages more slowly than do other species. Thus, on this alone, one would afford more proportional status to puppies or to baby lizards than to humans. Obviously, this is not the way we act. This is because we employ precautionary reasoning.

20. This interpretation of the personal worldview imperative comes about through the sense of consistency. It would be inconsistent to view oneself as being outside nature's laws. Therefore, to will exceptions for yourself is irrational (because it is inconsistent).

21. The notion of proportional rights stems from the individual's best assessment of the possible degree of agency that *may* exist. This goes well beyond any demonstrated agency (which may be as late as thirty months after birth). This attribution of rights is given not because of demonstrated capacity on the part of the fetus but because it seems possible that an individual may possess attributes that confer agency, viz., a sense of inductive and deductive logic along with the capacity to deliberate about action (even in a very minimal way) *before* this is operationally evident to some observer. Therefore, out of precaution, we act *as if* the individual has these capacities (even though there is no demonstrable evidence for this). As a result, we confer precautionary rights of agency. These differ from full rights of agency only in the fact that they are not *dialectically necessary* (Gewirth) or *apodictically necessary* (Kant). They are, in fact, contingently necessary (contingent because they are based on the assessment of that person who is making the attribution).

22. As well as those cases between A and B—as per note 15 (covering rape and incest and all other cases of involuntary sex that has resulted in a pregnancy).

23. Such a situation would be bizarre, and one would have to stretch his/her imagination to come up with a plausible case. Unfortunately, in my volunteer work experience, it is all too frequently the case that adults feel threatened by children. "They cry too much," or "They keep needing to have their diaper changed," or "They drive me nuts with their fussiness," and so on. Far too often the "threat" threshold is much too low for these adults. Beating, abusing, and even killing infants is justified in the minds of these adults because the needs of the child interfered with their life plans (as per F and G above). Such a response to the perceived threat is far too great. It is therefore morally impermissible.

3

Ethics of Surrogacy

A Comparative Study of Western Secular and Islamic Bioethics[1]

Sharmin Islam, Rusli Bin Nordin, Ab Rani Bin Shamsuddin, Hanapi Bin Mohd Nor, and Abu Kholdun Al-Mahmood

ABSTRACT

The comparative approach regarding the ethics of surrogacy from the Western secular and Islamic bioethical view reveals both commensurable and incommensurable relationship. Both are eager to achieve the welfare of the mother, child, and society as a whole but the approaches are not always the same. Islamic bioethics is straightforward in prohibiting surrogacy by highlighting the lineage problem and also other social chaos and anarchy. Western secular bioethics is relative and mostly follows a utilitarian approach.

SURROGACY: DEFINITION, REASONS, AND CLASSIFICATION

Surrogate literally means "substitute." In this case, a woman bears a child for another woman. The concept of surrogacy is a by-product of artificial insemination (AI) and in-vitro fertilization (IVF) techniques. In a surrogacy arrangement, a woman carries a fetus in her womb throughout pregnancy and, after delivery of the newborn, it is handed over to another family who is unable to have a child on its own. The surrogate mother will be free from all responsibilities to the child or its family.[2] Surrogacy is actually the most low-tech treatment to overcome infertility.

Surrogacy is of two types, genetic and gestational. In genetic surrogacy, the ovum of the surrogate is artificially inseminated by the donor's sperm (the father of the child). In gestational surrogacy, the ovum of a woman is fertilized by the sperm of a male in vitro and the resulting embryo is implanted in the uterus of the surrogate.

Married couples look to surrogacy when the wife is physically unable to conceive a child due to absence of the uterus or a disease or when the wife is just unwilling to carry a baby. She may have a genetic disease that she is unwilling to pass to her offspring. She may not want to become pregnant because of her busy schedule. The couple may choose surrogacy over adoption because the child will be at least half-related to them (in genetic surrogacy). Sometimes, unmarried couples look for a surrogate mother although the practice is not very common. Similarly, this practice is open for a single man willing to be a father or to a homosexual couple who want to have a child.[3]

When a woman is incapable of producing ova as a result of disease or normal aging, the surrogate can provide the ovum that is then fertilized by the woman's husband and then implanted in the surrogate's uterus to carry the fetus to term. The surrogate then delivers and hands the baby to the couple (genetic surrogacy).

This technique allows post-menopausal women or many women once considered hopelessly barren to become mothers even though they have no genetic link to the child.[4]

Surrogacy can be either commercial or altruistic. In the former case, the surrogate is paid for donating the egg, gestating the fetus or both. In altruistic surrogacy, the surrogate is unpaid and the resulting baby is regarded as a gift to the couple.[5]

SURROGACY: ISLAMIC BIOETHICS PERSPECTIVES

In making a legal ruling, Muslim scholars consider *Maqasid al- Sharfah* or purposes of the Law. *Maqasid al- SharTah* are *Hifz al- Din* (Protection of Religion), *Hifz al-Nafs* (Protection of Life), *Hifz al- Nasl* (Protection of Progeny), *Hifz al-'Aql* (Protection of Mind) and *Hifz al- Mal* (Protection of Wealth).[6] This classification describes clearly the paramount and basic necessities of human beings. These purposes need protection, preservation, and promotion.

The purpose of law that is most related to the topic of surrogacy is protection of progeny. As Islam encourages reproduction, it advocates treatment of infertility. Further, protection of progeny entails care for pregnant women and the health of the children. It further entails preservation of lineage. Each newborn should know and be related to both his/her mother and father.

Hiring a "womb" for procreation is a very recent phenomenon that contemporary jurists have to handle. Islamic bioethics cannot accept this practice because surrogacy is a clear form of using donor sperm, a foreign element, in the womb of a woman which results in the mixing of lineage. Mufti Sheikh Ahmad Kutty, an Islamic scholar, opines that the introduction of male sperm into the uterus of a woman to whom he is not married transgresses the bounds of Allah.[7]

In view of the term "transgressing the bounds of Allah" he mentions the following verses of the *Quran*:

وَالَّذِينَ هُمْ لِفُرُوجِهِمْ حَافِظُونَ
إِلَّا عَلَىٰ أَزْوَاجِهِمْ أَوْ مَا مَلَكَتْ أَيْمَانُهُمْ فَإِنَّهُمْ غَيْرُ مَلُومِينَ
فَمَنِ ابْتَغَىٰ وَرَاءَ ذَٰلِكَ فَأُولَٰئِكَ هُمُ الْعَادُونَ

and who are mindful of their chastity, [not giving way to their desires] with any but their spouses or what their right hands possess: for then, behold, they are free of all blame, whereas such as seek to go beyond that [limit] are truly transgressors.[8]

Again, a very basic component of *hifz al-nasl* is to protect lineage.

Consider a case of gestational surrogacy. If the surrogate mother is married, the resultant child would legally be that of her husband although the sperm was donated by another person. The case of genetic surrogacy is more critical and troublesome because here the woman is not only carrying the fetus but also donating her egg. So she is the actual mother of the child but cannot be given the status of a mother. In fact, surrogacy creates a dilemma regarding the identity of the offspring. In a word, the status of any baby born under the surrogacy contract would be illegitimate because the contracting man has not entered into matrimonial contract with the surrogate. "Even if a husband gave written consent that his wife could act as a surrogate, there is a religious problem that would prohibit this. Islam prohibits the semen of one man to touch a fetus that is a product of another man's semen. Will we issue a law prohibiting husbands from exercising their legal right [to sexual relations] with their wives when they are pregnant with another man's baby? And were such a law passed; how it will be enforced?"[9]

To quote G. I. Serour, professor of obstetrics and gynecology, and director of the International Islamic Centre for Population Studies and Research, al-Azhar University, Cairo, Egypt,

> The basic concept of Islam is to avoid mixing genes, as Islam enjoins the purity of genes and heredity. It deems that each child should relate to a known father and mother. Since marriage is a contract between the wife and the husband during the span of their marriage, no third party intrudes into the marital functions of sex and procreation. A third party is not acceptable, whether providing an egg, a sperm, or a uterus. Therefore, sperm donation, egg donation, and surrogacy are not allowed in Islam.[10]

Even in case of bigamy (a husband married to two wives) in which an ovum is taken from one wife and fertilized with the husband's sperm and carried till birth in the womb of the second wife, the pregnancy is carrying an alien seed, the ovum of the first wife which is outside the marriage contract binding the husband and his second wife. The child will belong to the second wife who carried it and gave it birth although she is not the child's biological mother. Thus surrogacy, even in that context, is not permissible.[11]

The Council of the Islamic Fiqh Academy holding its third session, in Amman, Hashemite Kingdom of Jordan, from 8 to 13 Safar 1407H (October 11-16, 1986), declared that surrogacy (the fertilization taking place in vitro between the sperm and the eggs taken from the spouses, and then the fertilized ovum being implanted into the womb of a volunteer woman) is Islamically forbidden and absolutely prohibited due to the consequences of the lineage confusion and loss of motherhood.[12]

Another Islamic concept that is to be considered is the clear identification of mothers as those who give birth to their children as stated in the Quran.

$$\text{إِنْ أُمَّهَاتُهُمْ إِلَّا اللَّائِي وَلَدْنَهُمْ}$$

None can be their mothers except those
who gave them birth.[13]

So a surrogate mother may claim to be the real mother even though she bears the egg of another woman in her womb. She may have a marriage bond in case she is a second wife to the embryo's father, but she does not have any genetic relation to the child in this case. So how could she claim to be the real mother? Similarly, how could the ovum donor have claim over the child even though she did not bear the child or give birth to the child as mentioned in the *Quran?*

Some Muslims argue for the permissibility of surrogacy in Islam by resorting to qiyas. However, rulings based on qiyas could be unreliable because the current issues of medicine are drastically different in nature and context to be analogous. They suggest that surrogate motherhood could be considered analogous to foster motherhood. Can this analogy be justified?

It is true that Muslims can transfer their child to a wet nurse to be breastfed by her and she will be a foster mother of the child by virtue of suckling. In the case of gestational surrogacy, the sperm and ovum of a legally married couple are fertilized in vitro and the embryo is replaced in the womb of the surrogate either on a volunteer or on a commercial basis. The woman who provided the ovum may be considered the real mother because the child will have a genetic link with her and the woman who carries the fetus in her womb and gives birth to it would be considered a foster mother. But this is a faulty analogy. In the first place the wet nurse does not have any relationship with the father of child of whose she is a wet nurse. But in a surrogacy contract, either the woman is artificially impregnated with the sperm of the father of the child or the embryo is produced by the father's sperm and then placed in her womb to carry it up to term and give birth to it.

Further, the wet nurse feeds the child only up to a certain period and does not have any biological relationship with him.[14]

COMPARISON OF WESTERN SECULAR
AND ISLAMIC BIOETHICS OF SURROGACY

A comparative study of Islamic and Western secular philosophical perspectives reveals some similarities and several dissimilarities. Both approaches are concerned about the well-being of both mother and child. Both are very concerned about the welfare of the society. Robertson looks for a very straightforward utilitarian interpretation to justify the practice of surrogacy. He opines that although surrogacy is a deviation from our cultural norms of reproduction, nevertheless it is good for the parties involved. His argument is that if the surrogacy arrangement can fulfill the desire of a barren couple, why should we deprive them from taking this opportunity? He argues that it also opens the way for financial gains of some needy women. In addition, some women enjoy pregnancy and the respect and attention that it draws. It is a blessing for the child because he/she would not have come to the light of the world except through this special arrangement.[15]

The approach of Islamic ethics is very different. Islam prohibits surrogacy because it interferes with proper lineage. To quote Mohammad Hashim Kamali, "The laws of *Shariah* are for the most part distinguishable in regards to their objectives *(maqasid)* and the means which procure or obstruct those objectives. If the means violate a basic purpose of the *Shariah,* then it must be blocked. The means are generally viewed in light of the ends they are expected to obtain and it is logically the latter which prevail over the former in that the means follow their ends, not vice versa."[16] According to Islamic ethics, if the means violate a basic purpose of the *Sharīah,* then it must be blocked. There is no place for surrogate motherhood within the Islamic system, for the evils that would accrue from it will far outweigh any good.

Western secular philosophers criticize surrogacy on different grounds. They frequently argue that, instead of making a better family tie, it threatens it. Even they worry about the family of the surrogate mother. For example, Krimmel thinks that through surrogacy arrangement, the family of the surrogate would face some hazardous situations. When the baby is handed over to the adopting parents, it is removed not only from the surrogate mother but also from her family. Are not the siblings of that baby hurt that their little baby sibling has been given away? Instead of having happiness, the adopting couple may engage themselves in conflict and ultimately the marriage bond may be broken. It may happen that the adopting mother has no biological link to the baby but the adopting father has. May not the father say to his wife, "Well, he is my son, not yours"? In any case, if the marriage ultimately breaks, will the custody be treated simply as a normal child custody dispute?[17]

Krimmel compares surrogate motherhood with second marriage where the children of one party by a prior marriage are adopted by the new spouse. As asymmetry in second marriage situations causes chaos in a family, surrogacy is also no exception.[18] Analysis of the above arguments in relation to Islamic ethical viewpoints reveals dissimilarities. While both argue against surrogacy, the arguments are different. Islamic ethics permits second marriage because it does not create any problem in the lineage of the offspring. But it vehemently prohibits surrogacy because it fails to preserve the principle of lineage of the resulting progeny.

Human nature is such that, when one pays money, one expects value. It is very disappointing for the parents when they learn that the child is born with some genetic or congenital birth defect. The surrogate mother might blame the biological father for providing defective sperms and, similarly, the adopting parents might accuse the surrogate for a defective ovum or for improper care of the fetus during pregnancy. So, the consequence is that neither the adopting parents nor the surrogate would like to keep the child. Like brushed fruit in the produce bin of a supermarket, this child would become a reject.[19] Is it not like treating the child as a commodity?

Islamic ethics strictly advises to form the family solely on the basis of biological ties. Islam condemns surrogacy because the child will be deprived of information about his lineage and may result, unknowingly, in half-sibling marriage which is a dangerous consequence for a society. But on the contrary, a Western secular bioethicist argues that family ties have never been only biological: a husband and a wife, to take the most obvious example, are not biological relatives. It is also argued that, if 'the family' is a good thing, then developing more children by different methods, including non-biological ones, to form a family should also be seen as a good endeavor.[20]

Paid surrogacy sometimes becomes a means of exploitation. Sometimes, poor women lease their wombs to carry the fetus for some money. Evidence shows that sometimes they are given a very small amount of money for their service; sometimes they are given no money at all. Supporters of surrogacy reject this point. Michael Kinsley argues that if women are forbidden to enter into surrogacy contracts, why not ban other kinds of services that women contract to perform? Why do we not forbid women to work as maids or nannies? Why not forbid them to work at all? He also argues that, if the product in question was food or telephones rather than children, a shortage would be seen as a failure of the system. For instance, when the Soviet Union forbade market contracts, shortages occurred. Similarly, if the United States banned procreative contracts, shortages would occur.[21]

Besides, there is at least some evidence that the opportunity to be paid for one's services in bearing a child has not been exploitative of poor women. Statistics show that the "average surrogate mother is white, attended two years of college, married young, and has all the children she and her husband want."[22]

Furthermore, some women enjoy this service with an altruistic vision. If we really want to protect those women who consider child-bearing for somebody else as degrading but are compelled to do so because of economic necessity, then we have another way. We can put restrictions on who can enter into contracted child-bearing arrangements, but need not prohibit the practice entirely. Some may object that such restrictions would be unjust because they would prohibit poor women from doing something that other women were permitted to do. But that would imply that the restrictions would be denying the poor women a good, rather than protecting them from a harm, which in turn means that the initial assumptions about exploitation itself was misguided.[23]

CONCLUSION

The discussion of ethics of surrogacy in a comparative perspective makes one point clear. It is that although in Western secular bioethics there are arguments and counter arguments in judging its moral worth, Islamic bioethics denounces the practice altogether as incompatible with the five purposes of the *SharīTah*.

The debate regarding surrogacy will continue as we are free to cultivate our own reasons to judge the morality of surrogate motherhood. The overall analysis shows that its benefits are less than its harm. It is bad both from the deontological and consequential points of view. If it would have been good from consequential point of view, then we should reevaluate its deontological position and try to justify its relevance to the society. But we see it can neither satisfy the deontologist nor the consequentialist nor the feminist nor society. So why should we support it?

NOTES

1. JIMA Vol 44 2012 and on Creative Commons. Reprinted with permission of Abu Kholdun Al-Mahmood for the authors and Creative Commons.

2. Schwartz L, Preece PE, Hendry RA. *Medical Ethics: A Case-Based Approach*. Edinburgh and New York: WB Saunders; 2002.

3. [Missing author] Reproductive technologies. In: Post SG (editor). *Bioethics for Students: How Do We Know What's Right?: Issues In Medicine, Animal Rights and the Environment*. Vol 1. New York: Macmillan Reference USA; 1999; I:177-99.

4. Munson R. Reproductive Control: In Vitro Fertilization, Artificial Insemination And Surrogate Pregnancy. In: Munson R, Hoffman C (editors). *Intervention and Reflection: Basic Issues In Medical Ethics*. 5th ed. Belmont: Wadsworth Publishing Co: 1996; 489–551.

5. Pence GE. *Classic Cases In Medical Ethics*. 2nd ed. New York: McGraw-Hill, 1995.

6. Kasule OH. Medical Jurisprudence between Originality and Modernity. Proceedings of the 5th Scientific Meeting of the Islamic Medical Association of Malaysia, Penang, May 28–29, 2004; and Kasule OH. A Critique Of The Biomedical Model From An Islamic Perspective. In: Fadel HE (editor). FIMA Year Book 2002. Islamabad: Federation of Islamic Medical Associations in collaboration with Medico Islamic Research Council (MIRC) and Islamic International Medical College; 2003: 95–108.

7. Kutty A. Does Islam Allow "Surrogate Motherhood"? Doha, Qatar: Islamonline.net. [Updated 2007-Jan-7; Accessed 2013-Apr-8]. http://bit.ly/ZJv6bp

8. The Glorious Quran, Chapter 23, Verses 5–7.

9. Farag F. Al-Ahram Weekly On-line. 17-23 May 2001, Issue No. 534. [Updated 2001-May-17; Accessed 2013-Apr-8] http://weekly.ahram.org.eg/2001/534/feat1.htm

10. Serour GI. Reproductive Choice: A Muslim Perspective. In The *Future of Human Reproduction: Ethics, Choice and Regulation*. Harris J, Holm S. Oxford and New York: Clarendon Press and Oxford University Press, 1998. http://bit.ly/ZIxwXr

11. Hathout H. Islamic *Perspectives in Obstetrics and Gynaecology*. Cairo: Alam al-Kutub; 1988. http://bit.ly/17nkR45

12. Al-Kawthari MA. What Is The Islamic Position on Surrogate Motherhood? Qibla [website on Internet]. [Accessed 2018-Apr-8] http://bit.ly/15bACM1

13. The Glorious Quran, Chapter 58, Verse 2.

14. Surrogate parenting. Islam: The Modern Religion [website on the Internet]. [Accessed 2013-Apr-8]. http://www.themodernreligion.com/misc/hh/surrogate-parenting.html

15. Robertson JA. Surrogate Mothers: Not So Novel After All. Hastings Cent Rep. 1983;13:28-34. http://dx.doi.org/10.2307/3560576

16. Kamali MH. Principles of Islamic Jurisprudence. Selangor Darul Ehsan: Pelanduk Publications; 1989.

17. Krimmel HT. The Case against Surrogate Parenting. Hastings Cent Rep. 1983;13:35-39. http://dx.doi.org/10.2307/3560577

18. Krimmel HT. The Case against Surrogate Parenting. Hastings Cent Rep. 1983;13:35-39. http://dx.doi.org/10.2307/3560577

19. Krimmel HT. The Case against Surrogate Parenting. Hastings Cent Rep. 1983;13:35-39. http://dx.doi.org/10.2307/3560577

20. Pence GE. *Classic Cases in Medical Eth*ics. 2nd ed. New York: McGraw-Hill; 1995.

21. Pence GE. *Classic Cases in Medical Ethics*. 2nd ed. New York: McGraw-Hill; 1995.

22. Malm H. Paid Surrogacy: Arguments and Responses. Public Aff Q. 1989 Apr;3:57-66. PMID: 11650275

23. Malm H. Paid Surrogacy: Arguments and Responses. Public Aff Q. 1989 Apr;3:57-66. PMID: 11650275

4

Euthanasia Could Be a Medical Duty

Carlos Verdugo Serna

ABSTRACT

Most people, including philosophers and physicians, would be willing to accept that human beings have some sort of moral rights to live not only with the highest possible level of autonomy, dignity, liberty, and well-being but also with the minimum level of unnecessary pain, suffering, distress, anguish, and physical or mental degrading conditions.

By accepting those rights, we can also claim that we have some duties to respect them and behave accordingly. In addition, since it is a fact that dying is part of the process of living, it is reasonable to believe that the rights and duties acknowledged above apply also to the process of dying.

I will attempt to show that, when physicians, under some restricted conditions, bring about a patient's death, they are acting in compliance with the moral rights and duties mentioned before.

INTRODUCTION

In his influential paper "The Scientist qua Scientist Makes Value Judgments" (1953), the late American philosopher Richard Rudner said:

> The question of the relationship of making of value judgments in a typical ethical sense to the method and procedures of science has been discussed in the literature at least to that point which E.E. Cummings somewhere refers to as "The Mystical Moment of Dullness." Nevertheless, albeit with some trepidation, I feel that something more may fruitfully be said on the subject. (540)

I have to confess that I am in a similar position writing about the morality of euthanasia. Nevertheless, with some trepidation, I think I can add (hopefully) something relevant and fruitful to the age-old and still vigorous euthanasia debate. Of course, I am fully aware that the very nature of philosophy and logic impedes giving conclusive arguments in "pro" or "con" of the morality of any form of assisted dying.

I also agree with Popper's idea that the method for dealing with philosophical problems, including of course ethical problems, is the method of stating a problem as clearly as possible and then assessing any solutions critically. But this method does not allow us to reach definite and conclusive true answers to our problems. In philosophy and science, all of our intended solutions are conjectural and can never be proved to be true.

Nevertheless, this does not imply that we have to abandon our search for truth in philosophy or science. We have only to accept, following Popper, that we do not have criteria for truth (i.e., for proving that we have reached truth) and that for logical reasons we can never prove that we are justified claiming that we have the right answers to some questions, especially in the field of philosophy. According to Popper, there exist no general criteria of truth not only in the realm of facts but also in the realm of values and standards or proposals, including moral ones:

> For though we should seek for absolutely right or valid proposals, we should never persuade ourselves that we have definitely found them, for clearly, there cannot be a *criterion of absolute rightness*—even less than a criterion of absolute truth. . . . But although we have no criterion of absolutely rightness, we certainly can make progress in this realm. As in the realm of facts, we can make discoveries. That cruelty is always "bad"; that it should always be avoided where possible; that the golden rule is a good standard which can perhaps even be improved by doing unto others, wherever possible, as *they* want to be done by: these are elementary and extremely important examples of discoveries in the realm of standards. (2013, 501)

I also want to indicate that we cannot simply abandon the use of arguments in dealing with some moral questions but only that it is very important to learn what are the functions, possibilities, and limits of arguments or inferences in general. The next section will be devoted to expanding briefly these working observations.

LOGICAL–METHODOLOGICAL PRELIMINARIES

Let's start by first remembering that, as a matter of elementary logic, we know that, in any valid deductive arguments, if the truth of a conclusion R logically follows from assuming the truth of premises P and Q, then we have to also accept that, if R is false (-R), then it is not possible that all premises are true.

For example, if we accept the truth of the following premises:
P: All forms of intentionally killing firstborn children by humans or God are inherently morally wrong.
Q: God killed all the firstborn Egyptians.

We can therefore conclude:
R: God did something inherently morally wrong.

Now, if someone does not want to accept the truth of the conclusion, he/she could also formulate the following valid deductive argument:
-R: It is false that God did something inherently morally wrong.
Q: God killed all the firstborn Egyptians.

Therefore:
-P: It is false that all forms of killing newborn children are inherently morally wrong.

An additional and deeper difficulty with giving conclusive arguments in general is the known fact that it can be shown that valid deductive arguments are circular: the truth of the conclusion has already been accepted in the premises; that is, they assume what they are trying to prove or supposed to prove.

This important logical point has been remarked by David Miller (2006) in *Out of Error: Further Essays on Critical Rationalism*:

> Since, as Mill noted, the conclusion of every valid syllogism, indeed of every valid argument, is included entirely within its premises, the premises cannot lend any weight at all to the conclusion. At an everyday level we may say that any purported proof or justification is *circular*, that is, *begs the question at issue*, or in a more philosophical jargon, commits the fallacy of *petitio principia* . . . if the premises of a deductive valid argument are not already proved, the argument will be insufficient to prove the conclusion (this is the objection of classical scepticism); but if the premises are already proved, then the conclusion, being a part of the premises, is also proved (though admittedly we need an argument to make this obvious to us). (70)

Nevertheless, there are two uses of arguments that will be relevant and fruitful for the ensuing discussion on the morality of euthanasia: Valid deductive arguments or inferences, as in formal and empirical theories, allow us to identify the logical consequences of what we assume to be true. Another use of arguments in deductive logic has been remarked on by Popper (1975):

> We can say: if all the premises are true and the inference is valid, then the conclusion *must* also be true; and if, consequently, the conclusion is false in a valid inference, then it is not possible that all the premises are true. In this way deductive logic becomes the theory of rational criticism. For all rational criticism takes the form of an attempt to show that unacceptable conclusions can be derived from the assertion we are trying to criticize. If we are successful in deriving, logically, unacceptable conclusions from an assertion, the assertion may be taken to be refuted. (98–99)

In other words, the role of logical arguments in deductive logic is to be the *organon* of criticism and should not to be taken as an instrument allowing us to prove or justify our theories in science or philosophy.

All these considerations will show their importance in the analysis and assessment of arguments against or in favor of the morality of euthanasia.

ARGUMENTS AGAINST EUTHANASIA

In an article entitled "The Wrongfulness of Euthanasia," bioethicist J. Gay-Williams gives three arguments to show that euthanasia is morally wrong: (a) the argument from nature, (b) the argument from self-interest, and (c) the argument from practical effects. Even though I think there are serious flaws in these arguments, I will concentrate my criticism on the first one.

The Argument from Nature

This argument is an attempt to show that euthanasia is inherently wrong and should be rejected because it violates the natural propensity to preserve our life (i.e., it is unnatural). Let's quote the argument:

Every human being has a natural inclination to continue living. Our reflexes and responses fit us to fight attackers, flee wild animals, and dodge out of the ways of trucks. In our daily lives we exercise the caution and care necessary to protect ourselves. Our bodies are similarly structured for survival right down to the molecular level. When we are cut, our capillaries seal shut, our blood clots, and fibrogen is produced to start the process of healing the wound. When we are invaded by bacteria, antibodies are produced to fight against the alien organisms, and their remains are swept out of the body by special cells. Euthanasia does violence to this natural goal of survival. It is literally acting against nature because all the processes of nature are bent towards the end of bodily survival. . . . By reason alone, then, we can recognize that euthanasia sets us against our own nature. (Gay-Williams 1987, 57–58)

It seems that, according to this quotation, Gay-Williams is formulating the following argument:

1. Every human being has a natural inclination to preserve their life or to continue living (premise).
2. Euthanasia acts against nature and sets us against our own nature (premise).
3. Therefore, euthanasia is morally wrong.

But this argument cannot be accepted. First, clearly, this argument is not an instance of a valid deductive argument. Even if the premises were true, the conclusion would not necessarily be true. Why? Because the information content of the conclusion is wider than the content of the premises. To imply the conclusion, you need to add another premise, such as

4. Everything that acts against nature and sets us against our own nature is morally wrong.

However, if Gay-Williams wants to claim that this premise is true, he would have to accept very undesirable consequences, among them that all self-sacrificial deaths would be morally wrong. It seems awkward to claim that firemen, soldiers, and policemen, when putting their lives at risk and thereby acting against their natural inclination to preserve their own lives and to continue living, are doing something morally wrong.

On the other hand, if he were trying, on the basis of premises 1 and 2 to infer the normative conclusion "We should not practice euthanasia" or "We have the moral duty to reject euthanasia" or "We ought not to perform euthanasia," he would be guilty of deriving a normative conclusion from descriptive premises (i.e., from premises stating facts). (Hume in the eighteenth century made the straightforward logical remark that no ought-statements are logically deducible from only factual are-statements.)

A similar criticism concerning the problem of *prima facie* unacceptable consequences of some premises can be applied to an argument against euthanasia put forward by the late Chilean philosopher Dr. Alfonzo Gomez-Lobo (1940–2011), who held the Ryan Chair in Metaphysics and Moral Philosophy at Georgetown University.

In his book entitled *Morality and the Human Goods: An Introduction to Natural Law Ethics* (2002) we find the following:

For there to be a genuine case of euthanasia (or "mercy killing," as it used to be called), the agent must first intend the death of the person; this is the main immediate goal or point of his action. The agent also must have the further goal, however, of relieving a dying person of great suffering. Without this further goal, the action would be classified as murder. If a patient is in severe pain but is likely to recover soon, or terminally ill but not suffering pain, killing such a patient will hardly count as causing a good death. The alleged mercy is simply misplaced.

In plausible cases of euthanasia, then, there is a conflict that becomes all the more acute if the pain becomes unbearable. Is that sufficient, however, to justify intentional killing? I argue that it is not. Here is the fundamental argument against active euthanasia (voluntary or otherwise):

(Premise 1): Any act whose goal is intentionally to attack, harm, destroy an instance of a basic human good is irrational and morally wrong. (This is the guideline of respect for basic goods under the Formal Principle of practical reason. How seriously wrong the act is will depend on the prudentially determined importance of the good under attack.)

(Premise 2): Life is a basic human good (the first supplementary principle of practical rationality).

(Premise 3): Active euthanasia is an action whose goal is intentionally to take the life of a terminally ill patient to alleviate great pain (definition of active euthanasia).

Conclusion: Active euthanasia is irrational and morally wrong.

Before evaluating this argument, it is important to understand exactly what he is asserting in premise 2, especially his use of the word "life." Here is Gomez-Lobo's (2002) definition:

> By "life" I mean here human life at the basic biological level, manifesting itself in the typical functions of a human organism (taking nourishment, growing, etc.). Whether a certain organism is human depends on whether it has the complete set of standard human chromosomes or a deviation therefrom that counts as a human genetic abnormality. An egg or a sperm by itself does not qualify. Neither of them, as we now know, has the complete set. (10, 101)

What can be said about this argument?

First, this argument is an instance of a valid deductive inference. If somebody accepts that the premises are true then, he/she has to accept that the conclusion is also true. (Although, as we know, a big debate still exists about the alleged truth or falsity of moral sentences, only for the sake of our discussion, let's also agree that the argument is not valid but that it is sound). But, as we emphasized before, a valid deductive argument is circular; therefore, you are assuming the truth of the conclusion has already been included in the premises. Thus, the truth of the premises cannot "justify" the truth of the conclusion.

Actually, we can formulate, as we also showed above, that we could put forward another instance of a valid deductive inference by affirming instead the falsity of the conclusion and therefore the falsity of at least one of the three premises accepted by Gomez-Lobo. In this case, I would claim that the first premise is false. Or, as we did before with the argument given by Gay-Williams, we can show that the first two premises seem to imply some consequences that are very difficult to accept.

Among these undesirable commonsense consequences we find that, according to these premises, war is irrational and morally wrong because it necessarily involves soldiers intending to kill human beings and, therefore, harming and destroying a basic good (i.e., life). Thus, it seems that we are obliged to be "absolute pacifists" for whom human life has an absolute value and therefore must not be destroyed. From this it follows that we could not defend at all the moral justifications in favor of going to war, not even in the case of national self-defense.

A similar problem would face someone adopting a less extreme view about the morality of war. One of them, known as "limited pacifism," considers as morally wrong only wars involving the killing of innocent "noncombatants" (i.e., people who are not members of the armed forces). We have to also point out that just-war theorists, while strongly defending the value of human life, are at the same time willing to accept that, under some conditions, a country has a moral right to go to war. Additionally, certain police actions, self-defense, and capital punishment would also have to be rejected as immoral.

All of these consequences show that the two first premises of Gomez-Lobo's argument against euthanasia claiming that life is a basic good and that any act whose goal is intentionally to attack, harm, or to destroy an instance of a basic good is irrational or morally wrong should be rejected. I will argue later that euthanasia should also be seen as another important exception or example of *force majeure*.

Now, let's critically examine another rejection of voluntary active euthanasia based on the doctrine that putting to death is always wrong because all human life has a especial worth, or dignity (or sanctity), and should be preserved.

This doctrine, called "the inviolability of human life," seems to be behind the claim that doctors have an absolute prohibition against killing patients. An illustrative example of this strong position is Leon R. Kass's (2014) article "Why Doctors Must Not Kill." Therein, he says:

> In forswearing the giving of poison, *when asked for it*, the Hippocratic physician rejects the view that the patient's choice for death can make killing him—or assisting his suicide—right. For the physician, at least, human life in living bodies commands respect and reverence—*by its very nature*. As its respectability does not depend upon human agreement or patient consent, revocation on one's consent to live does not deprive one's living body of respectability. The deepest ethical principle of restraining the physician's power is not the autonomy or freedom of the patient; neither is its own compassion or good intention. Rather, it is the dignity and mysterious power of human life itself, and, therefore, also what the oath calls the purity and holiness of the life and art to which he has sworn devotion. (181–82)

We cannot in this short space deal in-depth with the issue of the sanctity of life or the principle of the inviolability of human life. Nevertheless, I want to make a couple of short comments on this subject. It is rather difficult to understand what Kass means by "the dignity and mysterious power of human life itself." How do we understand the phrase "the dignity of human life itself"? What does he mean by "life"? And why "For the physician, at least, human life in living bodies commands respect and reverence—*by its very nature*"? Is he using this term in the same or close to the same sense that was used by Gomez-Lobo in his argument that we examined above (i.e., meaning the more basic biological functions)?

I think he does. Actually, Kass claims that our highest mental life and functions "are held up by, and are inseparable from, lowly metabolism, respiration, circulation, excretion" (Kass 2014, 182). Unfortunately, he did not provide any philosophical reasons for his claim on the "dignity and mysterious powers of human life itself."

Nevertheless, what is really surprising and difficult to understand is the fact that most of the people who strongly support the thesis or the principle of an intrinsic, inviolable value, dignity, sacredness of life, or a right to life principle, normally stress just the wrongfulness of killing. The question is, why stress only or mainly the medical duty of not killing, instead of the duty to do everything possible to save a patient's life? If life is so precious, it is a basic human good, has an intrinsic value, and is inviolable and even sacred. Why not act to protect and save it under all conditions and circumstances or to prolong it by all possible means?

This is the way that Gomez-Lobo and Keown (2015) answer this question when dealing with persistent vegetative state patients:

So, if the "right to die" means a right to end one's life, to commit suicide by refusing life-prolong-
ing treatment, it should be rejected. Or does the phrase connote a right to resist medical obstinacy
or vitalism? Does it mean a right to resist doctors who, forgetful that the core purpose of medicine
is to restore patients to health, practice "meddlesome medicine" and try to preserve life at all costs,
even by way of clearly disproportionate treatments that impose excessive burden on the patient or
her family? If this is what the "right to die" means, it is a legitimate right. (85)

Both philosophers support a natural law perspective on bioethics, and they emphasize that
their ethical claims and arguments are based on reason alone. A similar position has been
defended by the Catholic Church. Talking about the Bland case, the late Cardinal Winning
said in an interview in 1999 that "To give someone antibiotics in a vegetative state, with no
prospect of recovery, was extraordinary and, one would say, unnecessary. Perhaps he could
have been left to die on several occasions."

Thus, it is clear that concerning bioethics a natural law perspective is common to some
philosophers and religious people, such as the Catholic Church. But it is more important
for our discussion to realize that some of those who defend the principle of the sanctity and
inviolability of life also admit additional limitations in its application. First, even though life
can be considered a basic good and human life is invaluable, doctors are not morally obliged to
maintain this good at all cost. Second, according to the Catholic Church, sometimes, killing a
human being can be morally legitimate, as in Cardinal Winning's (1999) words: "Human life
is invaluable, innocent human life is inviolable and the only time the state can take human
life is to right an injustice—in other words when somebody's committed a crime where the
punishment is death" (142).

Clearly, according to Cardinal Winning, killing somebody can be a morally legitimate
means "to right an injustice." We also have to remember that there is another morally justified
killing not only for the Catholic Church but also for very important supporters of natural
law ethics, such as Thomas Aquinas. He is often cited saying, "He who kills a tyrant to free
his country is praised and rewarded" (Aquinas, *II Sentences*, 44.2.2., cited by Harty 2012).

With all these exceptions, it seems odd that many people, including doctors, religious
believers, and lawyers, who defend normative moral claims such as "We have the moral duty
to reject euthanasia," "We ought not to perform euthanasia," "Doctors must not kill," or "We
are always morally culpable for killing someone" could support those claims appealing to a
strict and absolute understanding of the principles of the "sanctity of life" or the "right to life."

Following, I argue that, contrary to the claim that a right to life makes euthanasia morally
wrong, the right to life principle—when human life is understood far beyond the basic
biological level—actually makes euthanasia not only a morally permissible medical act, but,
more importantly, under certain conditions, it could be considered a medical duty.

AN ARGUMENT FOR EUTHANASIA

One of the most common arguments advanced in favor of euthanasia is the existence of a
"right to die" or a right to choose death. Thus, it is argued that, if we have such rights, euthanasia and physician-assisted suicide are morally permissible. Now, due to the empirical biological fact that death is an inevitable event for any living animal, including human animals, it
seems to be quite odd to fight or defend this right. We are going to die anyway.

On the other hand, there are not many possibilities of how to die to choose from, with
the exception of a few cases, such as committing suicide; sacrificing your life for your family

so they can access a lifeboat (as we saw in the movie *Titanic* as it was sinking); or, in some war scenarios, such as leading an assault on a fortified enemy position. Nevertheless, you can sometimes choose how you want to go through the process of dying, the ending of one's life by death. In this case, you can claim that other people have the moral obligation to respect your autonomous and deliberate decision about some form of dying, for example, if you want to die without receiving a blood transfusion in order to save your life.

What I want to claim is that such a right to choose how to die should be included within the right to live (i.e., with the right to choose how we should live our own life).

I think that most people would accept that we have a right to live with the highest possible level of self-determination or autonomy; of freedom from any kind of illegitimate or unjustified coercion; and with the best possible functioning of our physical, psychological, emotional, and intellectual capacities. Of course, we also firmly believe that we have a right to live without unnecessary pain, suffering, and anguish and also with the least degrading and humiliating conditions.

Thus, I want to propose accepting that, if we believe that we are obliged to promote this kind of life or we have a right to live under the conditions mentioned above, this also applies to the process of dying. I also want to claim that any physician involved in an act of euthanasia is fulfilling this important duty.

All of the assertions made above can be formulated in the following arguments:

1. Every human being has the right to live with the highest possible level of autonomy or self-determination, freedom from any kind of illegitimate or unjustified coercion, and with the best possible functioning of our intellectual capacities. We also have the right to live with the minimum level of pain, suffering, and anguish and without any form of degrading and humiliating conditions.
2. Dying is a process included in the process of living.
3. Therefore, every human being has the right to die with the rights mentioned in premise 1.

Now, if we accept the conclusion 3 as a premise, and then we add this new additional premise:

4. Euthanasia allows human beings to die with the rights mentioned in premise 3.

We can conclude,

5. Therefore, any human being has a right to euthanasia.

Of course, those who are opposed to the morality of killing will claim that taking the life of a patient even when the patient is asking to end his life is wrong. But, as shown before, there are exceptions to the absolute principle of the sanctity of life or to the absolute inviolability of the right to live principle. What are the reasons for not considering euthanasia as a case of *force majeure* (i.e., as a reasonable and plausible exemption benefiting some patients)?

A logical objection has been formulated by some authors, including Kass (2014), who, in his article cited above, asks: "Can one benefit the patient as a whole by making him dead? There is of course, a logical difficulty: how can any good exist for a being that is not? But the error is more than logical: to intend and to act for someone's good requires his continued existence to receive the benefit."

I think that this logical criticism is unfounded. First, many people believe that they are morally obliged to take care of our environment for future generations, to the benefit of beings that are not existing today. They will think that they are doing something good for their future descendants. Of course, to enjoy some common goods (e.g., a healthy condition), you have to be alive. Neither can any bad exist for a being who is not.

But, in the case of euthanasia, we are talking of human beings who are alive and going through the process of dying. Thus, "making a patient dead" is a process and not an event. The good here is to relieve the unbearable and unnecessary pain while the patient is alive. And this is exactly the good that a patient enjoys as a benefit while still alive and conscious. Of course, it will be nonsense to try to relieve pain in a dead patient. Thus, it seems to me that Kass is ignoring the distinction between dying and death and that we do not have to solve his problem but rather just dissolve it.

Now, I would like to show that our argument can, with some modifications, be applied by some doctors who claim that it is not only a right for them to perform euthanasia but even a duty to do it. This is the case of Pieter V. Admiraal (2014), who, in his article "Euthanasia in the Netherlands: Justifiable Euthanasia," says:

> It is my opinion that every doctor has the right and the duty after prolonged and thorough delib-
> eration to carry out euthanasia; at the request of the other person and in its interest, knowing that
> he is responsible to himself, to the others, and to the law. Similarly, every doctor has the unassail-
> able right under any circumstances to refuse to carry out euthanasia, knowing that he is responsible
> to himself and to the other. (176)

Earlier, in 1999, in Admiraal's defense of the morality and legality of euthanasia, he had already stated: "It is my intention that the patient will die and his suffering will come to an end. It is my intention, my right and my duty to stop the suffering of a patient who has unbearable suffering" (2014, 129).

I think that Admiraal's claim that doctors have a duty to stop the unbearable suffering of their patients by carrying out euthanasia clearly demonstrates that, if doctors believe that they have the same rights mentioned in premise 1 above, then it is also their duty to see that other human beings also enjoy them.

In sum, it seems that, after all, euthanasia can be considered a doctor's duty.

CONCLUSION

Surely the contemporary debate concerning euthanasia will continue in the future as long as we have to admit that the nature of any rational discussion on philosophical issues, and espe-cially on ethical problems, cannot be resolved once and for all. The use of arguments can only help us to establish the logical consequences of some premises that are, in principle, always conjectural and subject to criticism.

I have tried to show that the ethical problem of euthanasia can be seen and examined from a new perspective when the basic fact has been accepted, being that the process of dying is part of the process of living, together with a set of conditions and values that seem reasonable to be proposed as belonging to a desirable human life.

Insofar as they have been accepted, euthanasia can be considered by doctors as a medical duty to carry out to the extent that one of the principal aims of medicine is to reduce and eliminate human suffering. Thus, euthanasia has to be seen as another important exception to the sanctity of life or a right to life principle.

ACKNOWLEDGMENTS

I am indebted to David Wayne for his helpful comments on the accuracy of my English translation of a previous presentation in Spanish. I am heavily indebted also to Rodrigo Lopez for his invaluable help in presenting my work according to international edition standards. I want also to thank Professor Michael Boylan for some valuable comments on a lecture given under the title "A Defense of Euthanasia," held at Marymount University in 2014.

REFERENCES

Admiraal, P. V. 2014. "Euthanasia in The Netherlands: Justifiable Euthanasia." In *Medical Ethics*, edited by M. Boylan, 171–78. West Sussex: Wiley Blackwell.

Gay-Williams, J. 1987. "The Wrongfulness of Euthanasia." In *Social Ethics: Morality and Social Policy*, edited by T. A. Mappes and J. S. Zembaty, 55–60. New York: McGraw-Hill.

Gomez-Lobo, A. 2002. *Morality and the Human Goods: An Introduction to Natural Law Ethics*. Washington, DC: Georgetown University Press.

Gomez-Lobo, A., and J. Keown. 2015. *Bioethics and the Human Goods: An Introduction to Natural Law Bioethics*. Washington, DC: Georgetown University Press.

Harty, J. 2012. "Tyrannicide." In *The Catholic Encyclopedia*. Vol. 15. New York: Robert Appleton Company. Accessed July 3, 2019. http://www.newadvent.org/cathen/15108a.htm.

Kass, L. R. 2014. "Why Doctors Must Not Kill." In *Medical Ethics*, edited by M. Boylan, 179–84. West Sussex: Wiley Blackwell.

Miller, D. W. 2006. *Out of Error*. Burlington: Ashgate Publishing Company.

Popper, K. R. 1975. "The Logic of the Social Sciences." In *The Positivist Dispute in German Sociology*, edited by Theodor W. Adorno et al., 87–104. London: Heinemann Educational Books.

Popper, K. R. 2013. *The Open Society and Its Enemies*. First single volume of Popper (1945). Princeton, NJ: Princeton University Press.

Rudner, R. 1953. "The Scientist qua Scientist Makes Value Judgments." *Philosophy of Science* 20, no. 1: 1–6.

Winning, C. 1999. "Interview." In *Euthanasia: The Heart of the Matter*, edited by A. Dunnett, 141–54. London: Hodder & Stoughton.

5

Is There a Global Bioethics?

End of Life in Thailand and the Case for Local Difference[1]

Scott Stonington and Pinit Ratanakul

ABSTRACT

The 21st century has seen a debate over whether there should be international standards in medical ethics and human rights. Critics worry that such standards risk overlooking important cultural differences in the way people conceptualize medical decision-making. The question for a global bioethics then is what bioethical guidelines and framework should guide developing countries that are building allopathic medical systems. This essay examines the issue—including the presumed universality of Western bioethics values like autonomy, beneficence, non-maleficence, truth-telling, and justice. It concludes that Western bioethics is inadequate to solve the problems in non-Western societies.

INTRODUCTION

Over the past decade, several scholars have advocated for international standards in medical ethics and human rights [1–3]. Others have countered that such standards risk ignoring important cultural differences in the way people conceptualize medical decision-making [4–8]. Within this debate hangs a question for international bioethics: As developing countries build allopathic medical systems, what should their bioethics be? In this essay, we explore possible answers to this question, ultimately arguing that Western bioethics is insufficient to solve the problems that arise in the practice of allopathic medicine in non-Western contexts.

As an example, we discuss recent conflicts over the use of mechanical ventilators in Thailand. Thailand is a center of cutting-edge allopathic medical care in Asia. It has a universal health-care system, which provides many Thais with access to mechanical ventilation. So many Thais are placed on mechanical ventilators at the end of life that it has become one of the largest drains on Thailand's universal health-care system [9]. Furthermore, the use of ventilators has become a source of vehement national debate, mostly as a result of several prominent political figures who received overly aggressive medical care at the end of life [10,11]. As in Western hospitals, the ascension of mechanical ventilation has introduced a host of difficult ethical dilemmas for doctors, families, and patients [12,13]. How will Thais go about solving these dilemmas? On which principles of bioethics will they rely?

To answer these questions, we start with a case that illustrates a common ethical dilemma about withdrawal of mechanical ventilation in Thai intensive care units. We then explore some concepts from Western bioethics to see if they help resolve this dilemma. Finally, we explain some of the local ethics behind the case and discuss the concept of a Thai bioethics to address the use of ventilators in Thailand.

A CASE SCENARIO

The following fictional case is based on 30 ethnographic interviews and two months of participant-observation fieldwork by one of us (SS) in 2005. The case contains themes that arose frequently during this research.

Gaew, a 39-year-old Thai construction worker, falls from a scaffold and hits his head on the pavement. He is unconscious by the time he arrives at one of Bangkok's cutting-edge emergency rooms. He is intubated and placed in the intensive care unit. Gaew's physician, Dr. Nok, informs Gaew's brother, Lek, that Gaew has little chance of recovery due to his lack of brain activity.

Lek does not know what to do—he wants to give his brother the best care possible, but he knows his brother is suffering. He would like to remove Gaew's ventilator. Dr. Nok replies that this is impossible because it is unethical to remove ventilators. Very few physicians in Thailand withdraw ventilators from patients [10]. They have a complex array of reasons for declining to withdraw ventilator support, including their medical training, fear of litigation, and belief in the sanctity of life.

As with most Thai physicians, Dr. Nok's refusal to withdraw the ventilator is explicitly Buddhist. The first precept of Buddhism forbids killing. Other Buddhist doctrines teach that the last part of the body to die is the breath. For a Thai Buddhist physician, pulling out a patient's ventilator may feel like pulling out the patient's soul. If Dr. Nok withdraws Gaew's ventilator, she will necessarily have "ill-will" or "repugnance" in her mind [14,15].

In Buddhist terms, Dr. Nok's own karma is at stake. Karma is a moral law, central to lay Thai Buddhism, which describes chains of cause and effect that result from individual behavior.

Actions generate either merit or demerit, and the balance of these two currencies determines one's spiritual future [10,15,16]. If Dr. Nok's mind contains ill-will or repugnance, she will accrue demerit, and this will negatively affect her in this and future lifetimes.

Neither Lek nor Dr. Nok asks what Gaew would have wanted in his current situation. They do not ponder this question because in lay Thai Buddhism, the self is seen as different from moment to moment—so Gaew is not the same person now as he was ten days ago. To Dr. Nok and Lek, an advance directive seems ludicrous. How could a person know what he would want years later, in a different state of consciousness [10]?

Dr. Nok is ready with a strategy for circumventing their dilemma. She tells Lek that together they must help Gaew "let go." She explains that it is Gaew's mental attachments that are keeping him alive and suffering on the ventilator. When Dr. Nok says "attachments," she uses the Thai word for "knot of problems" (bpom bpan ha), implying a gnarled set of worries tangling Gaew's mind and keeping him from achieving mental clarity and letting go of life. She asks Lek what Gaew might be worried about. Lek replies that Gaew wanted to be ordained as a monk before dying. Although they cannot know what is in Gaew's mind in his new state of consciousness, this is a possible element in his "knot."

Dr. Nok suggests that Lek go to Bangkok and ordain as a monk for several days in Gaew's stead, then return to tell Gaew what he has done. She explains that even though Gaew has little brain activity, when all of the senses subside, the spirit may still take in sound [15]. She hopes that when Gaew hears about his brother's ordination, he may let go and die with the ventilator still attached and running. This way, she and Lek can relieve Gaew's suffering without compromising their karma.

HOW WOULD WESTERN BIOETHICS HANDLE THIS CASE?

There has been a recent fervor of discussion in many Western medical schools about culture and bioethics [8]. Medical students and physicians are being trained in "cultural competence" to help them handle a culturally diverse society. This training usually focuses on prototypic cases meant to exemplify particular cultural or ethnic groups. In general, it is assumed that the principles of Western bioethics—autonomy, beneficence, non-maleficence, truth-telling, and justice—are universal. Different cultures are seen as emphasizing these principles differently, rather than as operating on unique principles of their own.

A classic example, taught in many United States medical schools, is the story of the "Asian" elder who comes into the hospital, and whose son says "please, do not tell my father that he has cancer." Most Western physicians would analyze this situation as follows: the son believes that knowing about the illness will hurt his father; the son values beneficence (doing what is best for the patient) over autonomy (the patient's prerogative to make decisions for himself) and thus wants to conceal the illness from his father. In this analysis, the principles of bioethics are held to be universal—the son's culture simply makes him value these principles in a unique proportion.

This approach proves unhelpful in understanding Gaew's case. Dr. Nok's refusal to remove the ventilator is not based on Gaew's wishes; it is not based on what is best for Gaew; and it is not about what is most truthful, or what is best for Thais as a whole. None of these fundamental principles of Western bioethics—autonomy, beneficence, non-maleficence, truth-telling, or justice—sufficiently explain Lek and Dr. Nok's dilemma. Even though the hospital taking care of Gaew is a center of allopathic medicine—a form of medicine grown out of the West—it is nonetheless a zone governed at least partially by non-Western bioethical principles.

A tool central to the practice of bioethics in Western hospitals is delineating between different kinds of dilemmas. The most widely read textbook of bioethics in the West, by Beauchamp and Childress, distinguishes between at least three kinds of dilemmas: (1) ethical dilemmas, where two ethical principles dictate opposite actions; (2) self-interest dilemmas, where the decision-maker's own self-interest conflicts with a decision dictated by an ethical principle; and (3) practical dilemmas, where something logistical prevents an ethical decision from being enacted [17]. Making these distinctions is often the first task that a physician must complete during an ethics consult. One must separate the entangled needs of doctors and family members from the ethical principles that determine how to treat a patient.

So what kind of dilemmas are Lek and Dr. Nok confronting? Are the principles governing their behavior ethical, practical, or self-interested? Take, for example, Dr. Nok's reason for not withdrawing the ventilator: to do so would be revoking a patient's life. At first, this sounds like an ethical principle, a kind of non-maleficence. But on closer inspection, the principle beneath her action diverges significantly from non-maleficence.

In a Buddhist framework, killing is ethically wrong because it defiles the mind of the killer. Even if Dr. Nok thinks that withdrawing the ventilator is the most compassionate thing for Gaew, it would be spiritually disadvantageous for her. As one Thai physician explained, "It may be the best thing for the patient [to withdraw the ventilator], but how could you find someone who would do it?" A Thai physician would not want to take the risk of acquiring spiritual demerit.

It would then be tempting to say that Dr. Nok's situation represents a self-interest dilemma. An ethical decision—compassionately relieving suffering by removing the ventilator—is in conflict with Dr. Nok's concern for her own spiritual fate. But this interpretation also breaks down because the precise thing that would generate demerit for Dr. Nok is ill-will toward Gaew.

In a Buddhist ethical framework, it is impossible to withdraw a ventilator with beneficent intent. In Dr. Nok's case, self-interest and ethical duty are so intertwined as to be indistinguishable. The distinction made between self-interest and ethical dilemmas collapses. The first task of a Western ethicist—to determine the type of dilemma at work—proves an impasse in Gaew's case.

The fact that a Western bioethical approach fails in Gaew's case may be a indication of the limitations of the "one-size-fits-all" bioethics used in Western hospitals as much as it is an illustration of local differences in ethical reasoning (Damien Keown, personal correspondence). Western bioethics is a young discipline, and draws on only a minority of the rich history of Western ethical philosophy [18]. Nonetheless, the conceptual tools of Western bioethics dominate policy, law, bureaucracy, and physician decision-making in Western hospitals. These concepts are beginning to have weight in policy making in Thailand [19]. Gaew's case makes it clear that one must examine local ethical concepts before uncritically importing Western bioethical tools.

DOES THAILAND NEED A THAI BIOETHICS?

Dr. Nok's solution to Gaew's end-of-life is instructive as an introduction to what a Thai bioethics might look like. Dr. Nok and Lek cannot remove Gaew's ventilator, and yet their compassion and duty demand that they relieve his suffering. They circumvent this dilemma by helping Gaew to let go of his life peacefully. This strategy has a positive effect on the karmic fate of everyone involved. They relieve Gaew's suffering. Lek acquires merit by ordaining as a monk.

These decisions are based on the logic of karmic morality. They also illustrate the Buddhist principle of interdependence. Interdependence means that doctors, patients and relatives must think about the emotions and interests of all parties involved in a medical decision. This is in contrast to the Western concept of autonomy, which allows a patient to make decisions without consideration of the feelings and responsibilities of other people concerned. Dr. Nok's solution to Gaew's end-of-life is not just for Gaew, it is also for herself and for Lek. It is an ethics of compassion that must relieve the suffering of all people concerned.

One of us (PR), as a member of a team of Thai scholars, has worked for the last ten years to develop an applied ethics using principles such as karma, compassion, and interdependence [20–23]. In the West, the main purpose of a country-wide policy is to resolve conflicts between individuals over medical decisions. However, because the concept of interdependence is so central for most Thais, Thailand's bioethical policies may differ dramatically from those found in the West.

CONCLUSION

The purpose of this exploration has been to illustrate the need for Thailand and other countries to develop bioethical systems using local concepts. It would be a mistake, however, to leave our analysis of Thai bioethics without considering the term "Thai." This has long been a problem with writings on "Asian values" or "Asian thinking."

In this article, we have emphasized Buddhism as a major ethical system, but it is one of many such systems engaged in decisions about the end-of-life in Thailand. Buddhist monasteries, lay Buddhist organizations, advocates of medical technology, public health officials, and lobbyists for the booming medical tourism industry are all engaged in vehement debate over what should guide Thailand in making medical decisions [10,11]. As with other countries, Thailand is not a place with a single ethics. In the same way that one cannot import concepts from the West to solve dilemmas in Thailand, one cannot haphazardly select a view within Thailand and label it as "Thai."

Nonetheless, there is an urgent need for solutions to the "ventilator problem"—both to patch the failing universal health-care system and to help Thais make difficult decisions about intervention at the end-of-life. Thailand is just beginning the long process of integrating its multitude of local voices and concepts into nationwide ethical standards. This new Thai ethics promises to be much more effective at solving Thailand's ethical problems than tools imported uncritically from the West.

ACKNOWLEDGMENTS

This research was made possible by the University of California Pacific Rim Research Program and the University of California San Francisco Office of International Programs. I would like to thank Warapong Wongwachara for translation, insight, and comments in all phases of fieldwork. I would like to thank Gay Becker, Vincanne Adams, China Scherz, Olivia Para, Sherry Brenner, and Damien Keown for help with this manuscript.

REFERENCES

1. Benatar SR (2005). Achieving gold standards in ethics and human rights in medical practice. PLoS Med 2: e260. DOI: 10.1371/journal.pmed.0020260
2. Kim JY (2000). Dying for growth: Global inequality and the health of the poor. Monroe (ME): Common Courage Press. p. 584.
3. Farmer P (2001). Infections and inequalities: The modern plagues. Berkeley: University of California Press. p. 419.
4. Adams V (2002). Randomized controlled crime: Post-colonial sciences in alternative medicine research. Soc Stud Sci 32: 659–90.
5. Butt L (2002). The suffering stranger: Medical anthropology and international morality. Med Anthropol 21: 1–24; discussion 25–33.
6. Cohen L (1999). Where it hurts: Indian material for an ethics of organ transplantation. Daedalus 128: 135–65.
7. Pellegrino ED, Mazzarella P, Corsi P (1992). Transcultural dimensions in medical ethics. Frederick (MD): University Publishing Group. p. 221.

8. Turner L (2005). From the local to the global: Bioethics and the concept of culture. J Med Philos 30: 305–20.
9. Alpha Research (2005). Thailand public health 2005–2006. Nonthaburi (Thailand): Alpha Research. pp. v.
10. Ratanakul P (2000). To save or let go: Thai Buddhist perspectives on euthanasia. In: Keown D, editor. Contemporary Buddhist ethics. Richmond, Surrey (United Kingdom): Curzon. pp. 169–82.
11. Jackson PA (2003). Buddhadasa: Theravada Buddhism and modernist reform in Thailand. Chiang Mai (Thailand): Silkworm Books. p. 375.
12. Kaufman SR (2005). And a time to die: How American hospitals shape the end of life. New York: Scribner. p. 400.
13. Klessig J (1992). The effect of values and culture on life-support decisions. West J Med 157: 316–22.
14. Keown D (1998). Suicide, assisted suicide and euthanasia: A Buddhist perspective. J Law Relig 13: 385–405.
15. Keown D (2005). End of life: The Buddhist view. *Lancet* 366: 952–55.
16. Keown D (1995). Buddhism and bioethics. New York: St. Martin's Press. p. 208.
17. Beauchamp TL, Childress JF (2001) Principles of biomedical ethics. New York: Oxford University Press. p. 454.
18. Jonsen AR (1998). The birth of bioethics. New York: Oxford University Press. p. 431.
19. Lindbeck V (1984). Thailand: Buddhism meets the Western model. Hastings Cent Rep 14: 24–26.
20. Ratanakul P (1988). Bioethics in Thailand: The struggle for Buddhist solutions. J Med Philos 13: 301–12.
21. Ratanakul P (1990). Thailand: Refining cultural values. Hastings Cent Rep 20: 25–27.
22. Ratanakul P (1999). Love in Buddhist Bioethics. Eubios J Asian Int Bioeth 9: 45–46.
23. Boyd A, Ratanakul P, Deepudong A (1998) Compassion as common ground. Eubios J Asian Int Bioeth 8: 34–37.

NOTE

1. © 2006 *Journal of Public Library of Science* and open access. Used with permission.

6

Confucianism and Killing versus Letting Die

Cecilia Wee

ABSTRACT

Much of the Western contemporary debate on the permissibility of active euthanasia centers on whether there is any morally significant distinction between killing and letting die. Those who would prohibit active euthanasia but permit passive euthanasia point out that the former involves a direct *act* of killing, whereas the latter involves an *omission* (i.e., omitting to do that which may prolong life). This argument turns on a commonly accepted view in the West that there is a morally significant difference between an act and an omission (even in contexts where the eventual outcomes are the same).

This paper will argue that this distinction between act and omission may not carry the same moral weight in Confucianism. I begin with an outline of Confucian role-morality. Drawing in part from classical Confucian texts, I then argue that, on such a role-based morality, the distinction between acting and omitting to act may be largely irrelevant to moral decision-making. This is then brought to bear on end-of-life decisions: I suggest that, to the Confucian, the distinction between killing and letting die may not play the same role in end-of-life decisions that it has in the West.

INTRODUCTION

Medical ethics, particularly in Western countries, has traditionally held that there is a clear distinction between passive and active euthanasia, that is, between withholding treatment from a patient so as to allow her to die and taking direct action aimed at killing the patient. While the former is held to be permissible in certain circumstances, the latter has been seen as wholly impermissible. Put another way, while it is acceptable in some cases to let a patient die, it is never acceptable to kill a patient.

The difference in the perceived ethical permissibility of active and passive euthanasia is at least partly rooted in another previously entrenched distinction, namely, the moral (and in many cases also legal) distinction between an action and an omission to act. Consider Person A who wants to see a person dead and, hence, deliberately shoots and kills that person. Person A would be deemed to have direct moral culpability for that person's death and might well be guilty of murder. In contrast, consider Person B who also wants a particular person dead and accordingly decides to stand by and not save her from being killed, although she could easily have done so without harm to herself. Person B would generally be deemed to be less morally culpable than A (if morally culpable at all) for the death. She would not be seen as having murdered the person. This suggests that there is a moral difference between acting to obtain an outcome and (knowingly) failing to act in order that the outcome obtains. This distinction underpins the permissibility of withdrawal of treatment in end-of-life situations and the nonpermissibility of an act that is designed to directly kill the patient.

In view of these debates (many of which have yet to receive final resolution), it would be helpful to put in some caveats concerning the scope and concerns of this paper. First, note that the distinction between active and passive euthanasia used here is rather broad. The actual range of options pertaining to end-of-life situations should perhaps more appropriately be classified as follows:

1. Passive euthanasia
2. Indirect euthanasia (namely, pain-relieving treatment under the nonintended risk of abbreviation of life)
3. Abetment to suicide (e.g., procurement and provision of deadly medicine)
4. Active euthanasia

For the purposes of argument, however, this paper will merely contrast active euthanasia with passive euthanasia, including (3) and (4) broadly under active euthanasia and (1) and (2) broadly under passive euthanasia. Indeed, the primary focus of the paper will be a contrast of (1) with (4).

Second, while the distinction between action and omission is widely (and most likely correctly) accepted as underpinning the distinction between active and passive euthanasia, the two distinctions may not stand in a one-to-one relation with each other. To begin with, suppose that one distinguishes passive euthanasia from active euthanasia on the basis that the former involves an omission and the latter an action. One objection is that the term "passive euthanasia" is a contradiction in terms. This is because euthanasia, by definition, causes death and omissions, by definition, cannot cause anything. Passive euthanasia would then be that which causes death but cannot cause anything.[1] The viability of this objection hinges on the question of whether omissions can have causative effect. Recent commentators have suggested that omissions in specific contexts can in fact do so.

The discussion above assumes that passive euthanasia always involves an omission to act. Another objection as to why active and passive euthanasia do not stand in a one-to-one correlation with action and omission comes by way of the point that passive euthanasia does not always involve an omission to act. For example, we usually encompass under passive euthanasia the case of "pulling the plug" on a patient's ventilator, which involves an *action* by some agent. A reply here is that pulling the plug and thus allowing the patient to die as she would have done if Nature were allowed to take its course is different from the direct killing that occurs when, say, one stabs someone to death. In the latter case, the outcome would be death regardless of whether the individual in question is healthy or ill. In the former case, the outcome is the death *specifically* of a terminally ill person. Frances Kamm (2008)[2] has likened the case of pulling the plug on a patient whose life is being prolonged solely by the ventilator to a situation where one has been saving someone from drowning and then decides to stop (perhaps by pressing a button on one's side). Both cases thus count as omissions to save (despite one's action).

Another case where passive euthanasia involves an action would be the case where such euthanasia involves extraordinary treatment (e.g., putting the patient on a ventilator) being discontinued while ordinary treatment (e.g., providing nutrition) is continued. In such a situation, passive euthanasia arguably involves not just pure omission but action (in the provision of nutrition). However, the relevant contrast in the present debate concerning end-of-life situations is that of the action of *killing* versus the omission of letting the patient die. The action of providing nutrition is aimed at the (ordinary) *sustenance* of life and, hence, is not directly germane to the specific action–omission contrast at issue here.

The distinction between active and passive euthanasia may not map directly onto the distinction between action and omission. Nevertheless, there are reasonable grounds, and some intuitive plausibility, to holding that passive euthanasia is an omission, in relevant contrast to active euthanasia, which is an action. In this paper, I shall take it that passive euthanasia is indeed an omission to act, while active euthanasia is an action.

Let me now come to the third caveat. As can be seen above, it is not always easy to distinguish clearly between actions and omissions. (Pulling the plug on the ventilator that keeps a patient alive can be both an action and an omission.) But, even if one assumes there is a distinction between an action and an omission, there remains the question as to whether there is any significant *moral* difference between action and omission.

The debate here too has been huge. For example, it has been argued that the moral distinction between an action and an omission derives from the fact that an action can cause an outcome but an omission cannot. The agent is causally responsible (and hence morally responsible) for the outcomes of his actions, but he cannot stand in a relation of causal responsibility (and hence of moral responsibility) with respect to his omissions. However, as indicated above, some commentators argue that in fact omissions can be causal as well, and we can thus be morally responsible for our omissions. Whether one accepts that there is a moral difference between an action and an omission to act may also ultimately depend on the ethical theory that one holds. The utilitarian, for instance, would hold that there is no relevant moral difference between an action and an omission to act because utilitarianism enjoins that one should always pursue (whether by action or omission to act) that which maximizes the overall balance of pleasure over pain.[3]

In this paper, I shall not engage with the recent debate and controversy on the distinction (moral, metaphysical, or both) between actions and omissions. The moral distinction between action and omission is likely a pervasive feature of the moral perspective of the average person, even if he or she is seldom clear about the actual bases for making such a distinction. That the American Medical Association has maintained that passive euthanasia is permissible but active euthanasia is not goes to show how entrenched is the assumption of the moral difference between action and omission.[4]

I shall try to show here that the pervasive Western assumption of moral difference between action and omission is much less likely to obtain in a person who comes from a role-based morality like Confucianism. As a result of this divergence, the distinction between active and passive euthanasia (plausibly taken to be underpinned by this action–omission distinction) continues to play an important role in determining end-of-life medical decisions in the West but would likely not have the same role in such decisions in societies with a strong Confucian background.

Bioethical decision-making in countries influenced by Confucianism differs markedly from that which obtains in Western countries. On this basis, some writers have advocated the development of a distinctive Confucian bioethics that draws on the fundamental metaphysical and moral beliefs of the tradition (see, e.g., Fan 1999; Lee 2007). If indeed there is no morally significant difference between active and passive euthanasia in Confucianism, this can be addressed when developing a Confucian bioethics.

This paper begins by giving a brief account of Confucian morality as a role-morality. I then discuss role-moralities in the context in which they are most frequently associated in the West, namely, the professions. In contexts where there are well-specified professional role-obligations, there is sometimes no moral distinction to be drawn between an act and an omission to act. Confucianism is then shown to be similar to the professions in having highly specific sets of role-obligations. It is then argued that the distinction between act and omission is similarly absent in such Confucian contexts. This is used to explain why end-of-life decisions in Confucian societies may differ from those in the West.

CONFUCIANISM AS A ROLE-MORALITY

The view that Confucianism is essentially a role-morality is well accepted and pervasive. (Rosemont 1986 and Nuyen 2007 provide succinct accounts of this view.) Apart from this view, various commentators have argued that there are important similarities between Confucianism and Aristotelian virtue ethics (e.g., Sim 2007), feminist care ethics (e.g., Li 2000), and Kantian deontology (e.g., Wawrytko 1982). It is not clear whether the view that Confucianism is a role-morality is ultimately incompatible with any of these other positions (e.g., Roger Ames and Henry Rosemont [2008, 2009] have argued that it is not thus compatible). This issue is evidently one that cannot be settled here. What is certainly true is that the view of Confucianism as a role-morality has considerable textual and historical support and that it is very likely an accurate representation of Confucianism *as it is actually practiced* (see Ho 1998).

According to Confucius, there is one true path ("the Way") that all humans should try to follow and attain. Following this true path has as its crucial component the cultivation and development of the appropriate inward attitudes and feelings toward others, which are then expressed in appropriate outward behaviors. However, unlike the rival Mohist school, which had advocated the development of an attitude of universal and impartial concern toward all mankind, Confucians held that the appropriate attitudes and behaviors toward others should be subject to gradations and should in general differ according to the relation in which one stands to the person in question. Confucianism is well known for emphasizing the importance, indeed the primacy, of the family. More generally, what is accorded to any given person would depend on the *role* one inhabits with respect to that person: what is appropriately accorded to one's father, elder brother, friend, political leader, etc. would thus be quite different.

There are of course certain general virtues or attributes that Confucius and his followers thought the ethical person should possess and should make an effort to cultivate. These virtues would include sincerity (*cheng*), trustworthiness (*xin*), conscientiousness (*zhong*), and especially benevolence (*jen*), held to be the key or overarching virtue, without which one cannot be an effective political leader or attain moral sagehood. But these attributes or virtues may be expressed in different behaviors and may receive somewhat different emphases, depending on the role that one occupies with respect to the person in question. There are also virtues that tend to be role specific; for instance, the virtue of filiality (*xiao*) obviously applies specifically to sons and daughters.

It has been argued that Confucian role-morality has its roots in the Confucian conception of the self, which sees the self as relational and embedded within a set of social, and more especially, familial relations.[5] This conception of the self differs from the standard Western conception of the self or person as an independent individual with autonomy, choosing freely to enter into the various associations she enters.[6] The Confucian conceives herself primarily as a part of a larger whole(s). She is a *member* of a particular family, a particular institution, a particular society, and, hence, embedded in a wider network of specific relationships. It then behooves her to cultivate the appropriate internal attitudes and outward behaviors in respect of each of these roles.

I now turn to professional ethics, which accepts that how a person should act is to some extent regulated by the specific role that she has undertaken as a professional. It will be argued that, in the context of such professional roles, the moral or ethical gap between act and omission to act is usually less than in ordinary nonprofessional contexts.

PROFESSIONAL ROLES AND THE MORAL DIFFERENCE BETWEEN ACTION AND OMISSION

Writers on professional ethics have emphasized the link between the specific role that a professional plays and what is ethically or morally expected of her in virtue of occupying that role. Being in a certain profession generates certain role-obligations, which are often embodied in a code of ethics. While such obligations may include the observance of professional etiquette, they would also, and importantly, include the moral and ethical obligations that a professional has in virtue of being a member of that profession (Beauchamp and Childress 1989, 6).

A substantial portion of the literature on professional role-morality concerns the potential conflicts that might arise between the specific moral obligations that a professional has in her professional role and the (more) universal moral norms that should be observed. We will not be concerned here with how the moral obligations of particular professions stand in relation to the wider set of moral norms, whether genuine conflicts may arise between the two, and if so, what the potential means of resolution are.[7] These issues lie beyond the scope of the paper. Instead, that these issues arise at all makes evident that the moral obligations of the professional are different from—extend beyond—the broader moral norms that people are expected to observe in the community. In this section, I highlight two ways in which the presence of such professional role-obligations can affect the moral assessment of omissions to act by the professional.

The first is that an omission or failure to observe a professional role-obligation is often taken to be a more significant moral failure than other comparable omissions to act in contexts that do not involve such role-obligations. Consider a doctor who, in the course of treating a patient for a minor problem, discovers a tumor needing urgent excision. The doctor fails to inform the patient of the tumor and the need for urgent surgery. Compare this with someone who notices that there are some loose tiles on their neighbor's roof, which should be fixed urgently, as they could be dislodged and cause serious injury. The person fails to inform the neighbor of the loose tiles.

We would tend to assign the doctor a higher degree of moral culpability for her failure to inform than we would the neighbor. This is because the doctor in her professional role has well-specified role-obligations toward her patients. The same does not apply to neighbors, where the issue of what one owes to, or ought to observe in respect of, a neighbor is much less specific. One's attitude toward a neighbor can acceptably range from the stance of "Am I my brother's keeper?" to one of some degree of concern and responsibility. This contrasts with the doctor, who, in embarking on her profession, is required to have a reasonably clear idea of what is or is not morally acceptable in a doctor–patient relationship.

The second way in which omissions to act by professionals differ from omissions in a nonprofessional context can be made clear through the following example. Suppose Doctor C conspires with a patient's relative to ensure the patient's demise so that the latter can inherit her vast wealth. To bring about this demise, she deliberately prescribes a drug that she knows full well will, given the patient's condition, result in the latter's certain death. Now, Doctor D is similarly in conspiracy with a patient's relative to ensure the patient's demise. To bring about this demise, she deliberately withholds a drug, knowing full well that, given the patient's condition, this will result in her certain death.

In the situation outlined above, *both* doctors would be seen to be morally culpable for their respective patients' deaths. Moreover, it is not intuitively evident that there is any clear difference in the *level* of moral culpability in the two doctors, although one doctor brings about the death by deliberately acting and the other by deliberately omitting to act. While physicians are bound by the obligation to not kill, but are allowed to let die in end-of-life contexts, they are also bound by the obligation to prolong the life and well-being of the patient. All other things being equal, the deliberate transgression of this obligation, whether by omission or commission, would be counted as a moral failure.

The cases of Doctors C and D thus stand in some contrast to the cases mentioned in the introduction, where the level of moral culpability between A and B is intuitively judged to be quite different. What underpins the difference in our intuitions in the two cases is again that the doctors here are acting in their professional roles and in that capacity have a particular set of obligations that A and B, judged to be acting in their personal capacity, do not.

"Ordinary" morality, underpinned by "ordinary" intuitions, generally assigns less culpability to one who fails to act to bring about an outcome than one who acts to bring it about. A direct action aimed at a negative outcome is a much more serious overall threat to the peace and security of humans in a society than an omission to act to bring about that outcome (see Nesbitt 1999).[8] However, matters are different when one is acting in a professional capacity and hence is governed by well-specified role-obligations. In such contexts, transgressions of such obligations, whether by omission or commission, are, *certeris paribus*, regarded quite equally as transgressions.

In sum, professional roles generally come with specific obligations embodied within and emphasized by a code of ethics. In such a context, an omission to act would clearly count as an ethical failure, where an omission in ordinary, nonprofessional contexts might not.

PROFESSIONAL ROLE-MORALITY AND CONFUCIAN ROLE-MORALITY

I now turn back to the role-based ethics of Confucianism, which enjoins the cultivation of the appropriate inward attitudes, which will then be expressed as appropriate outward behaviors. These appropriate attitudes and behaviors would differ according to the specific relationship that obtains between oneself and the person in question.

Suppose that Mei-ling is both a daughter and a sister. As a daughter, she would be expected to cultivate certain attitudes and behaviors in respect of this role; they would not be quite the same as the attitudes and behaviors that should be cultivated in her role as a sister. Moreover, the respective behaviors by which Mei-ling expresses her filiality and sisterhood would include not only general sorts of behaviors that manifest concern for parent and sibling. Confucianism also indicates that her appropriate inward attitudes would also be expressed by the fulfillment of some well-specified requirements, including the observance of various rituals and rites.

There are thus similarities between professional role-morality and Confucian role-morality. First, both emphasize the role that an individual inhabits in relation to an other and on the role-obligations that obtain as a result. Second, these role-obligations are well-specified in Confucianism, as in professional role-morality.

These features suggest that Confucian morality would differ significantly from "ordinary" morality in the West. Consider the question of what a son should morally owe to his father. In "ordinary" morality, there seems to be relatively wide latitude for one's answers to this question, just as there is for one's answers to what one owes to a neighbor. One son may maintain that he owes it to his father to turn up annually for Thanksgiving; another might think he is obliged to regularly visit his parent once a month; and so on.

In contrast, the role-obligations of a son are quite clearly specified in the Confucian tradition. As Ho notes, the "stringent demands" that must be fulfilled for one to be filial include "providing for the material and moral well-being of one's aged parents, performing the ceremonial duties of ancestral worship . . . ensuring the continuity of the family line, and in general conducting oneself so as to bring honor and avoid disgrace to the family name" (Ho 1998, 11). Inhabiting the role of son thus brings with it very specific role-obligations, and the tradition is quite emphatic on the need to observe these specific obligations. In these respects, Confucian morality is more akin to professional morality than "ordinary morality."

There is also a degree of latitude as to how a Confucian child should manifest filiality, just as there is a degree of latitude as to how a professional, such as a doctor, should meet her obligation to her patients. For example, a Confucian child may manifest filiality by deciding to take her parents on an overseas holiday; similarly, a doctor may decide on prescribing one specific course of treatment for a patient rather than another. Also, specific obligations that a Confucian child is expected to fulfill to her parents could change over time in accord with changes in tradition, just as a doctor's specific obligations can change over time in accord with changes in the accepted code of medical ethics. Nevertheless, both the Confucian child and the doctor are subject, at any given point in time, to very specific obligations in many areas in which "ordinary" (Western) morality does not enjoin any specific obligation.

Given these similarities, one might expect to find that there is less of a moral distinction in Confucianism between actions and omissions to act, particularly in contexts where these are transgressions of a particular role-obligation. And, indeed, there is textual evidence in classical Confucian texts that this is the case. While there are certainly examples of moral transgression that involve a specific action in Confucian texts, there are a number of texts in which an *omission to act* is treated as moral failure. In 4A:26 of the *Book of Mencius*, Mencius notes: "There are three ways of being a bad son. The most serious is to have no heir."

Here, it is the *omission* of providing an heir that is considered a transgression of one's role-obligation as a son. Again, Mencius also notes that: "No one considers the *neglect* of parents and the *denial* of relationships between prince and subject, and between superior and inferior as laudable" (*Mencius* 7A:34, emphasis mine).

Once again, moral transgression is expressed in terms of what one has omitted or failed to do. The failure to look after one's parents and to observe the role-obligations that obtain in the relations between prince and subject and superior and inferior are deplored because one has *omitted* to behave in the morally appropriate way. Confucius notes: "Faced with what is right, to leave it undone shows a lack of courage" (*Analects* 2:24). This encapsulates the general

Confucian position that an *omission* to do what is right (which of course includes what is demanded by one's various role-obligations) is morally wrong.

There are significant similarities between professional role-morality and Confucian role-morality. Both emphasize role-obligations that pertain to the particular role one inhabits, and in both cases, these role-obligations are fairly well specified. Finally, both would hold that transgression of these role-obligations constitutes a moral breach, whether the transgression is caused by a direct action or an omission to act.

In the next section, because the Confucian sees no moral distinction between a transgression of one's role-obligation by omission and one by direct action, she will not see any moral difference between letting die and killing in end-of-life situations. Letting die in this context is quite as bad as killing for the Confucian.

END-OF-LIFE ISSUES AND THE CONFUCIAN MORAL PERSON

Empirical studies have suggested that, in countries with a strong Confucian background, families are often reluctant to withdraw life support for family members in end-of-life situations. (Hui 1999). To understand why this may be so, we need to take into account not just the role-obligations of family members but the overall Confucian attitude toward the body.

The Confucian, and more generally East Asian, understanding of "body" is shaped by a different metaphysical framework than that which obtains in the West. The predominant conception of the person in the latter as an autonomous individual rests on a dichotomy between mind and body. After all, the autonomous decisions by the individual are often seen as *mental* decisions, as taking place in the individual's mind, and this is seen as (at least) conceptually distinct from what takes place in the body. This distinction does not obtain in Confucianism. There is no corresponding concept in Confucianism of what we would call the individual "mind" insofar as that is seen as the locus not only of one's autonomous choices but also as the repository of a lifetime of thoughts, feelings, experiences, and memories (Rosemont 2007).

Part of what underwrites the movement to define "death" as brain death is the assumption that, with the cessation of brain function is a cessation (or, if one believes in an afterlife, a departure from the body) of the *ego*, or "I." That is, there is an end or departure of a particular consciousness with its own specific thoughts, choices, life experiences, memories from the body, and, therefore, for all intents and purposes, an end to a *lived* life in that particular body.

But Confucians do not have an equivalent concept of mind *qua ego*, or discrete experiencing "I," conceptually distinct from body. Thus, brain death, commonly seen as concomitant with the end or departure of a consciousness in the West, may not be accorded the significance that it holds in the West. Absent the contrast of mind and body, the individual live body of someone in a vegetative state is not seen as an empty husk; it remains significant despite this cessation of brain function. Confucianism also enjoins in general a reverent attitude toward the body: "Being reverent about the body (*shen*) is of the greatest importance. The body is a branch of one's parents, so how could one be irreverent in this regard?"[9]

The Confucian body is seen as a branch whose foundational trunk are the parents. The reverence for one's body is seen implicitly as a form of family reverence. Failure to take care of one's body is a dishonoring of one's parents. Failure to take care of one's parents' bodies might well be seen as a dishonoring of one's ancestors or family line. Given this Confucian attitude toward the body, we can now come back to the role-obligations of the Confucian family member.

Confucianism emphasizes the primacy of family: patient autonomy does not receive the same emphasis that it does in the West (Fan and Tao 2004). Many significant medical decisions, including end-of-life decisions, are made by family members rather than the patients (Fielding and Hung 1996; Li and Chou 1997). Patient confidentiality also takes a back seat. Bad medical news is usually conveyed by the doctor, first, to family members, who then decide whether the patient should be told of her condition. In the context of such medical decisions, a family member is expected to honor her role-obligations to the patient. Thus, if one is making a decision for a parent, the attitude that one should bear when deciding is that of filiality, or *xiao*.

One significant role-obligation of a Confucian child (especially a son) is to ensure his parents' well-being and to take care of them in their old age. This is often held to include keeping one's parents alive for as long as possible. For example, *The Twenty-Four Paragons of Filial Piety*, written by the Yuan dynasty scholar Guo Jujing, abounds with stories of paragons who went to extreme lengths to prolong their parents' or in-laws' lives.[10] To keep one's parents, and, more specifically, parents' bodies, alive on life support is an expression of filiality (Hui 1999; Tse and Tao 2004).

For the Confucian (as for the professional), an omission to meet one's role obligation is a significant moral transgression. Given that the Confucian's primary obligation is to her parent or other family member, *not* keeping the latter alive is a serious moral transgression, even if the family member is brain dead or in a persistent vegetative state. This is because there is, first, no clear conception here that the family member's life is over because her lived, experienced life is over, and, second, because of the general Confucian reverence for body. Withdrawal of a ventilator or life-support system—the letting die of one's family member—would be seen as a failure or omission to keep that member alive. This would be a transgression of one's role-obligation and might indeed be almost as bad as if one were directly to kill a family member in similar circumstances.

Where the West has had a tendency to assume that there is a morally significant difference between killing and letting die, the tendency in Confucianism is to see no difference in the two in such contexts. Moreover, in the West is the line of argument that, if it is morally permissible to let die in appropriate contexts, it should also be morally permissible to kill in those contexts. In Confucianism, the assimilation apparently goes in the other direction. The Confucian assimilates letting die to killing, maintaining that, inasmuch as it is morally impermissible to kill one's parents, it is also impermissible (given one's role-obligations) to let them die.

In November 2008, a Seoul Western District Court ordered doctors to remove life support from a woman who was "in a persistent vegetative state." This made international news because, prior to this, South Korean courts, and indeed, the general populace, had generally been against the withdrawal of life support for such patients. This in turn has been widely attributed to the Confucian background of South Koreans. This was thought to be similar to a 1997 case in which a father had requested the removal of a ventilator, an extraordinary means of life support, from his son who was similarly in a vegetative state. The doctors who acceded to his request and took the patient off life support were subsequently convicted of "abetment to murder."

The withdrawal of life support, and the consequent *letting die*, of the patient, was deemed to be a (direct) act of *murder*, and the doctors were guilty of abetting the father in murder. While none of the parties involved were jailed, the very conviction of "abetment to murder" does at least suggest the lack of a clear-cut distinction between omission to keep alive and direct action to kill in respect of this particular end-of-life decision. Confucianism, as I showed, is a role-morality with well-specified moral obligations in respect of end-of-life situations. In such contexts, an omission to preserve life could be seen as impermissible as, and not entirely distinguishable from, a direct killing.[11]

REFERENCES

Ames, R., and H. Rosemont. (2008). "Family Reverence (*xiao*) as the Source of Consummatory Conduct (*jen*)." *Dao* 7, 9–19.

Ames, R., and H. Rosemont, trans. (2009). *Xiaojing: The Chinese Classic of Family Reverence.* Hawai'i: University of Hawai'i. (See esp. 34–59.)

Andre, J. (1991). "Role Morality as a Complex Instance of Ordinary Morality." *American Philosophical Quarterly* 28, no. 1: 73–80.

Beauchamp, T. L., and J. F. Childress. (1996). "Rachels on Active and Passive Euthanasia." In *Ethical Issues in Death and Dying.* 2nd ed. Edited by T. L. Beauchamp and R. M. Veatch. Upper Saddle River, NJ: Prentice Hall.

———. (2001). *Principles of Biomedical Ethics.* New York: Oxford University Press.

Bowie, N. E. (1982). "Role as a Moral Concept in Health Care." *Journal of Medicine and Philosophy* 7: 57–63.

Confucius. (1979). *The Analects.* Edited by D. C. Lau. Harmondsworth: Penguin.

Fan, R., ed. (1999). *Confucian Bioethics.* Dordrecht: Kluwer.

Fan, R., and J. Tao. (2004). "Consent to Medical Treatment: The Complex Interplay of Patients, Families and Physicians." *Journal of Medicine and Philosophy* 29: 139–48.

Fielding, R., and J. Hung. (1996). "Preferences for Information and Involvement in Decisions during Cancer Care among a Hong Kong Chinese Population." *Psycho-Oncology* 5: 231–329.

Foot, P. (2002). "Killing and Letting Die." In *Moral Dilemmas.* Oxford: Clarendon Press.

Garrard, E., and G. Wilkinson. (2005). "Passive Euthanasia." *Journal of Medical Ethics* 31: 64–68.

Gibson, Kevin. (2003). "Contrasting Role Morality and Professional Morality: Implications for Practice." *Journal of Applied Philosophy* 20, no. 1: 17–29.

Ho, D. Y. F. (1998). "Interpersonal Relationships and Relations Dominance: An Analysis Based on Methodological Relationalism. *Asian Journal of Social Psychology* 1, no. 1–16.

Hui, E. (1999). "A Confucian Ethic of Medical Futility." In *Confucian Bioethics,* edited by R. Fan. Dordrecht: Kluwer.

Kamm, F. (2008). "Physician Assisted Suicide, Euthanasia and Intending Death." In *Physician Assisted Suicide: Expanding the Debate.* Edited by M. Battin, R. Rhodes, and A. Silver. New York: Routledge.

Kuhse, H. (1999). Why Killing Is Not Always Worse—and Sometimes Better—Than Letting Die. In H. Kuhse and P. Singer (ed.), *Bioethics: An Anthology* (227–30.) Oxford: Blackwell.

Lee, S. C. (2007). *The Family, Medical Decision-Making and Biotechnology: Critical Reflections on Asian Moral Perspectives.* Dordrecht: Kluwer.

Legge, J. (1894). *The Chinese Classics.* University of Hong Kong reprint of Shanghai edition.

Li, C. (2000). *The Sage and the Second Sex: Confucianism, Ethics and Gender.* Chicago: Open Court.

Li, S., and J. L. Chou. (1997). "Communication with the Cancer Patient in China." *Annals of New York Academy of Sciences* 809: 243–48.

Mackenzie, C., and N. Stoljar, eds. (2000). *Relational Autonomy: Feminist Perspectives on Autonomy, Agency and the Social Self.* New York: Oxford University Press.

McLachlan, H. V. (2008). "The Ethics of Killing and Letting Die: Active and Passive Euthanasia." *Journal of Medical Ethics* 34: 636–38.

McMahan, J. (2002). *The Ethics of Killing.* New York: Oxford University Press.

Mencius. (1970). *Mencius.* Translated by D. C. Lau. Harmondsworth: Penguin.

Nesbitt, W. (1999). "Is Killing No Worse than Letting Die?" In *Bioethics: An Anthology*. Edited by
H. Kuhse and P. Singer, 231–25. Oxford: Blackwell.

Nuyen, A. T. (2007). "Confucian Ethics as Role-Based Ethics." *International Philosophical Quarterly* 47,
no. 3: 315–28.

Rachels, J. (1999). "Active and Passive Euthanasia." *Bioethics: An Anthology*, H. Kuhse and P. Singer,
227–30. Oxford: Blackwell.

Rosemont, H. (1986). "Kierkegaard and Confucius: On Finding the Way." *Philosophy East and West* 36,
no. 3: 201–12.

———. (2007). "On the Non-Finality of Physical Death in Classical Confucianism." *Acta Orientalia
Vilnensis* 8: 2.

Sim, M. (2007). *Remastering Morals with Aristotle and Confucius*. Cambridge: Cambridge University
Press.

Singer, P. (1979). *Practical Ethics*. Cambridge University Press.

Tse, C., and J. Tao. (2004). "Strategic Ambiguities in the Process of Consent: Role of the Family in
Decisions to Forgo Life-Sustaining Treatment for Incompetent Elderly Patients." *Journal of Medicine
and Philosophy* 29: 207–23.

Veatch, H. (1972). "Models for Ethical Medicine in a Revolutionary Age." *Hastings Center Report* 2: 5–7.

Wawrytko, S. (1982). "Confucius and Kant: The Ethics of Respect." *Philosophy East and West* 32, no.
3: 237–57.

NOTES

1. See, for example, Garrard and Wilkinson (2005) for a discussion of this particular claim.
McLachlan (2008) provides a response.

2. See also McMahan (2002). McMahan provides some fine-grained distinctions with respect to the
question of whether withdrawal of ventilator support counts as a killing or a letting die.

3. See, e.g., Singer 1979, 147–53. It is also likely that adherents of other moral theories, such as
Kantians and virtue ethicists, would accept that (at least under specific conditions) there may be no
relevant moral difference between an action and an omission. I thank an editor for this point.

4. Helpful further readings on the issues I have discussed above can be found in Beauchamp and
Childress 1996, Foot 2002, Rachels 1999, and Singer 1979.

5. Confucian scholars argue that the Confucian self is *metaphysically constituted* by the roles that she
inhabits with respect to the various others in her life (see, e.g., Rosemont 2007).

6. This conception of the self is also being reevaluated in the West (see Mackenzie and Stoljar 2000).

7. See, e.g., Andre 1991, Bowie 1982, Gibson 2003, and Veatch 1972.

8. Nesbitt's point here occurs in a response to Rachels (1999). Rachels's seminal paper uses a specific
example (usually called the example of the "nasty cousins") to argue that, under appropriately specific
conditions, there is no moral difference between killing and letting die. Nesbitt responds by revisiting
the example and arguing that the example does not show that there is no moral difference between killing and letting die. A response to Nesbitt is to be found in Kuhse (1999). Kuhse argues that Nesbitt's
conclusions from the example are not germane to the case of active versus passive euthanasia, and she
provides other examples that she thinks are more closely analogous to the latter.

9. See Legge (1894, 288).

10. These include the Emperor of Han, who unfailingly tasted the daily prescriptions for his sick
mother himself, and Lady Tang, who saved her ailing mother-in-law from death by daily expressing her
own milk for the latter.

11. I would like to thank C. L. Ten, Henry Rosemont Jr., and the editors of this volume for their very
helpful comments on earlier drafts of this paper.

7

Global versus Local

The Use of Lethal Injection in China

Cher Weixia Chen

ABSTRACT

Lethal injection has not yet been commonly discussed in China. This chapter seeks to expand the existing literature by focusing on one of the most recent development of the death penalty in China—lethal injection. Lethal injection is something scholars have for the most part failed to examine. In this paper I will look at its use from the perspectives of human rights and bioethics, both of which lethal injection by nature is intimately intertwined with. Two concerns will be given particular consideration: the participation of medical personnel in lethal injections and in the harvesting of organs from executed prisoners. I will also offer some recommendations as to the need for guidelines.

INTRODUCTION

In the past two decades, China has accounted for a large portion of executions throughout the world. For example, in 2008, China carried out 1,718 out of 2,390 executions (72 percent) worldwide (Amnesty International 2008). China's death penalty system has always been seen as a violation of human rights. Its socialist government is said to utilize capital punishment to maintain its social order, to oppress its political opposition, and to curb the rising crime rate (Lim 2013).

There is truth to these reports. However, Western media reports and academic research on the death penalty in China tend to be one dimensional and oversimplified. They typically lack sufficient detail and overlook the complex nature of the issue. In addition, Western legal academics pay little attention to the most recent developments in China's practice of capital punishment.

Lethal injection has not yet been examined in China to the extent it has in the West. It merits a much more thorough analysis than it has received. In this chapter I seek to expand the existing literature by focusing on one of the most recent developments of the death penalty in China's use of lethal injection. In particular, I will discuss its use from the perspectives of human rights and bioethics.

LETHAL INJECTIONS AND HUMAN RIGHTS

In the twentieth century, lethal injection was included in the international human rights movement against methods of executions. This movement has been a restraining influence on China, a country that has been frequently cited as a violator of human rights because of its extensive use of the death penalty. It is the concern for a better global image that propelled China to research lethal injections as a preferable method of executions and led China to adopt lethal injection in 1997 (Li 2008).

The use of lethal injections in China shares many elements with other countries while having some distinctive local peculiarities. Given that the United States regularly uses lethal injection to execute convicts, its use will be addressed as a point of reference.

China previously used shooting as the sole legal method of execution, but added lethal injection in 1997. A key contrast to shooting or other methods of execution is that lethal injection simulates a *medical procedure*. This has fundamentally transformed the practice. From the violent nature of conventional executions such as shooting, China introduced a method that potentially utilizes medical personnel on a regular basis. To undergo lethal injection, the inmate is typically put in an environment like an "operating" room. Medical or designated personnel are present to place a needle in the arm of the prisoner to induce sleep. The next step in the process is a drug-induced cardiac arrest, followed by the inmate's death (Maggio 2005, 48).

On the basis of research China developed its own combination of drugs that would be used in lethal injections (Li 2008). The drug combination used in China is similar to that in the United States. It is composed of three ingredients: one is to cause loss of consciousness (pentothal), one is to paralyze the heart and suspend pulmonary activities (Pavulon), and the third (potassium chloride) is to induce cardiac arrest (Yang 2008).

I should note, however, that there are differences between China and the United States with regard to the use of lethal injection. One major distinction is that lethal injection in China takes place in an "execution van" or "mobile execution chamber." In 1997 these execution vans were developed and utilized for the first time in Yunnan. They are windowless units. Amnesty International (2004) gives this report:

> The windowless execution chamber at the back contains a metal bed on which the prisoner is strapped down. Once a technician attaches the needle, a police officer presses a button and an automatic syringe injects the lethal drug into the prisoner's vein. The execution can be watched on a video monitor next to the driver's seat and can be recorded if required.

The Human Rights Committee has urged that "The death penalty . . . must be carried out in such a way as to cause the least possible physical and mental suffering" (ICCPR 1992, 6). It has been argued that lethal injection inflicts less physical and mental pain than its alternatives (Lifton and Mitchell 2000). In this sense, China's use of lethal injection is in conformity with the international human rights standards. But the implementation of such international human rights standards concerning the method of execution is rather localized.

To some degree, the notion of an execution van is used by China to balance its international obligations and local realities. On the one hand, China sought to humanize its method of execution. Because of the influence of the global human rights movement, it adopted the method of lethal injection. On the other hand, the cost of building execution grounds for lethal injection could put a financial strain on the local courts. Thus, execution vans were developed in part to relieve the local courts of such financial burdens (Yang, 2008).

Though there is a concern among human rights activists that execution vans and their secrecy may cause the process to be less transparent, they are preferred over conventional execution grounds for at least three reasons. First, execution vans elicit much less resistance from the public than execution grounds. This is because most people do not want to be living close to an execution ground. It is deemed inauspicious in Chinese culture (Xu and Tang 2003, 33). Secondly, execution vans are windowless and, thus, do not involve a public spectacle. The vans prevent the widely condemned public executions rampant in the 1980s and 1990s (Amnesty International 2004).

Finally, execution vans are more cost effective. They require less manpower and allow local courts to share and save on the cost. In light of the fact that execution grounds are expensive to be built, the lower-priced execution vans find favor in financially stricken local courts ("Execution Van," 2009). Even so, execution vans pose a fiscal burden on local communities. As a result, some experts have called for a special fund to assist local courts in building execution vans (Yang 2008). For these reasons, execution vans are more suitable than the conventional execution grounds for the local settings in China and have, therefore, been encouraged.

Historically speaking, embracing the global human rights movement and adopting lethal injection signify a philosophical shift of the domestic criminal justice system in China. It is fair to say that the imperial law in China was primarily a prescription of punishments. For example, under the Code of Qing, there were 3,987 punishable offenses (Da Qing Hui Dian). By performing physical torture and mutilation, and very often in public, the state ensured that law was literally implicated into the body politic. When convicts were decapitated, mutilated, or disemboweled, pain was inflicted and it was thought that justice was served. Lethal injection, in contrast, is viewed as painless (Pan and Wang 2008). It is intended to be more humane and to minimize the suffering of both inmates and executioners (Zheng 2008). Not only have the policy makers valued the painless lethal injection, but the public also agreed that humane methods of execution are preferable. For this reason it was concluded that lethal injection should replace the traditional execution methods (Yuan 2009). From this standpoint, using less painful lethal injection is a historical landmark in the evolution of the Chinese criminal justice system.

China is seeking to expand the use of lethal injection on a nationwide basis. In 2008 there were about half of the 404 intermediate courts using lethal injection. One major obstacle to the expansive use of lethal injection is cost considerations. Consequently, in order to lower the cost and to expedite the reform, the Supreme People's Court took a bold step: it decided to provide the lethal cocktail utilized in the injection to the local courts for free (Bezlova 2008). The next step for China's death penalty is to legalize lethal injection as the sole lawful method of execution. There are various reasons to recommend this reform. First, it results in less suffering. Compared to shooting and other methods of execution, lethal injection inflicts much less pain on convicts (LeGraw and Grodin 2002, 387). It is the method of execution least likely to constitute "cruel and unusual punishment."

Secondly, there are human rights' concerns. Lethal injection conforms to international human rights standards. As far as prisoners' rights, it is in accordance with inmate preferences. According to a Supreme Court poll, death row inmates overwhelmingly prefer lethal injection (Yang 2008). In this sense, to use lethal injection, a more humane method of execution favored by prisoners, is to respect prisoners' rights.

Thirdly, the invention of execution vans has effectively addressed local concerns throughout China. That is to say, they have provided a unique approach for China to implement global human rights standards within its own social context. For this reason, China should discontinue the use of shooting and establish lethal injection as the sole method of execution.

Lastly, by making lethal injections the only form of capital punishment, discrimination and corruption among officials will be reduced. Public opinion polls indicate a concern about the fair use of lethal injections. Several media reports indicate that lethal injection has become the "privilege" of wealthy convicts, while others receive shooting instead (Bezlova 2008). Some experts argue that this phenomenon is not because of corruption but an "economic" reason instead. Since the use of lethal injection proves to be too costly for many less developed areas, it is plausible that corrupt officials allow lethal injection more often for wealthy criminals than those who are more disadvantaged.

Nonetheless, a consistent and detailed implementation guideline that explicitly prescribes who receives lethal injection and how it should be carried out is imperative (Yang 2008; Bezlova 2008). This is not simply a matter of honoring the last wish of the convicts, but an issue of fairness and integrity of the criminal justice system as a whole.

LETHAL INJECTIONS AND BIOETHICS

In general, the use of lethal injection is a positive step forward in China's reform of its death penalty system. Its "humane" feature identifies with the spirit of the international human rights standards. Nevertheless, the "medical" nature of lethal injection demands that any discussion of its use should involve bioethics.

In China the implementation of lethal injection has raised several bioethical concerns with some distinctive local features. Currently, there are two key bioethical issues that need to be attended to. These are the role of the medical profession and the harvesting of organs from executed prisoners. Let us look at both of these concerns.

The Role of Medical Professionals: One source of the controversy surrounding lethal injection is the involvement of medical professionals. Before 1997, China used shooting as the sole legal method of execution. No other medical personnel other than forensic officers took part in the process. But to carry out lethal injection, medical knowledge is essential. As a result, medical professionals or personnel with medical training have to take part in the implementation of lethal injection. Whether such involvement violates medical ethics is subject to debate (Amnesty International 1994, 8).

In the United States, the medical profession has expressed mixed views on participating in the process of lethal injection (Maggio 2005, 48). One argument is that it violates the Hippocratic Oath of "first do no harm." However, there is no agreement yet as to what exactly constitutes "participation" in an execution, even though physicians, nurses, and other medically trained personnel "play a vital role" in lethal injection at least in the United States (LeGraw and Grodin 2002, 384). Participation of medical professionals in lethal injection is considered to be morally impermissible by some scholars. They are accused of using their medical knowledge to assist in state-sanctioned killing—"judicial homicide." Furthermore, it is argued that they facilitate the process and glorify the death penalty by taking part. One concern is that this then shields capital punishment from legal challenge (LeGraw and Grodin 2002, 386).

Some scholars in China have argued that "do no harm" is a relative concept. It does not necessarily entail humanitarianism. Under certain circumstances, only relative humanitarianism can be achieved (Zhou 1997, 26). Generally speaking, the role of medical professionals in the process of lethal injection has yet to become as much a source of debate in China as in the United States. One way to solve the ethical dilemma for the medical profession is to abolish the death penalty so that lethal injection will not be needed. After all, the death penalty itself has long been challenged as a violation of human rights (Méndez 2012).

There has been a worldwide movement toward the end of capital punishment (Schabas 2002). Such international trends have pressured the Chinese government to compromise (Cohen 1987, 532). While acknowledging the international trend toward the abolition of the death penalty, it is crucial to be aware of the important role that local culture can play.

Overall, the death penalty law in China is headed in the right direction, namely, toward conforming to international human rights law. With ongoing reform, China will abolish the death penalty altogether ("China Questions Death Penalty," 2005). Until then, it appears that "killing fewer and killing carefully" will be the new policy. If so, this will be a step closer to the ultimate abolition of capital punishment and is more applicable to the social reality of China (Stetler 2008, 27).

It helps to look at the issue in a historical context. The use of capital punishment constitutes "cruel and unusual punishment" is a fairly new and modern concept. There had been general acceptance of the necessity of harsh punishments for thousands of years in China (Moore 2001, 731; Zhang 2008, 166). Drastic change might be counterproductive. Nonetheless, among Chinese policy makers and academics is an increasing willingness to reconsider the use of the death penalty. There is also an increasing eagerness to reform their death penalty system.

We can see a dramatic rhetoric change in examining the discussion on the death penalty among the Chinese policy makers since the economic reform took place in 1978. This change indicates less and less stress on the local context over time. In 1987, Gao Mingxuan, a prominent legal scholar and official claimed that the death penalty was indispensable in China "to protect the fundamental interests of the state and people, to safeguard our socialist construction and to secure and promote the development of productive forces" (Fitzpatrick and Miller 1993, 278; Wyman 1997, 561).

In 1993, a top Chinese official asserted at the World Conference on Human Rights that "countries at different development stages or with different historical traditions and cultural backgrounds . . . have different understanding and practice of human rights" (Schabas 2002; Wyman 1997, 561). But in 2008, Xiao Yang, the former chief justice of the Supreme People's Court, reported to the National People's Congress. He stated that executions in China were now limited to an "extremely small number of extremely serious and extremely vile criminals posing a grievous threat to society" (Bodeen 2008). Evidently there is a growing interest in the issue of the death penalty among Chinese authorities. They are more receptive to the global trend of an abolitionist movement and have adjusted their local policies accordingly. It seems that the death penalty in China will continue to be reformed and seems likely that it will be abolished in the future.

The debates on the death penalty among Chinese legal scholars have shifted the focus from the justification of its use to how to eventually abolish it (Sun 2009, 106). With the global abolitionist movement in mind, fewer Chinese legal scholars believe in the permanent necessity of capital punishment in China. More and more agree that it is just a matter of when and how to abolish it. They have proposed a strategy for the gradual abolition of the death penalty in an attempt to maintain a balance between the international trend and the local reality (Wei 2008, 57).

To a large extent, a gradual abolition is a workable and realistic proposal. It could be dangerous to become abolitionist overnight, especially if that country is known for its overuse of the death penalty (Sharoni 2001, 284). "Killing fewer and killing carefully," as a transitional policy toward the ultimate abolition of capital punishment in China, should be allowed. Until China abolishes the death penalty, lethal injection is a relatively humane method of execution to use. Thus, as long as lethal injection is used in capital punishment, the ethical dilemma for the medical profession remains.

China has found an uncommon way to moderately solve this ethical dilemma by sheltering the entire medical profession, including physicians and nurses, from the process. In China local prison officers are trained to carry out lethal injection, and forensic officers are present only to pronounce the death of prisoners (Zhuang 2005, 24). Essentially, this practice minimizes the involvement of medical personnel and to a certain extent frees them from the ethical predicament. Undoubtedly, it will require strict protocols to avoid any botched executions. But at least the medical profession can somewhat be exempted from the ethical dilemma that their American colleagues face with lethal injections. However, even though according to the current practice in China the medical profession does not have to participate directly in the process of actual lethal injection, other issues arise. They still have to be involved in the process, such as training prison officers and developing a safe formula for drugs to be used in lethal injection. The latter two activities may or may not constitute "participation in execution."

According to the the AMA (American Medical Association) definition, to train prison officers to carry out lethal injection is "an action which would assist, supervise, or contribute to the ability of another individual to directly cause the death of the condemned." To develop a safe drug formula to be used in lethal injection could also constitute "participation in execution" (AMA Code of Medical Ethics, Opinion 2. 06). In this sense, the current practice in China has not completely excused the medical profession from the ethical dilemma.

In addition to the ethical predicament of the medical profession, harvesting organs of death row inmates is another major bioethical issue associated with lethal injection. Both shooting and lethal injection offer the opportunity to harvest organs of prisoners, as these two methods of execution allow most organs to remain intact.

There has been an outcry that China practices harvesting prisoners' organs without their consent (Brown 1996, 1073–74). Human rights activists worried that the use of lethal injection and execution vans makes the body undamaged and therefore might promote the actual organ harvesting of prisoners in China (Bezlova 2008).

The issue of harvesting organs of prisoners is multifaceted. First, death row inmates should be allowed the opportunity to *donate* their organs. When an organ is transplanted, the donor may perceive that his/her life has been continued in the recipient (Shen 1997, 102). This act of altruism is the ethical foundation for organ transplants (Guan and Li 2001, 8). As members of the society, death row inmates should be granted organ donation if they explicitly express that wish. Conversely, death row inmates should have the right to refuse to donate their organs. Because the practice of harvesting prisoners' organs without their consent has occurred in China, this side of arguments should be emphasized to prevent any injustice.

Second, if prisoners do not give consent, harvesting their organs is morally wrong and should be illegal. The percentage of the Chinese favoring organ transplants is around 70 percent, but the donation rate is much lower (Wang, Su, and Liu 2002, 21). Such discrepancy reflects the impact of the traditional culture. According to Confucianism, our bodies are received from our parents, and donation is the most unfilial act. Many people still think that to keep a dead body intact is a respectful act and hope they can have an unbroken body after death (Xie, Huang, and Liu 2000, 39). This is to say that a significant number of Chinese people culturally oppose the idea of donating their organs. Thus, to lure or force death row inmates to donate their organs or to harvest their organs without their consent is considered repugnant (Caplan 2011).

Third, harvesting organs requires medical knowledge. One way to thwart illegal harvesting is to have a strict ethical code prohibiting medical professionals from engaging in any illegal harvesting of organs of executed prisoners (Brown 1996, 1073–74). In response to such concern, the Ministry of Health in China issued a ban on the sale of organs ("Execution Van" 2009). In addition, the People's Supreme Court issued an order stipulating that only with the consent of death row inmates or their families can their organs be harvested (Liu 2006). The effect of these orders remains to be seen.

In order to address those two bioethical dilemmas—medical personnel participating in lethal injections and harvesting executed prisoners' organs—a detailed implementation guideline on lethal injection is imperative. This guideline ought to be based on widely accepted principles of bioethics, such as those proposed by Beauchamp and Childress (2008). Their transformative four principles are those of autonomy, nonmaleficence, beneficence, and justice. All are strongly relevant to the issues described above. For example, their theory of "autonomy" could be useful to look at the meaning of consent with respect to condemned prisoners donating their organs in China. How to apply these principles to the specific policies is challenging, but seems very fruitful.

China has incorporated international standards into its major national bioethics regulations that explicitly refer to the international bioethics documents, such as the Declaration of Helsinki (WMA 2004). Nevertheless the principal concern is that these regulations lack specifics, a problem that the new guideline on lethal injection should overcome (Hennig 2006). A guideline with specifics will also help prevent the occurrence of botched lethal injections, as happened in the United States. In particular, the administering of the drugs in the United States has been found problematic. The botched executions of Raymond Landry, Stephen McCoy, and Billy Wayne White raised the question on how to improve the safety of administering lethal injection and to minimize the pain inflicted on prisoners (Maggio 2005).

So far in China no such cases have been reported. Nevertheless, China could learn from what has occurred in the United States. The People's Supreme Court of China issued the Notice on Using Lethal Injection in Executions in 2001 to standardize the procedures (Liu 2006). But the notice itself lacks details and lags behind in addressing some critical issues, such as the role of the medical profession and organ transplants.

It is worth mentioning that the psychological impact on executioners has been duly noticed in China. In Chinese culture, it is normally considered inauspicious to administer an execution. Because of such a heavy psychological burden, some prison officers were reluctant to carry out lethal injections (He and Li 2008, 77). How to seek professional psychologists' aid for those involved in lethal injections should also be included in the guidelines (Yang 2008). If lethal injection is to be effectively applied in China, there needs to be the satisfactory implementation of global human rights and bioethical norms, as well as cultural considerations noted above.

CONCLUSION

To sum up, the use of lethal injections represents a progressive development of the death penalty in China. It is an attempt to balance China's international obligations with its own social and cultural realities. The practice of lethal injections in China indicates that, when abstract international human rights and bioethical norms are implemented in local contexts, there exists a degree of variation. Such variation is inevitable and ought to be tolerated. The use of execution vans is a case in point. As the Universal Declaration on Bioethics and Human Rights justly puts it, "the importance of cultural diversity and pluralism should be given due regard" (UNESCO 2005, art. 12).

Lethal injection requires a continuous reform to ensure its safe and fair use. Such reform should consider local details while incorporating the global standards. Practical application of global norms necessitates deep knowledge of local conditions. Neglecting local conditions and cultural factors influencing values and perceptions could be disastrous.

Two major related bioethics challenges—the role of the medical profession and organ harvesting of condemned prisoners—call for legislative and judiciary action. A detailed implementation guideline of lethal injection based on the local specifics should be developed to adequately address these challenges. It is not easy to find a balance between global norms and local reality, especially when the global norms are new to the local culture. But it is not impossible.

REFERENCES

American Medical Association. Code of Medical Ethics, Opinion 2. 06. Retrieved from http://www.ama-assn.org/ama/pub/physician-resources/medical-ethics/code-medical-ethics/opinion206.shtml.

Amnesty International. (2004). Undermining Global Security: The European Union's Arms Exports. Retrieved from http://www.amnesty.org/en/library/info/ACT30/003/2004.

Amnesty International. (2008). Death Sentences and Execution. Retrieved from http://www.amnesty.org/en/death-penalty.

Beauchamp, T., and Childress, James F. (2008). *Principles of Biomedical Ethics* (6th edition). Oxford University Press, USA.

Bezlova, A. (2008, June 16). China: Will The People Choose the Death Penalty? Retrieved from http://ipsnews.net/news.asp?idnews=42810.

Bodeen, C. (2008, March 1). China Hails Reform of Death Penalty. Retrieved from http://www.usatoday.com/news/world/2008-03-10-975780323_x.htm.

Brown, K. M. (1996). Execution for Profit? A Constitutional Analysis of China's Practice of Harvesting Executed Prisoners' Organs. *Seton Hall Constitutional Law Journal*. 6. 1029–82.

Caplan, A. (2011). The Use of Prisoners as Sources of Organs—An Ethically Dubious Practice. *American Journal of Bioethics*. 11:10. 1–5.

China Questions Death Penalty. (2005). Retrieved from http://www.chinadaily.com.cn/english/doc/2005-01/27/content_412758.htm.

Cohen, Roberta. (1987). People's Republic of China: The Human Rights Exception. *Human Rights Quarterly* 9.

Da Qing Hui Dian (Collected Institutes of the Great Qing Dynasty), 54:1a-b.

Execution Van. (2009). Retrieved from http://en.wikipedia.org/wiki/Execution_van.

Fitzpatrick, J., and Miller, A. (1993). International Standards on the Death Penalty: Shifting Discourse. *Brooklyn Journal of International Law*. 19. 273–366.

Guan, Wenxian, and Li Kaizong. (2001). Kaizhan huoti qiguan yizhi de lunli xue sikao. Yixue yu Zhexue (*Medicine and Philosophy*), 22-6, p. 8.

He, Chengbing, and Li, Jiaxian. (2008). Kaowen zhushe sixing de sanda nanyan zhiyin. Fazhi Yanjiu (*Legal Research*). 10, 75–79.

Hennig, Wolfgang. (2006). Bioethics in China. Retrieved from http://www.nature.com/embor/journal/v7/n9/full/7400794.html

ICCPR. (1992). General Comment 20, U.N. HRC, 44th Session, U.N. Doc ccpr/c/21/Add.3.

LeGraw, J. M., and Grodin, M. A. (2002). Health Professionals and Lethal Injection Execution in the United States. *Human Rights Quarterly.* 24:2. 382–423.

Li, Jingrui. (2008). Zhushe sixing. Retrieved from http://www.thebeijingnews.com/news/reform 30/2008/11-03/011@100438.htm.

Lifton, Robert, and Mitchel, Greg. (2000). *Who Owns Death? Capital Punishment, the American Conscience, and the End of the Death Penalty.* William Morrow.

Lim, Zi Heng (May 9, 2013). Why China Executes So Many People. *The Atlantic.*

Liu, Xiaoxiao. (2006). Zhejiang jiuyue yiri qi zhushe daiti qiangjue zhixing sixing. *Legal Daily.*

Maggio, E. J. Esq. (2005). A Violent Roman Tradition. *Digest.* 13:35. 35-49.

Méndez, Juan E. (2012). The Death Penalty and the Absolute Prohibition of Torture and Cruel, Inhuman, and Degrading Treatment or Punishment. Human Rights Brief. 20:1. 2–6.

Moore, B. Jr. (2001). Cruel and Unusual Punishment in the Roman Empire and Dynastic China. *International Journal of Politics, Culture, and Society.* 14:4. 729–72.

Pan, X., and Wang, X. (2008, April 10). Zuihou yiqiang-zhongguo jiasu puji zhushe sixing. Nanfang Zhoumo (*Southern Weekend*). A03.

Schabas, W. A. (2002). *The Abolition of the Death Penalty in International Law* (3rd ed.). Cambridge: Cambridge University Press.

Sharoni, Michelle M. (2001). A Journey of Two Countries: A Comparative Study of the Death Penalty in Israel and South Africa. *Hastings International Comparative Law Review* 24.

Shen, Mingxian. (1997). Shengsi JuShan, Rendao Biyi. Shanghai Shehui Kexue Yuan Xueshu Jikan (*Academic Seasonal Journal of Shanghai Academy of Social Science*), 2.

Stetler, R. (2008). Killing Fewer, and Killing Carefully: Death Penalty Defense in China on the Eve of the Beijing Olympics. *Champion.* 32:22. 27.

Sun, W. (2009). Sixing cunzai de beilun yu feizhi de genben dongle. Huadong Zhengfa Daxue Xuebao (*Journal of the East China University of Political Science and Law*). 2. 106–12.

UNESCO. (2005). Universal Declaration on Bioethics and Human Rights. Retrieved from http://portal .unesco.org/en/ev.php-URL_ID=31058&URL_DO=DO_TOPIC&URL_SECTION=201.html.

Wang, Hua, Su, Bo, and Liu, Jianwen. (2002). Guanyu Woguo Qiguan Yizhi de Youguan Falv he Lunli Wenti. Zhongguo Yixue Lunli Xue (*Chinese Medical Ethics*), 4, 21.

Wei, Y. (2008). Qiu xinglong he 96ming sixingfan tongjian. Nanfang Renwu Zhoukan (*Southern People Weekly*). 12. 57–59.

WMA. (2004). *Declaration of Helsinki: Ethical Principles for Medical Research Involving Human Subjects.* Ferney-le-Voltaire, France: World Medical Association.

Wyman, J. H. (1997). Vengeance Is Whose?: The Death Penalty and Cultural Relativism in International Law. *Journal of Transnational Law and Policy.* 6. 543–67.

Xie, Miao, Huang Chun, and Liu Xingchun. (2000). Guanyu Woguo Qiguan Yizhi yu Qiguan Juanxian de Sikao. Zhongguo Yixue Lunli Xue (*Chinese Medical Ethics*) 6, 9.

Xu, R., and Tang, J. (2003). Yunnan tuiguang zhushe sixing: guannian zuai. Xinwen Zhoukan (*News Weekly*). 9. 32–33.

Yang, X. (2008, January 3). Expert: China Is Fit for Lethal Injections. Retrieved from http://www.china .org.cn/english/GS-e/237842.htm.

Yuan, B. (2009). Woguo minzong sixing jinben guannian shizheng fenxi. Xingfa Luncong (*Criminal Law Review*). 1. 36.

Zhang, Y. (2008). Woguo sixing zhidu xianzhuang zhi fansi yu chonggou. Fazhi yu Shehui (*Legal Systems and Society*). 8. 166.

Zheng, J. (2008). Zhushe sixing de rendao zhuyi tanxi. Sheke Zongheng (*Social Sciences Review*). 4. 263.

Zhou, Chengxiao. (1997). Yixue lunli shengsi guan de kunjiong yu chongjian. Jingzhou Shizuan Xuebao (*Academic Journal of Jingzhou Normative College*). 4. 26.

Zhuang, Xujun. (2005). Qianxi woguo zhushe sixing zhifu. Xinan Keji Daxue Xuebao (*Journal of Southwest University of Science and Technology*). 22. 24.

Part III Discussion Topics

Wanda Teays

1. How can we balance the needs of pregnant women, infants, and children with the needs of the aging?
   - What steps should be taken to address the medical—and ethical—issues at the beginning and end of life?

2. Should children be able to participate in—if not decide—treatment in life/death medical decisions?

3. Share your concerns regarding the autonomy of minors seeking an abortion.
   - A 2013 report on the state of Arizona stated that 25 percent of abortion requests by minors that go before the Juvenile Court are denied, for example, because of her "maturity." Share your thoughts on the cultural or other influences on maturity and how that might impact this issue.

4. Is there a way to resolve concerns around late-term abortions?

5. The Internet has changed access to abortions. See Catherine Trautwein, "Medical Abortions Have Changed Abortion Access—And They're Available on the Internet," *Frontline*, April 23, 2019, https://www.pbs.org/wgbh/frontline/article/self-managed-induced-medication-abortion/. Read the article and share your thoughts about the ethical issues raised.

6. Should parents be able to use the sperm of their dead son to have grandchildren? Set out your position in response to this case: Matter of Zhu, Justia, May 16, 2019, https://law.justia.com/cases/new-york/other-courts/2019/2019-ny-slip-op-29146.html.

7. Consider the case of the NASA scientist who used in vitro fertilization (IVF) with a nineteen-year-old embryo in her quest for a child. Nancy Josephson (2013) reports:

   > [NASA scientist Kelly Burke used] a donated embryo that is believed to be the second old-est cryopreserved human embryo in history. Baby Liam has biological siblings born many years earlier. They were created from the same embryo cycle, using IVF. Those sibs are fraternal twins. Liam's sibs will able to vote by the time the new arrival turns one later this year. Liam's story actually began more than 19 years ago when a young woman donated her eggs at the Reproductive Science Center (RSC) in San Francisco. At that time, doctors transferred two donated embryos into the uterus of an Oregon woman who was seeking fertility treatment. Fraternal twins resulted from that cycle. Doctors froze the remaining embryos for use later on.

   - What limits—if any—do you think should be put in place?
   - Given the unknown risks of using embryos, eggs, and sperm that have been frozen for years or even decades, at what point should societal interests be factored into policies regarding such assisted reproduction?

8. Do you think it is right to restrict or even prohibit egg donation or sales? Read the following excerpt from *Science Daily* (2011), and then share your thoughts:

   > Women who have become pregnant after egg donation should be categorized as high-risk patients. . . . Ulrich Pecks and co-authors . . . support their assessment with data from recent publications and with a case series they encountered in their own hospital. . . . they found that within the past 4 years, 8 women who had received donated eggs had to be treated for pregnancy-induced hypertension. Three of these pregnancies had to be terminated prematurely because of the threat to the mother's life. The other 5 cases showed a milder course of pregnancy-induced hypertension.
   >
   > Egg donation has been in use for more than 25 years to treat unwanted childlessness. Since the German law on the protection of embryos explicitly forbids the procedure, couples often use medical institutions in neighboring European countries. After successful embryo transfer, the pregnant women are subsequently cared for in Germany in accordance with statutory maternity provision. Because of the risk of a hypertensive disorder of pregnancy, the authors recommend that the patients are closely monitored by doctors with a specialization in maternofetal medicine. ("Egg Donation: The Way to Happy Mother-hood, with Risks and Side Effects," January 25, 2011, https://www.sciencedaily.com/releases/2011/01/110124074013.htm).

9. If a patient cannot speak for himself or herself and has no advance directives, but the hospital knows the patient's religious affiliation, should doctors be allowed to turn to a representative (priest, minister, imam, rabbi, etc.) about patients' medical care in end-of-life decisions?

10. Scott Stonington and Pinit Ratanakul, as well as Cecilia Wee, examine cultural issues in decision-making around euthanasia.
    - What do you think might be a way to factor in cultural considerations when looking at such important medical issues as those centered on the end of life?

- Would some form of cultural sensitivity suffice to bridge the differences between caregivers and the patient and his or her family? If not, what else could be put in place, for example, in terms of cultural protocols?

11. Should doctors participate in lethal injections?

12. Amnesty International objects to lethal injections in capital punishment and raises concerns on its website about the involvement of medical personnel when it comes to harvesting organs from condemned prisoners.
    - State one argument *for* and one argument *against* harvesting organs from executed prisoners.

Part IV

PUBLIC HEALTH

1

Issues in Global Health Ethics

Udo Schüklenk

ABSTRACT

This chapter provides a brief overview of major ethical challenges in international health. This overview aims to demonstrate that current health inequities are not simply an unfortunate incident but that they are unjust and ought to be addressed. Among the issues reviewed is the question of whose moral responsibility global health resourcing is. What are the moral obligations, if any, of nation-states, international institutions, transnational NGOs, and large multinational corporations in this context. Infectious disease control poses its own ethical challenges. HIV/AIDS and influenza will be used as examples of paradigmatic pandemic diseases that require a concerted global response. It is, for instance, conceivable that the provision of a forthcoming pandemic influenza vaccine would preserve more lives if it were deployed in certain developing countries first. What are the moral obligations of developed world governments under such circumstances?

The next section of this chapter provides an overview of some of the salient ethical issues in infectious disease control, focusing initially on HIV/AIDS, before investigating the issues of standard of care in clinical trials in the Global South, as well as the question of access to experimental drugs in public health emergencies, such as recent Ebola virus disease outbreaks.

This chapter will proceed to a moral evaluation of health workers' migration issues. It is well known that, for instance, more Malawi trained health care workers work in countries other than Malawi. What are the moral obligations of health workers to the societies that enabled their training? What are the obligations of net recipient countries (usually located in the developed world)? Is free-riding on developing countries' training of health care professionals ethically acceptable? Issues in global health ethics will conclude with a cursory discussion of at least some pertinent issues in international multicenter clinical research studies. Questions to be addressed include standards of care in a trial, as well as post-trial care with regard to both therapeutic and nontherapeutic clinical research.

PREVENTABLE SUFFERING AND GLOBAL HEALTH

Gross inequities in health treatment and health outcomes exist throughout the world. These inequities are determined by a complicated combination of local circumstances and international policies, and it is beyond the scope of this chapter to examine in detail the specific statistics relating to them. However, there is a clear geographic pattern: health outcomes, health care systems and access to health care in the developing world fall far below the standards that are enjoyed by the developed world. This provides important questions for all manner of academic disciplines, from economics to immunology to anthropology to public policy and beyond. Many of the issues that arise have clear ethical dimensions, and we will consider some of the most topical.

Inequities between countries are inevitable. Some countries are stronger than others in terms of geographic area, natural resources, location, and population size. Such differences are unavoidable and in broad terms are morally neutral. However, inequities in health outcomes and access to health care do not fall into the same category. Rather, many if not all of them are the direct and indirect products of historical and contemporary exploitation in the form of colonialism and oppressive economic policies.[1]

Why should we be concerned about health in the first place? Why does health matter? Even though having good health is not synonymous with living a happy or worthwhile life, there is a strong link between good health and the ability to pursue one's preferences: the satisfaction of preferences is made easier by good health and more difficult by illness. Improving health and access to health care, therefore, must be one priority for any initiative designed to prevent suffering and improve the quality of people's lives. Those living in the developing world are disadvantaged in comparison to those living in the developed world.

This is typically characterized by poorer health generally and by diminished life expectancy.[2] However, it must be borne in mind that poor population health is not simply a symptom of substandard health care systems, but it is also almost invariably indicative of extreme poverty. Social inequality in societies with two-tier health care systems or private health care delivery infrastructure translates into significant differences in terms of health outcomes, and these differences are usually to the detriment of the poorer members of society.

Similarly, while investment in health services is obviously crucial to improving health outcomes, interventions in other policy areas can lead to dramatic health improvements. For example, education, social inclusion, and safe and sanitary built environments have beneficial impacts on individual and public health. In some circumstances, these can improve health outcomes to a greater degree than clinical interventions. Similarly, basic primary care facilities in many developing countries can be more effective in terms of health outcomes than state-of-the-art facilities, such as high-tech transplant centers. However, it is important to recognize that, even when adjustments are made to account for population size and cost of living, developed countries spend approximately thirty times more per person on health care than developing countries.[3]

These international disparities are largely a consequence of the global economic system. A minority of the world's population lives with material abundance while a significant proportion suffer severe harm as a result of extreme poverty. It is morally significant that this harm—of which poor health outcomes are only one manifestation—is preventable: the resources necessary to address global poverty and thereby to reduce substantially the suffering it causes exist.

The relationship between global economics, poverty, and suffering was brought into sharp focus by the events following the earthquake that struck Haiti in January 2010. This earthquake caused devastating damage to towns, villages, and cities, and more than 150,000 Haitians were killed.[4] Much of the destruction, death, and suffering, however, was preventable. Due to the extreme poverty in Haiti, its building safety standards are much lower than in the developed world, and buildings are therefore less resilient; if an earthquake of the same magnitude had struck Japan, for example, less damage would have been done to the built environment, and fewer people would have died or been injured. The poverty in Haiti is preventable. At its root is interference by its formal colonizers and the United States.[5] When seen in this light, much of the suffering caused by the earthquake was not merely unfortunate; it was unjust. It was not so much a result of the—unavoidable—earthquake but of the poverty that meant that building safety standards in Haiti were so low.

There is now widespread acceptance that the developed world has a moral obligation to address the suffering caused by extreme poverty by providing aid to the developing world. As we shall see later in this chapter, different models of moral reasoning support this conclusion. There is disagreement about the nature and extent of this obligation, which specific harms should be addressed, and how aid interventions ought to be prioritized. Competing answers to these questions can translate into enormously divergent policy solutions. But before we take a closer look at these policy issues, it will be useful to examine and discuss the competing theoretical frameworks that underpin them.

POLITICAL VERSUS HUMANITARIAN RATIONALES

A large proportion of aid to the developing world is delivered by means of intergovernmental transactions. These transactions involve the transfer of money, resources, or expertise by a government or intergovernmental organization in the developed world to a government or governments in the developing world. The actors involved in delivering this type of aid are governments, but there is continuing disagreement among political philosophers about whether the obligation to provide aid has its roots at the governmental level or whether this obligation actually belongs to individual citizens in the developed world.

These competing ideas take a variety of forms, and they have been loosely categorized into two discrete strands.[6] The first line of reasoning is the political rationale, which holds that the obligation to provide aid lies essentially with governments or nation-states. Pogge has suggested that governments or nation-states are responsible for providing aid as a form of reparation or compensation for historical wrongs.[7] This can be taken to mean, for example, that certain European countries have an ethical obligation to provide assistance to certain West African countries due to the manifold social, economic, and environmental harms inflicted on one country by another during colonialism. Furthermore, the political rationale goes beyond just compensation for past wrongs. It also addresses ongoing wrongs, such as foreseeable extreme poverty caused in the developing world by present global economic arrangements.

Some objections to the political rationale have been made. Firstly, the idea of international aid as reparation for specific, definable harms, if applied strictly, might exonerate or severely reduce the obligations of some nations in the developed world. That is, while some developed countries have a clear history of colonialism or exploitation, others do not. This latter group, with no clear history of exploitation, could claim that they are therefore not morally required to provide aid to the developing world.

Secondly, major changes to geopolitics mean that some of the nation-states involved in historical injustices no longer exist. This raises the problem of how aid transactions should be carried out on behalf of now nonexistent developed countries or as compensation to now nonexistent countries in the developing world. Thirdly, it might be possible to define some countries as being both the victims and the perpetrators of exploitation. This is particularly relevant in the case of countries with rapidly growing economies, such as China or South

Korea, which once were part of the developing world but whose status in the global economy is now more accurately defined as "emerging" or "developed."

The political rationale is laudable in its intention to provide a theoretical basis upon which affluent governments in the developed world could be persuaded to alleviate suffering by providing support to underresourced governments in the developing world. If accepted by developed governments, the political rationale would yield overseas aid policies that could have an enormous impact on the well-being of people living in the developing world, and this would undoubtedly be desirable. However, although the political rationale is capable of producing favorable outcomes, its scope is necessarily limited by its premises, and this is probably the most serious objection to it.

The political rationale holds that aid transactions should be seen as compensation for historical malfeasance on the part of developed world governments. But while it is certainly true that there are good reasons for governments in the developed world to adopt this attitude, the political rationale alone cannot provide a sound theoretical basis for the type of aid necessary to alleviate suffering effectively.[8] For example, some suffering has not come about as a result of colonialism or subjugation on the part of countries in the developed world. There are numerous instances in which developing countries have been devastated by natural disasters, civil war, or gross political mismanagement.

While it could be argued that the causes of some of these might actually be traced back to the developed world—climate change or oppressive foreign and economic policies, for instance—the causes of at least some of them are purely local. Earthquakes, tsunamis, volcanic eruptions, civil wars, and failed political systems can all result in extremely poor health conditions and desperate but preventable suffering. But the political rationale states that, unless these conditions are linked to the behaviour of developed world governments, there is no justice-based obligation to provide aid or assistance in such circumstances.[9]

The governments of developed countries, according to the political rationale, have an obligation to provide aid to the developing world because of what has caused people's suffering, not simply by virtue of the fact that they are suffering. Those people who are starving as a result of political subjugation or military occupation should be afforded medical aid, but those who are starving because their crops have been obliterated by an earthquake should not. This picture seems incomplete and indicates that the political rationale alone cannot provide a sufficiently plausible theoretical basis for the provision of medical aid to those who need it most. Instead, it requires that injustices should only be addressed when their causes can be traced to the behavior of governments in the developing world. But frequently the circumstances that are arguably most deserving of aid have no such cause.

Moreover, the political rationale fails to offer any kind of guidance for the crucial task of prioritizing health aid. Severe health inequities exist within countries, as well as between them. Even in developed countries, there can be vast differences in health outcomes and health conditions between citizens. For example, the average life expectancy at birth of a man living in Kensington, an affluent area in London is 84.3 years, whereas a man living in Glasgow, also in the United Kingdom, can on average expect to live 70.7 years.[10]

Since the central tenet of the political rationale is that governments have an obligation to address the inequities brought about by their behavior, domestic inequities must also be considered. The political rationale offers no guidance on how competing domestic and overseas demands on public funds should be resolved and therefore leaves an important policy question unanswered. It is possible that the political rationale could require the prioritization of domestic needs ahead of overseas needs, perhaps even to the outright exclusion of any overseas interventions. It is probably fair to suggest that, although the suffering prevalent in developed countries can be serious and should be addressed, it is rarely as serious as the suffering experienced by those in absolute poverty in the developing world.[11]

The political rationale offers no comprehensive account capable of adequately addressing the problem of global suffering. The scope of the political rationale is far narrower than that which can reasonably be expected of a comprehensive approach to global health ethics. It provides no satisfactory answers to the question of how aid should be prioritized.

The humanitarian rationale, on the other hand, sees individual citizens as the relevant moral agents in obligations to provide overseas aid. At first glance, this approach might seem counterintuitive: although individuals can and do make contributions to charities, currently the main actors in the provision of global aid are governments. But perhaps this is simply a matter of practicality. The size and complexity of overseas aid payments means that they ought to be decided and negotiated by governments and the transactions involved should be carried out by governments, but this does not mean that the relevant moral actors are governments. The humanitarian rationale argues this very point and suggests that governments are acting as a necessary proxy for transactions between individual citizens in the countries involved.

According to this logic, when the Australian government makes an aid payment to support a public health initiative in Sudan, for example, this is a manifestation of a payment by the citizens of Australia to the citizens of Sudan. The obligation to provide aid in this scenario does not belong to the Australian government but to the Australian people, and the obligation requires that aid is provided to the people of Sudan, not to the Sudanese government. The fact that the transaction is carried out by governments is merely a matter of expediency.

The humanitarian rationale has at its root the principle of moral equivalence, or "universal undifferentiated moral standing."[12] This principle, simply put, asserts that every person has an equal claim to moral consideration. This thought is at the heart of the liberal tradition and has been central to many civil rights agendas. The humanitarian rationale asserts that in principle each person has a moral relationship with every other person, regardless of nationality or country of residence. This notion is strongly associated with the utilitarian tradition. It sees suffering or the prevention of the pursuit of preferences as harmful and therefore as having negative moral value.

We have a moral obligation to relieve suffering or barriers to preference satisfaction whenever doing so does not involve comparable risks to ourselves. When applied to the issue of global suffering, this logic requires that those living in the developed world are morally obliged to prevent harm to those living in the developed world until the point that by doing so they would not cause comparable harm to themselves. However, the present distribution of resources is so distorted that such a tipping point is very unlikely to come about any time soon. Interestingly, some empirical estimates assert that sufficient resources could be diverted to address global poverty without bringing about any appreciable difference to the quality of life of those living in the developed world.[13]

It has been argued that geographic or political borders provide useful and ethically significant demarcations in deciding the boundaries of moral groups.[14] This view is supported by the fact that evolutionary pressure seems to support a preference for assisting members of one's family or one's immediate community over assisting strangers or people living on the other side of the world. However, although there are undoubtedly strong evolutionary reasons for human beings holding this kind of instinctive attitude, it does not stand up to much ethical scrutiny; good ethics does not always conform to our moral instincts, but explores them and sometimes requires us to act in opposition to them.

Some of the biggest ethical triumphs in recent history were cases in which the instinct to attribute special moral status to those in our immediate social groups was overcome: the abolition of slavery, universal franchise, and the vast majority of civil rights movements. Our moral group is expanding and becoming more inclusive; people who were historically excluded because of sex, skin color, sexual orientation, or worldview have been gradually admitted to the group. The rationale used for making these changes is applicable to those who as yet are not part of the established moral group. In the case under consideration, it is an argument against exclusion based on geographic location and requires that we do not recognize geographic or political borders as having special moral relevance.

Poor access to health resources, prolonged sickness, and premature death are very common phenomena in the developing world, and clearly these involve suffering and are often barriers to preference satisfaction. Furthermore, they constitute important hindrances to economic development. In the developing world, much sickness and premature death is easily preventable. It is caused by treatable conditions, many of which are very effectively contained in the developed world. The question of providing aid to the developing world is therefore largely one of resource allocation: Could the developed world provide medical assistance to the developing world without incurring a comparable risk to itself? We believe that it could.

The political rationale cannot provide a sufficient theoretical basis for the type of interventions required to address global suffering satisfactorily. By reconceptualizing the nature of the moral obligation, however, the humanitarian rationale does not encounter this problem. The humanitarian rationale proposes that inhabitants of the developed world have an obligation to provide aid to the inhabitants of the developing world who are suffering preventable harm regardless of the particular political or economic explanations for the suffering in question.

But the humanitarian rationale must also deal with problems concerning scope. For example, how much aid is the developed world obliged to provide to the developing world? Perhaps this question can be answered by calculating the degree of need in each case: the obligation is to provide as much aid as is necessary to alleviate the problem, so long as doing so does not create a comparable disadvantage to those living in the developed world. If this model were to become policy in the developed world, it would yield overseas aid interventions on a far larger scale than anything that has been implemented to date. Despite the persuasive case for this type of aggressive redistribution, it is difficult to envisage an immediate radical change to overseas aid. In the case of government spending, for example, even the most generous nations currently allocate only a tiny proportion of their GDP to overseas aid.[15]

INTERNATIONAL FINANCIAL ARRANGEMENTS

Aid payments to the developing world must be considered in the global economic context. Of particular relevance is the system of governmental loans which was implemented in the 1970s and 1980s, ostensibly to help developing world countries to alleviate acute health and wider social problems by investing in their domestic infrastructure. A number of countries in Latin America and the Caribbean took substantial loans from various international financial organizations, such as the World Bank and the International Monetary Fund, for this purpose, but there were specific conditions attached to the loans that affected the ways in which they could be used.

These conditions were primarily concerned with policy reforms in the recipient countries and required them to adopt neoliberal economic policies and to implement corresponding political and economic instruments. These conditions attached to the World Bank loans have in many cases crippled clinical and public health services in the recipient countries and have prevented the kind of reform and investment for which the loans were initially intended; in fact, in some cases the current system is no better than the old system. While it might in some circumstances be desirable to attach such conditions for structural or policy reform to aid payments, these conditions must be sensitive to existing local cultural and political systems.

Perhaps the most damaging consequence of these conditions was the requirement that health services in the recipient countries became privatized. This undid much good work that had previously been done, particularly in containing endemic diseases. Furthermore, recipient governments were required to employ expensive overseas consultants in order to establish and manage the new privatized health systems, which was a particularly inefficient use of the loan. In certain countries, a long-term effect of the privatized health care requirement imposed by the loans has been the emergence of vastly unequal multitiered systems, in which all patients must pay for health care.

In such systems, the rich minority of the population have access to health resources that are far superior to those available to the poor majority. It is difficult to see how such situations— or the policies underpinning the loans that created them—can be ethically justified, although there have been various unsuccessful attempts to do so.[16]

ACCESS TO TREATMENT

While differences in terms of health outcomes and provision exist both between and within countries in both the developing world and the developed world, there is a clear division between even the best-performing developing countries and the worst-performing developed countries. It is possible to make a few general observations about the differences between the two. The average life expectancy of someone living in the developing world is shorter than that of a person living in the developed world.

Moreover, a person living in the developing world is more likely to spend a greater proportion of his or her life in ill health. Medical conditions that are easily treatable in the developed world go untreated in the developing world, and access to vaccines, medicines, and other medical treatment is poor in comparison.

The types of illnesses encountered and the particular social contexts in which they exist make approaches to health policy in the developing world different from approaches in the developed world in significant respects. Preventable diseases, such as diarrhea and influenza, kill millions of people every year in the developing world. So why are vaccines and medicines not made available to those who need them in the developing world? The answer to this question has two parts.

The first part has to do with affordability. Some treatments are simply too expensive for those living in the developing world. Governments cannot afford to purchase enough drugs for their citizens, and the citizens themselves cannot afford to pay for their own treatment. The second part has to do with logistics: in many cases the health care infrastructure required to distribute medicines and organize mass vaccinations does not exist. Poor people in under-resourced countries either have no access to or cannot afford the simple treatments taken for granted in more affluent countries. Infectious diseases that are controlled or effectively eradicated in the developed world are rampant in the developing world because vaccines are too expensive and vaccination programs are not in place.

Drug prices are set by the pharmaceutical companies that develop the drugs. When a successful drug has been developed it is protected by a patent that prevents the drug being copied or produced by others. This system means that the company responsible for investing in the research and development of a successful drug can recoup the investment necessary to bring the drug to market and make a profit. For a pharmaceutical company to survive, its profits must at the very least cover the costs of all of its research and development programs, including those that are ultimately unsuccessful.

In fact, it is the incentive of substantial profits that motivates the pharmaceutical companies to undertake expensive research and development in the first place. Predictably, the pharmaceutical industry defends the system of patents and pricing by arguing that it serves the public interest: the development of new and better medical products depends upon commercial incentives for pharmaceutical companies to undertake drug research and development. While this might seem reasonable at first glance, the idea that pharmaceutical companies are motivated by the public interest does not bear much scrutiny. Pharmaceutical companies which hold patents on new medicines refuse to supply customers who cannot afford to pay their prices, thus effectively precluding access in much of the developing world.

Furthermore, patent holders frequently refuse to grant licenses to other companies that would produce and supply the same drugs at a reduced cost and vehemently pursue legal action against companies that breach patents to do so.[17] The result is usually that a new drug does not become available in the developing world until after the patent has expired, normally ten or more years after it has been granted. The patent holders cannot expect to make much profit from sales in large parts of the developing world while they hold the patent, and they certainly will not do so once the patent has expired.

The profit on new medicine comes almost exclusively from its sale in the developed world, and it is unclear how making patented drugs available in the developing world could harm the profit margins of its developer. Perhaps the pharmaceutical industry could reasonably be concerned that forgoing the patents in the developing world might mean that unlicensed versions of a drug become available in the developed world, thus impacting on profits. However, strict regulation of production and supply could prevent this from occurring. Pharmaceutical companies genuinely motivated by notions of public interest might reasonably be expected to make patented drugs available in the developing world, albeit under strict regulatory conditions.

But it would be unreasonable to expect pharmaceutical companies to act altruistically. It is not clear that shareholders of pharmaceutical companies should subsidize research that, according to both the humanitarian and political models, is the responsibility of all well-off citizens in the developed world. Pharmaceutical companies have fiduciary responsibilities to their shareholders to maximize profits and to prioritize the public interest ahead of commercial interest might be to overlook these responsibilities. If pharmaceutical companies were concerned more with the public interest than with profits, shareholders might prefer to invest in other industries, thus inhibiting the pharmaceutical industry.

Perhaps we should not expect them to undertake drug research on diseases most prevalent in the developing world unless those diseases are also prevalent in wealthy markets, or unless there are clear advance purchase commitments from motivated buyers. The lesson to be drawn from this analysis is this: if we think medicines ought to be developed for diseases prevalent in the developing world then we should consider paying for it. We cannot expect pharmaceutical companies to undertake this work purely altruistically.

The nature of existing health care infrastructures in many developing countries would make large scale treatment or vaccination initiatives very difficult and perhaps in some cases impossible. The establishment of workable health care infrastructures would go some way to allowing the kinds of preventive and reactive treatment programs that could make a significant contribution to addressing the health problems in the developing world. However, some governments in the developing world consistently fail to invest in health care and often prioritize military spending ahead of health care spending.

This practice is currently going on in Zimbabwe, North Korea, and Myanmar, among others. This behavior is sometimes used as an argument against providing medical aid to these countries: if their own governments choose not to prioritize health spending, the developed world should not provide assistance. This point of view is consistent with the political rationale, as described above. However, as we have seen, the obligation to provide aid exists between individuals, and the humanitarian rationale, while justifiably condemning the prioritization of military spending over health spending, would require the developed world to provide health aid to people living in those countries whose governments neglect to do so.

INFECTIOUS DISEASE CONTROL

Infectious diseases pose a threat to individual as well as public health in any given population. In the developed world, health care systems are generally quite efficient in managing and controlling the spread of common infectious diseases. However, in the developing world, with health care systems that are less sophisticated and less comprehensive in their coverage, infectious diseases are much more difficult to control.

HIV/AIDS is a paradigmatic example of this, and we need only compare the infection rates in Western and Central Europe with those in sub-Saharan Africa to see the extent of this problem.[18] If HIV/AIDS is allowed to continue to spread in the developing world, its already harmful consequences will continue or worsen. The natural spread of HIV/AIDS has been reinforced in some parts of the developed world by unhelpful government interventions, such as the disastrous treatment and education policies of the Mbeki administration in South Africa.[19] In the absence of a preventive vaccine for HIV, any successful initiative to control the disease would involve testing populations, treating those who are HIV positive and taking measures to prevent further infection.

Incidentally, treating those who are HIV positive with highly active antiretroviral medicines would have another desirable effect: for all intents and purposes they would be rendered noninfectious. AIDS treatment would not only provide them with the care necessary to survive, it would also have effects comparable to a preventive vaccine in terms of the effective protection it provides to the sexual partners of infected people. Such initiatives could potentially require significant infringements on the autonomy of those who are tested. Historically, these violations of autonomy were considered too serious to preclude the option of mandatory HIV testing.

Part of the rationale at the time was that even if those who were affected could have been identified, there was no effective treatment to reduce the fatalities caused by the disease.[20] However, today's treatments for HIV/AIDS are capable of preserving the lives of people with HIV/AIDS and reducing their risk of infecting others. The existence of these treatments casts serious doubt upon the autonomy objection. Identifying those who are infected by HIV/AIDS and treating them could bring about enormous improvements to individual and public health, and this might well be sufficient to override concerns about the potential violation of infected individuals' autonomy.

Let us consider a more complex version of this scenario, namely, the question of whether or not it might be good policy to introduce mandatory HIV testing for pregnant women. There is a 35 percent chance that an infant born to an HIV-positive woman will also be HIV positive. The number of children infected by this process worldwide was estimated to be between 2.1 and 2.8 million in 2004.[21] However, a fairly simple treatment program for the mother and child exists that can produce a reduction in mother-to-child transmission of 67.5 percent.[22]

Unfortunately, in many parts of the world where this type of intervention would be most effective due to a high prevalence of HIV, such as Botswana, being HIV positive carries a stigma that can have fairly severe social consequences. It is conceivable that pregnant women in these circumstances would feel sufficient social pressure that they would avoid attending clinics where they would be mandatorily tested for HIV, thus defeating the purpose of mandatory testing. These social and cultural phenomena might make a policy of mandatory testing difficult, but not impossible, to deliver.

For example, a mandatory testing program could aim to guarantee the confidentiality of the HIV status of mothers and newborns in an attempt to minimize such stigmatization and its concomitant negative consequences. Unfortunately, on current treatment modalities it would be difficult for those women who are HIV positive to preserve their anonymity while undergoing treatment.

While such operational challenges are certainly important, there is a prior debate regarding the ethical acceptability of mandatory HIV testing for pregnant women. A rigorous set of conditions have been proposed[23] that must be met in order for mandatory testing to be ethically justifiable. A pregnant woman must first of all have voluntarily decided to carry her fetus to term, in full knowledge of the available alternatives including abortion. A pregnant woman is not morally obliged to carry and deliver a fetus that she does not want.

However, when a pregnant woman does voluntarily decide to carry a fetus to term, she arguably accepts an obligation not to injure the fetus and to take reasonable steps to prevent it from being subjected to serious risk of bodily harms, such as life-threatening infections. Pregnant women therefore could be seen to have an obligation to ensure that they do not transmit HIV to their fetus, and this would first require the HIV status of the mothers to be ascertained.

Poor health resources and fragmented medical advice and treatment might make such a policy difficult to implement in the developing world. Pregnant women in developing countries might not have sufficient access to alternatives to pregnancy, and therefore a decision to carry a fetus to term might not always be voluntary. The obligations that apply to genuinely voluntary pregnancies would not apply in such cases. Moreover, while abortion can be an ethically acceptable alternative in the early stages of a pregnancy, it is more difficult to justify it for later-stage pregnancies. Substandard health care in the developing world could mean that pregnant women engage with health professionals too late in their pregnancies for abortion to be viable. This, again, might alter the voluntariness of a pregnancy and therefore any obligations that it implies.

The second condition for justifiable mandatory testing is that HIV-positive women who undergo mandatory testing and successfully deliver their children must be given access to life-preserving antiretroviral medication for themselves. This would mean that the mothers would be more likely to be well enough to look after their children, considerably improving the children's chances of survival. Furthermore, it would reduce the pressure on developing societies already struggling to cope with huge numbers of AIDS orphans.

However, participation in such an initiative would have to be voluntary since it would be impractical to enforce or supervise the women's adherence to antiretroviral treatment. Women who undergo some antiretroviral treatment but who do not continue to receive it can develop drug-resistant strains of HIV. This could have serious health consequences not only for the women concerned but also any future children that they may choose to have and indeed their sexual partners if they practice unsafe sex. Furthermore, there are significant public health implications of introducing drug-resistant strains of HIV.

The third condition is that the anonymity of pregnant women and their children should be maintained throughout and after the pregnancy, for the reasons outlined above. This would be likely to provide a formidable operational challenge to health authorities.

Antiretroviral treatment has the potential to make a significant impact not only on MTCT (mother-to-child transmission of HIV), but also on the overall global spread of HIV/AIDS. Enormous amounts of time and resources have been invested in trying to develop a preventive vaccine for HIV, but to no avail. However, as well as preserving the lives of those who are HIV positive, long-term treatment with modern antiretroviral medications can render them effectively noncontagious.[24] The combination of better health and a reduced chance of infecting others is likely to be a strong incentive for at-risk individuals to seek testing and, for those who are HIV positive, treatment.

This incentive would be stronger still if it was accompanied by changes to the legality of unsafe sex and a shift in the cultural attitudes toward HIV-positive individuals in both the developed and the developing world. By removing these legal and cultural barriers, at-risk individuals would be more willing to be tested. This in turn would allow health care agencies to quantify and track the incidence of HIV/AIDS and to contain it by rigorous treatment with modern antiretroviral medication. Projections published in 2009 suggest that such a policy could have a dramatic impact upon the AIDS epidemic within ten years of implementation and could reduce the prevalence of HIV in the world's worst-affected areas to 1 percent by the middle of this century.[25] However, the price of medications remains a significant obstacle to the implementation of effective control of infectious diseases.

MEDICAL RESEARCH AND CARE FOR RESEARCH PARTICIPANTS

A substantial amount of research into the development of new medical products takes place in the Global South and involves citizens of developing countries as research participants. Such research is almost always carried out by pharmaceutical companies based in the developed world, and the imbalance in wealth between these countries and the communities and individuals involved in research raises a number of ethical concerns about the potential exploitation of research participants in the developing world.

One of the most controversial issues in international research ethics concerns the standard of clinical care that should be afforded to research participants. The central issue is whether participants in the control arms of an international, multicenter trial should be given the same treatment, regardless of their geographic location, or whether they should be given the best locally available treatment. This issue triggered more than a decade of heated debate among the international bioethics community, following ACTG 076, an AIDS clinical trial that set out to establish whether an affordable treatment that would reduce the incidence of MTCT could be developed for use in the developing world.

Previous trials in the developed world had demonstrated that pregnant mothers who used particular treatment regime of the drug Zidovudine were much less likely to pass HIV on to their offspring than those pregnant women who took no antiretroviral medication. At the time of ATCG 076, therefore, the Zidovudine regime was the gold standard in the developed world, but it was unaffordable to most pregnant women in poorer countries. The investigators in ACTG 076 tested a lower, and therefore less expensive, dosage of Zidovudine. The trial sought to find out whether a lower dosage was more effective than no treatment at all, not whether it was more effective than the higher dosage used in the developed world. Those in the treatment arm of the trial received the lower dosage while those in the control arm received no treatment.

The trial was heavily criticized by medical scholars and ethicists.[26] It directly contravened one of the provisions of the World Medical Association's Declaration of Helsinki,[27] which requires that those in the control arm of biomedical trials are given access to the best available therapeutic and diagnostic techniques. This would require that everyone in the control arm, regardless of their geographic location, should receive the gold standard treatment; only in the absence of a gold standard does a placebo control become acceptable as a means to test the null hypothesis. But some people defended the trial methodology and suggested that the Declaration of Helsinki should in fact be revised to allow this type of trial.

The trial methodology has also been defended by arguing that, since pregnant women in the developing world had no access to Zidovudine or any other antiretroviral therapy, the women in the control arm were no worse off than they would have been if they had not participated in the trial while those in the treatment arm were likely to be better off. However, this justification is insufficient. It makes little sense in clinical terms since the purpose of most drug trials is to see how the trial drug performs against the gold standard drug, not poorer treatments.

Critics of the Helsinki Declaration argue that, if it were followed strictly, all new treatments would have to be tested against the best medication available anywhere in the world, even if such a medication was unaffordable for a large proportion of the global population. This would effectively prohibit trials designed to develop treatments that would be affordable in poorer countries. However, both of these defenses rely on an assumption that drugs are necessarily too expensive for people in the developing world to afford them. The reality, however, is that they are only too expensive because of the high prices demanded by pharmaceutical companies. The distinction between local and global standards of care is artificial, and any argument based on it is flawed.[28]

A related issue concerns the posttrial clinical care that should be provided to research participants in the developing world. After all, part of the ethical rationale of clinical research in developed countries is that patients, including those in the trial in question, would be afforded access to the drug that was tested successfully in a trial. Due to the cost issues mentioned earlier in this chapter, the same cannot be said for trial participants in the developing world. This raises the possibility of exploitation, as well as the question of whether special provisions ought to be made with regard to posttrial access to medicines.

The Declaration of Helsinki requires that any benefits resulting from clinical research should be made available to the individuals and communities that are involved in the research. This could be taken to mean that research participants should remain on that medication that the trial finds is the most effective, whether it is the trial drug or the best existing alternative. However, it has been argued that such a policy would be unaffordable and that it might prevent research that is taking place. The economics involved are complicated, but there is reason to believe that this argument is inaccurate.[29]

It perhaps says something about the commercial motivations of the pharmaceutical industry that the debates about standards of care can often—if not always—be reduced to calculations of profitability. But, as we have seen, it would be unreasonable to expect the pharmaceutical industry to stop behaving in accordance with these commercial motivations.

MEDICAL RESEARCH IN PUBLIC HEALTH EMERGENCIES

The issue of placebo controls in clinical research returned with a vengeance during the Ebola virus outbreak in Liberia, Sierra Leone, and Guinea during 2014–2015. At the time of writing, no successful therapeutic means exist to treat people with high viral load Ebola virus disease (EVD). The infection results in a fast-acting catastrophic illness, rendering patients during the final stages of disease progression highly infectious. Unlike in the case of the HIV-infected pregnant women in sub-Saharan Africa, a placebo control in clinical trials involving such patients is more readily defensible given that no gold standard of care exists. So one would need to find out whether a particular unregistered medical intervention that is tested is better than doing nothing, achieves the same, or might even be worse than doing nothing. Catastrophically ill patients could still be harmed by a drug that does more harm than good to them.

A contested ethical issue has been whether it is ethically defensibly to offer patients access to such experimental agents as a last attempt at preserving their lives. The stakes are high, and the odds are also high that such drugs fail.[30] A panel convened by the WHO during the outbreak at least agreed that it would be ethically justifiable to use such drugs.[31]

It is one thing to argue that it would be justifiable to *offer* such drugs to patients, provided they offered true first person voluntary consent as an indication of their willingness to take their chances with such agents. It is quite another thing to claim that such patients also have a moral claim to access such experimental drugs. Some authors have argued that catastrophically ill patients have a moral claim right to such drugs because in the absence of such a claim right they could not be considered true volunteers in placebo controlled trials. The ethical argument here, much abbreviated, goes like this: it is a cornerstone of research ethics (and research regulations the world all over) that patients, if they have the capacity to do so, must be asked for their first person voluntary informed consent to trial participation. If the only way for catastrophically ill patients is to access an experimental—last chance—agent in a placebo controlled clinical trial, they are arguably made a coercive offer; namely, if you want to get a 50/50 chance of accessing the experimental agent tested in this trial you must accept the randomization procedure that is part of the trial design. This offer is arguably coercive because patients are unable to access the experimental drug without trial participation. Many patients would likely not wish to be randomized into the placebo arm, knowing what essentially nontreatment for the underlying infection means for their survival probabilities. To ensure that those patients who opt to participate in the trial are true volunteers, it has been argued, it is necessary to provide them with an alternative access route to the experimental agent.[32]

Against such a view count several considerations, chief among them that medical progress would likely be delayed, because it would take longer to recruit a sufficient number of patient volunteers for trial participation. Of concern is also that such experimental drugs are typically in short supply, unless they are off-label uses of existing cheap medicines, so if a drug manufacturer had to produce additional quantities to provide to nontrial participants they might decide that the costs are too high for such an endeavor, given the high probability that the drug will fail.

MIGRANT HEALTH WORKERS

The problem of global health inequities is largely one of affordability and resource allocation. Developing world governments usually do not have the fiscal resources to provide health care that is comparable to those countries, such as Canada or the United Kingdom, whose public health care systems are able to provide a high standard of health care for their citizens. Sometimes, these governments might have the requisite resources, but they prioritize spending in other areas ahead of health care. A significant part of the problem is that developing countries do not have enough health care workers to be able to deliver the requisite services.

One of the biggest contributors to this situation is the widespread migration of health workers from developing countries to developed countries. This cannot be surprising given the economic factors at play. Even the United States does not train a sufficient number of nurses to cover its needs but relies on recruiting nurses from other parts of the world. Nurses, doctors, and other health professionals who train in the developing world frequently go on to spend the majority of their career working in developed countries. Fewer than one fifth of the total number of doctors and nurses in the world work in developing countries, and one in five doctors who received their training in the developing world works in the developed world.[33]

The incentives for health care workers are clear: developed countries promise an overall better standard of life for them and the family members who travel with them, and higher wages mean that they can send a proportion of their salary back home to support their wider family. Furthermore, a large proportion of health spending in the developed world focuses on the control of HIV/AIDS and other infectious diseases, so health care workers whose specialism is not infectious disease have a better chance of finding work overseas than at home. There are also economic advantages for the host countries: a stronger labor market characterized by skilled workers who will accept lower wages and whose training has been provided overseas. But when viewed in a global context, this situation is harmful: it exacerbates rather than addresses the disparities in global health.

One proposed solution to the problem of the migration of health care workers places an obligation on three distinct groups: recruiters and policy makers in the developed world, international medical aid organizations, and health care workers from the developing world themselves.[34] Each of these groups has voluntarily contributed to the problem and is therefore morally responsible for addressing it. The contribution of developed-world governments and policy makers lies both in their willingness to freeload by accepting cheap skilled labor from the developing world and in allowing shortages of health care professionals in their labor markets.

Responsible governments in the developed world should train enough health care professionals to populate their own health care systems, thus removing the need to source labor from the developing world. Arguably, developed world governments should compensate developing nations for the health care workers poached from them, for example, by supporting an educational infrastructure that produces an oversupply of health care workers. While some governments in the developed world recognize this moral responsibility and have taken steps to address it,[35] the problem remains.

The obligation of recruiters in the developing world lies in not contributing to the overall harmful consequences already caused by the migration of health care workers. Responsible recruitment policies would rule out proactively recruiting from countries with critically low numbers of health care professionals. Rather, recruitment should be limited to recruiting individuals only when there is a surfeit of professionals with comparable skills or specialisms in their home countries.

To suggest that the health care workers themselves have an obligation not to migrate seems at first glance problematic: it places a moral restriction on their ability to pursue a better life for themselves and their families. However, perhaps migration should be allowed only after health care workers have spent a certain time working in their home countries, perhaps giving enough service to pay back the cost of their training. Such policies exist in some countries, such as South Africa, and are similar to those that operate in some European countries whose armed forces pay for the training of doctors in return for a period of military service when they qualify.

A sensible system of migration for health care workers would ensure that there was a net gain, at least in the short and medium terms, to the developing world. It would also incorporate a system of compensation, whereby the countries that benefit from migration provide financial or in-kind reparations to the developing countries that provide the workers. This might include exchange programs for students and early-career professionals; access to equipment, facilities, training, and scholarly resources; and a commitment to direct more research into those medical issues affecting the developing world.

CONCLUSION

This chapter has covered some of the most challenging issues in global health ethics. However, it should not be seen as an exhaustive. Space constraints have forced us to omit some very important issues, such as transplant tourism and resource prioritization during global pandemics. We have shown that numerous injustices exist in global health care and that they are characterized by a clear and consistent recurring division between the resource-poor developing world and the more affluent developed world.

These problems are not simply accidents of nature. They are to a large extent the product of the historical exploitation of developing countries that is reinforced by unfair current global economic policies. This is not to suggest that globalization has not also brought benefits to people living in the developed world. It seems clear, however, that whatever ethical analysis one wishes to avail themselves of, people in the resource-rich parts of the world—and this now includes large numbers of citizens in countries such as India and the People's Republic of China—have moral obligations to assist those in the developing world by providing health aid and, arguably, by restructuring global trade and financial arrangements.

NOTES

1. T. W. Pogge, *World Poverty and Human Rights*, 2nd ed. (Cambridge: Polity, 2008).

2. C. Mathers, et al, "Global Patterns of Healthy Life Expectancy in the Year 2002," *BMC Public Health* 4 (2004): 66, doi:10.1186/1471-2458-4-66.

3. G. J. Schreiber, P. Gottret, L. K. Fleisher, and A. A. Leive, "Financing Global Health: Mission Unaccomplished," *Health Affairs* 26, no. 4 (2007): 921–34, doi:10.1377/hlthaff.26.4.921.

4. "Haiti Capital Earthquake Death Toll 'Tops 150,000,'" *BBC News*, January 25, 2010, http://news.bbc.co.uk/2/hi/americas/8477770.stm.

5. P. Farmer, M. C. Smith, and P. Nevil, "Unjust Embargo of Aid for Haiti," *Lancet* 361 (2003): 420–23.

6. C. Lowry and U. Schüklenk, "Two Models in Global Health Ethics," *Public Health* 2, no. 3 (2009): 276–84, doi:10.1093/phe/php032.

7. Pogge, *World Poverty and Human Rights*.

8. Lowry and Schüklenk, "Two Models in Global Health Ethics."

9. J. Narveson, "We Don't Owe Them a Thing! A Tough-Minded But Soft-Hearted View of Aid to the Faraway Needy," *The Monist* 86, no. 3 (2003): 419–33.

10. Office for National Statistics, "Big Variation in Life Expectancy," modified October 21, 2009, http://news.bbc.co.uk/1/hi/health/8317986.stm.

11. P. Singer, *The Life You Can Save: Acting Now to End World Poverty* (London: Picador, 2009), 8.

12. Lowry and Schüklenk, "Two Models in Global Health Ethics."

13. Singer, *The Life You Can Save: Acting Now to End World Poverty*, chapter 10.

14. P. Collier, "A New Alms Race to Help the World's Poor," *Observer*, March 15, 2009, http://www.guardian.co.uk/books/2009/mar/15/poverty-life-save-peter-singer.

15. Singer, *The Life You Can Save: Acting Now to End World Poverty*, chapter 7.

16. U. Schüklenk, M. Kowtow, and P. A. Sy, "Developing World Challenges," in *A Companion to Bioethics*, edited by H. Kuhse and P. Singer, 404–16 (Oxford: Wiley-Blackwell, 2009).

17. G. Anand, "Drug Makers Decry Indian Patent Law," *Wall Street Journal*, modified February 11, 2010, http://online.wsj.com/article/SB10001424052748703455804575057621354459804.html?mod=WSJ_World_MIDDLENews.

18. UNAIDS, *AIDS Epidemic Update 2009*, November 2009, http://data.unaids.org/pub/Report/2009/JC1700_Epi_Update_2009_en.pdf.

19. P. Chigwerdre, G. R. Seage III, S. Gruskin, T.-H. Lee, and M. Essex, "Estimating the Lost Benefits of Antiretroviral Drug Use in South Africa," *Journal of Acquired Immune Deficiency Syndrome* 49, no. 4 (2008): 410–15; U. Schüklenk, "Professional Responsibilities of Biomedical Scientists in Public Discourse," *Journal of Medical Ethics* 30 (2004): 53–60.

20. U. Schüklenk, "AIDS as a Global Health Emergency," in *A Companion to Bioethics*, edited by H. Kuhse and P. Singer, 441–54 (Chichester: Wiley-Blackwell, 2009).

21. UNAIDS, *AIDS Epidemic Update 2005*.

22. E. M. Connor, R. S. Sealing, R. Gelber, et al, "Reduction of Maternal Infant Transmission of Human Immunodeficiency Virus Type 1 with Zidovudine Treatment," *New England Journal of Medicine* 331 (1994): 1173–80.

23. U. Schüklenk and A. Kleinsmidt, "Rethinking Mandatory HIV Testing during Pregnancy in High HIV-Prevalence Regions: Ethical and Policy Issues," *American Journal of Public Health* 97, no. 7 (2007): 1179–83.

24. P. Vernaza, B. Hirschel, E. Bernasconi, and M. Flepp, "Les personnes séropositives ne souffrant d'aucune autre MST et suivant un traitement antiretroviral efficace ne transmettent pas le VIH par voie sexuelle," *Bulletin des Médecins Suisse* 89, no. 5 (2008): 165–69.

25. R. M. Granich, C. F. Gilks, C. Dye, K. M. De Cock, and B. G.Williams, "Universal Voluntary HIV Testing with Immediate Antiretroviral Therapy as a Strategy for Elimination of HIV Transmission: A Mathematical Model," *The Lancet* 373 (2009): 48–57.

26. P. Lurie and S. M. Wolfe, "Unethical Trials of Interventions to Reduce Perinatal Transmission of the Human Immunodeficiency Virus in Developing Countries," *New England Journal of Medicine* 337, no. 12 (1997): 853–56; U. Schüklenk and R. Ashcroft, "International Research Ethics," *Bioethics* 14, no. 2 (2000): 158–72.

27. World Medical Association, "World Medical Association Declaration of Helsinki," 2008, http://www.wma.net/en/30publications/10policies/b3/17c.pdf.

28. U. Schüklenk, "The Standard of Care Debate: Against the Myth of an 'International Consensus Opinion,'" *Journal of Medical Ethics* 30 (2004): 194–97.

29. Schüklenk, "AIDS as a Global Health Emergency."

30. M. Hay, D. W. Thomas, and J. L. Craighead, "Clinical Development Success Rates for Investigational Drugs," *Nature Bio-Technology* 32, no. 1 (2014): 40–51; J. Arrowsmith, "Trial Watch: Phase 3 and Submission Failures 2007–2010," *Nature Reviews: Drug Discovery* 10, no. 2 (2011, February): 87.

31. WHO, "Ethical Considerations for Use of Unregistered Interventions for Ebola Virus Disease (EVD)," August 12, 2014, http://www.who.int/mediacentre/news/statements/2014/ebola-ethical -review-summary/en/. See also WHO, "Ethical Considerations for Use of Unregistered Interventions for Ebola Virus Disease (EVD): Report of an Advisory Panel to WHO," accessed August 7, 2017, http:// apps.who.int/iris/bitstream/10665/130997/1/WHO_HIS_KER_GHE_14.1_eng.pdf.

32. U. Schüklenk and R. Smalling, "The Moral Case for Granting Catastrophically Ill Patients the Right to Access Unregistered Medical Interventions," *Journal of Law, Medicine & Ethics* 45, no. 3 (2017): 382–91.

33. M. A. Clemens and G. Pettersson, "New Data on African Health Professionals Abroad," *Human Resources for Health* 6, no. 1 (2008), doi:10.1186/1478-4491-6-1, http://www.human-resources-health .com/content/pdf/1478-4491-6-1.pdf.

34. Schüklenk et al., "Developing World Challenges."

35. Department of Health, *Guidance on International Nursing Recruitment* (London: Department of Health, 1999), http://www.dh.gov.uk/prod_consum_dh/groups/dh_digitalassets/@dh/@en/documents/ digitalasset/dh_4034794.pdf.

2

A Bioethics for Global Mental Health

Zenon Culverhouse

ABSTRACT

Global mental health (GMH) is a rapidly growing movement supported by the World Health Organization that aims "to improve treatments . . . and reduce human rights abuses of people experiencing mental disorders," particularly among the most vulnerable populations in the global South (Patel et al. 2014, 3). Because of GMH's reliance on Western psychiatry, this movement is criticized for engaging in a form of colonialization by imposing Western concepts and treatments of mental disorder on "other" cultures, often on the assumption that local cultural norms of disorder are inferior to the scientifically rigorous concepts of psychiatry. There is, therefore, a great need to reassess the moral principles that guide psychiatric interventions in non-Western cultures. Yet bioethics as a profession has paid relatively little attention to mental health, much less to mental health in a global context. In addition, the values of mainstream bioethics are the very values encoded in GMH and criticized by its opponents. I argue that a bioethics for GMH must avoid the twin horns of colonization and ethical relativism. Proposed solutions from GMH and bioethics are on the right path by incorporating guidelines for culturally sensitive treatment, but do not go far enough. To make up for this, I utilize the framework of epistemic injustice, which identifies a fundamental harm that other solutions miss and offers a solution for avoiding it.

THE PROMISE AND PERIL OF GLOBALIZED MEDICINE

GMH developed as a movement as a result of several alarming statistics on the burden of mental health worldwide. The World Health Organization's (WHO's) *World Health Report* stated in 2001 that approximately 7.5 percent of the world's population suffers from mental disorders, with increases projected (2001, 23, 26).

It also indicates that poverty-, war-, or disaster-stricken populations bear a disproportionate burden of mental disorder (2001, 40). This report spurred the creation in 2008 of the Mental Health Gap Action Programme (mhGAP).[1] Given that low- and middle-income countries, particularly in the global South are especially burdened by mental disorder due to a relative shortage or outright lack of resources, the primary objective of WHO was, and still is, to close the "treatment gap." Providing adequate treatment in countries with limited resources has the added challenge of having to rely on "*task-sharing*, whereby non-specialist health workers are trained to take on the more routine aspects of interventions" (Cohen et al. 2014, 16).

GMH is not without its critics. While the work of psychiatrists is well intentioned and often helpful, there is a concern that as a field dominated by Western values, psychiatry imposes these values on cultures and persons as though they are the only correct values. GMH is accused of a form of colonialism or "psychiatric imperialism" (Summerfield 2013, 1) by "exporting Western illness categories and treatments that would ultimately replace diverse cultural environments for interpreting mental health" (Bemme and D'Souza 2012). Many of the examples of testimony from those involved with GMH echo the complaints of psychiatric patients in the West: psychiatrists favor objective, scientifically verifiable evidence to make a diagnosis and therefore do not take seriously the patients' own subjective assessments of their distress (Mills 2014, 1).

Excessive reliance on pharmacological treatments is also problematic, especially when it supersedes or negates religious, spiritual, or culturally specific treatments (Fernando 2010; Mills 2014, 3). Most damning is the claim that psychiatry not only undermines a person's agency but is a threat to their very identity: "Western psychological discourse is setting out to instruct, regulate, and modernise, presenting as definitive the contemporary Western way of being a person" (Summerfield 2008, 992).

Framing these criticisms of GMH in terms of principle-based bioethics, the problem is that medical practitioners override a patient's autonomy in the name of beneficence, on the assumption that the two principles conflict. If these efforts at diagnosis and treatment are harmful, then GMH is really just paternalism in disguise. The problem is made more difficult given the cross-cultural context of GMH work. The right to autonomy (i.e., the right to self-determination and individual freedom) is arguably a distinctly Western value of liberal individualism, rather than a principle universal to all persons.

Many cultures that receive aid from GMH prioritize communal decision-making over individual autonomy. In effect, GMH is accused of failing to respect individual autonomy, on the one hand, and on the other, failing to acknowledge the relevance of cultural norms in diagnosing and treating mental disorders. A bioethics for GMH will therefore have to adapt its expertise to ensure that the individual patient has a voice in managing her own mental health and that the beliefs and practices of the culture in which that patient lives are given due respect.

However, anyone looking for a thorough assessment of the ethics of global mental health will not find it in mainstream bioethics alone. The Hastings Center series produced *What Price Mental Health?* in 1995. Though this work briefly acknowledged the unique difficulties that set mental health apart from general medicine, it mainly focused on how to allocate limited health care resources between the two in the United States (Boyle and Callahan 1995, 4–5). At the same time, there was a proliferation of entries on mental health in the second edition of the *Encyclopedia of Bioethics*, with updates and additions to the third edition (Post 2003). In spite of this and several publications urging the profession to devote more attention to mental health, a survey of popular bioethics texts published over the past decade contain very little devoted to ethical issues in mental health, much less in GMH.[2] To get a clearer picture of the potential challenges to a bioethics of GMH, it is necessary to consider the ethical decision-making tools currently utilized in mainstream bioethics.

AUTONOMY-DRIVEN BIOETHICS
OF MENTAL HEALTH, PAST AND PRESENT

When the Hastings Center began to establish itself as a premier center for bioethics, mental health (at the time labeled "behavioral control") was one of five areas of focus. This focus was short-lived due to bioethics' prioritization of autonomy and its preoccupation with physical medicine and technology. One of the center's cofounders, Daniel Callahan, writes that "bioethics is a child of American individualism," which favored "principlism," prizing respect for individual freedom and autonomy above all (Callahan 1999, 58). Emphasis on the right to self-determination and resistance to paternalism in medicine was not balanced with attention to the ways in which society and culture shape individual experience (Callahan 1999, 59). In other words, the focus on autonomy neglected the fact that an individual's values are embedded in a cultural context and are given meaning by that context.

Drawing from her review of bioethics literature from this time period, Nelson states that the conception of autonomy that emerges is a "rationalistic model of decision making," in which the patient is viewed as "an independent agent faced with essentially either/or choices to be made in the context of health care" (Nelson 2003, 186). This is implied by Callahan when he laments that the focus on autonomy marginalized the value of beneficence. When it comes to medical decisions that could override a person's own desires, beneficence looks like a crude form of paternalism or, as Callahan puts it, "deciding what's good for others" (Callahan 1999, 58). At the same time that bioethics was emerging, the public was reminded of horrific conditions in mental institutions, accelerating the move from institutionalization to community-based mental health services precisely because outpatient care was deemed more conducive to autonomy.[3]

Given that the psychiatric community moved on its own toward a more autonomy-friendly model of mental health care, bioethics left psychiatry to its own devices in determining the ethics of mental health care and turned its attention back to emerging issues in physical medicine and technology (Nelson 2003, 183; Williams 2016, 224). Given all of this, it is easy to see how ethical issues regarding mental health in other countries and cultures were even less of a priority. Furthermore, it is clear that the accusation of medical colonialization against GMH could not be countered by the principlism of bioethics. Bioethics' prioritization of individual autonomy could serve as a counter to GMH's medical paternalism, but, given the neglect of social and cultural factors, bioethics would have had little to say to critics of GMH who maintain that liberal individualism is among the values dogmatically imposed on other cultures.

More recent assessments of bioethics for mental health echo this prioritization of autonomy, despite their sensitivity to ethical challenges to medicine in a global context. Nelson argues that one of the reasons bioethics has not paid enough attention to mental health is professional isolation from those who work in the mental health profession and suggests that, in engaging with them, bioethicists ought to "educate themselves, not only on the medical techniques and practices involved, but on the full range of legal, political, cultural, and above-all social aspects of mental health care. [Bioethicists] need to develop a social bioethics rather than a narrowly analytic one that disregards a person's social identity" (Nelson 2003, 192–93).

In spite of this call for "social bioethics," she ultimately prioritizes autonomy in spite of her criticisms of it: "Bioethics discourse, drawing upon a richer conceptual framework of . . . autonomy, and self-determination in relation to recovery and inclusion, could significantly contribute to a deeper understanding of the stigma surrounding mental illness" (2003, 193). Williams, who draws from Nelson, also suggests that "such a union [of bioethics and mental health] may have the greatest implications for international human rights if American bioethicists can re-energize an understanding of autonomy" (Williams 2016, 225). Again, this may serve as a counter to medical paternalism, but this alone is insufficient to meet all the charges of medical colonialization. For that, it is necessary to have a bioethics that is more culturally sensitive.

A bioethics that is culturally sensitive must address the following dilemma. When faced with conflicting cultural values, one is often caught between two possibilities, namely, that there are universal moral principles that underlie some cultural variances but are at odds with others, or that there are no such universals: morality is relative to a given culture or society. There are pitfalls in both possibilities. Ethical relativism renders impossible cross-cultural judgments of harmful practices, such as female genital mutilation. Insistence on universal moral principles runs the risk of colonialism. One need not commit to either. In her work on culture and bioethics, Gbadgesin advocates for "cultural pluralism" (Gbadgesin 2012, 32).

To avoid the twin horns of paternalism and relativism, she argues that the pluralist ought first to seek out a "consistent and intelligible" standard that may underlie various beliefs and practices. To do this, Gbadgesin proposes that one make a serious effort to understand a culture by engaging in intercultural dialogue to identify potential commonalities. In doing so, she says, cultures can establish shared moral principles that may serve as the basis for intercultural bioethics. Only then can some judgment be made about whether or not to accept the belief or practice across cultures.

Gbadgesin's pluralism is not quite *moral* pluralism. Moral pluralism, for present purposes, is the view that there is no shared, universal moral foundation that underlies diverse moral practices and beliefs (Chang 2015). For Gbadgesin, by contrast, moral practices ultimately rest on an objective foundation, namely, a "principle of human flourishing" in which "the moral weight of culture in ethics and bioethics is *relative* to its effect on human flourishing," and flourishing is fundamentally "when an individual . . . is capable of participating in the affairs of the community as a free person with human dignity" (Gbadgesin 2012, 33–34). Should a cultural norm violate that dignity, then one is justified in rejecting it.

A bioethics for mental health in a global context, by extension, should examine the practices of mental health providers to ensure that they are sensitive to cultural norms while also steering clear of those that hinder human flourishing. Again, however, Gbadgesin's notion of human flourishing prioritizes individual autonomy and implies that the person be left alone to pursue her own interests without interference from society, a hallmark of liberal individualism. If a non-Western culture does not share this value, then to avoid the risk of colonization it is necessary to revise what human flourishing is. Furthermore, Gbadgesin's argument is aimed at a bioethics of physical illness. If flourishing requires having a sound mind, a diagnosis of mental disorder may carry with it an implicit and misguided conception of human flourishing or, worse, the view that the afflicted lacks the capacity to flourish at all.

ETHICAL CHALLENGES IN GLOBAL MENTAL HEALTH

Advocates of GMH see little controversy in their aims and methods. Vikram Patel, one of the leaders in the GMH movement, says that the cross-cultural work of GMH has "put to rest any notion that mental disorders were a figment of a 'Western' imagination and that the imposition of such concepts . . . amounted to little more than an exercise in neocolonialism" (Patel 2010, 1976; Patel 2012, 6–7). Framing the notion of mental disorder as a "figment of . . .

imagination" is a straw man argument. Despite strenuous efforts by Thomas Szaz and others, very few today think that mental disorder is a complete fiction designed to pathologize normal life challenges (Szaz 1961). But there is significant resistance to the idea that mental disorders are uniform across cultures, much more to the idea that the Western concept of mental disorder is the right one (e.g., Mills 2014).

Patel states that there is consensus on a middle ground: "despite the important contextual influences on how mental disorders were experienced, explained, and acted upon, these health conditions affected people in all cultures and societies" (Patel 2012, 8). In other words, mental disorders are fixed or universal in their ontology, though diverse in their expression. For Patel, this claim has normative implications: if mental disorders are universal, then the psychiatric community is justified in locating them across cultures and basing their treatment plans on them.[4] A corollary is that the rejection of any universally valid distinction between mental disorder and health runs the risk of ethical relativism: there is no justification for favoring Western modes of psychiatric diagnosis and treatment over a culture's own, ostensibly harmful practices.

To address this problem, GMH advocates have proposed some guidelines for interacting with patients from cultures different from the provider's own that avoids appropriating local medical practices and imposing Western ones. Kirmayer and Swartz (2014), for instance, acknowledge that human beings "live within culturally constructed systems of meaning that are shared by local and global communities" (41). Thus, they also acknowledge "the central role of culture in providing local explanations for suffering and impairment" (2014, 42). They propose an "ecosocial approach that characterizes mental health problems in terms of interactions with the local social environment" that aims to "translate interventions into culturally appropriate language" and "use specific intervention methods that draw from local cultural traditions," among other things (2014, 50).

This approach is promising: it is closely parallel to Nelson's call for "social bioethics" discussed above, and the guidelines mirror Gbadgesin's suggestions to understand a given culture's values, promote intercultural dialogue, and find common ground on which to establish ethical principles for medical treatment.

These guidelines address many of the charges of colonialism made by critics of GMH, particularly its lack of sensitivity to cultural norms and practices. But, if we attend closely to the language of the guidelines, it is clear that the fit between pathology and its cultural expression is one way: rather than questioning the validity of core concepts of mental disorder in light of cultural idiosyncrasies, these concepts are imported, "translated" into or characterized in terms of culturally specific language. In doing so, the dilemma posed by bioethics between ethical relativism and paternalism rears its head again. Kirmayer and Swartz (2014) and many advocates of GMH *reject* the view that mental disorders—at least the more severe ones—are entirely "culture-bound" (45).

What emerges is a form of pluralism parallel to that proposed by Gbadgesin. In this case it is primarily ontological pluralism of mental disorder that is nonfoundational. Mental disorders are diverse in their expression but universal in their pathology. That is, these interventions assume that understanding the plurality of experience of mental disorders ultimately aims to reduce them to their underlying, universal pathology in order to prescribe appropriate treatment. If they did not, the practice of psychiatry may have to give way to ontological relativism, or the view that there is no universal pathology by which to diagnose and treat an individual.

Given the ethical implications of diagnosis and treatment, ontological pluralism of this sort can also avoid ethical relativism: there are grounds to justify treatment in opposition to cultural norms. But in doing so, it risks being impaled by the other horn: in attempting to preserve objectivity, culturally sensitive interventions that rely ultimately on Western psychiatric concepts still risk colonialization. For instance, Kirmayer and Swartz rely ultimately on the view that cultural beliefs and practices—as well as disorders—are "inscribed in the brain" (2014, 44–45, 43), which fits squarely in the dominant, Western view of mental disorders that characterizes psychiatry today.

Even if it is not disputed whether mental disorders are fixed or universal, problems can still arise in how mental disorders are conceived by the psychiatric community at large and endorsed by GMH. The effort to "translate" psychiatric interventions into cultural idioms of distress does little to address problems at the source. Some explanation is needed to show that attention to cultural idiosyncrasies in the diagnosis and treatment of mental disorder is not simply a reductive exercise, in which cultural differences are stripped away to get at the underlying, universal pathology. This effort is rendered moot if the *proposed* universal pathology turns out not to be universal after all. It is therefore necessary to consider GMH's conception of mental disorder and its underlying values.

GMH is dominated by Western psychiatry, as is evident from the definition of mental disorder stated at the start of WHO's trend-setting *World Health Report* (2001, 21): "Mental and behavioural disorders are understood as clinically significant conditions characterized by alterations in thinking, mood (emotions) or behaviour associated with personal distress and/ or impaired functioning."

Though this report explicitly refers to WHO's (1992) standard manual for diagnosis of mental disorders, namely, the *International Classification of Diseases* (*ICD*), the phrase "clinically significant" also echoes the definition of mental disorder found in all editions of the American Psychiatric Association's (1994) *Diagnostic and Statistical Manual of Mental Disorders* (*DSM*).[5] The phrase effectively makes the medical practitioner the sole arbiter of what counts as a mental disorder. Put in a global context, this problem is compounded by conflicts between the *DSM* and the *ICD*, now in its eleventh edition (2018). Fulford highlights one such conflict, in which a person receives a diagnosis of schizophrenia from the *ICD-10*, but not the *DSM-4*, precisely because the latter, and not the former, requires that the symptoms of schizophrenia significantly impair social functioning (Fulford 2003, 1790–91). While the person in question suddenly behaved in ways that were unusual, he thrived in his work and life.

In light of such an example, which is by no means rare, it is difficult to accept Patel's dismissal of the idea that mental disorders as defined by the *DSM* and *ICD* are not constructs imposed on individuals and societies. Furthermore, while Patel may be right to claim that there is a universal ontology of mental disorder, it does not follow that the *DSM* or the *ICD* provides the correct one. The values that inform psychiatric approaches to mental disorders in these manuals suggest it is not.

The discipline of psychiatry is still embroiled in controversy over whether mental disorder is a natural kind or a social construct. Both the *DSM* and *ICD*, despite efforts to acknowledge the role culture plays in shaping the experience of mental disorder, are mainly reductive. Particularly relevant is the *DSM*'s "hyponarrativity" of a given syndrome. In his analysis of values in the *DSM*, Sadler observes that "[t]o diagnose a person under the *DSM* is to reveal little of the person's biography . . . and, most importantly, how the illness experience interacts with these narrative aspects" (Sadler 2005, 177). To treat a person's disorder solely in terms of a set of symptoms marginalizes that person's own voice and effectively strips the patient of agency: the patient's subjective assessments of her own distress add little of value to an accurate diagnosis that relies on a general classification of symptoms (e.g., "distressing thoughts" or "avoidance") or, as psychiatrist Jonathan Shay puts it, "sorting the patient's words into mental bins" (Shay 1995, 10). This makes provider–patient interaction and any subsequent treatment plan effectively paternalistic. While practitioners may acknowledge shortcomings of their practice, the *DSM* and *ICD* do not provide—nor are intended to provide—any guidance on the role of patient agency and voice in diagnosis.

Hyponarrative assessments of mental disorders are largely due to the psychiatric profession's adherence to values that Sadler describes as "disease naturalism," "individualism," and "empiricism" (Sadler 2005, 177–78). Put roughly, mental disorders are universal, neurobiological pathologies that occur in an individual and are subject to scientific verification. The phenomenology of a disorder, particularly how an individual perceives her own experience, is deemed less important than the underlying ontology of the disorder, given that the underlying ontology is identified via empirical science.

On this model, treatment again focuses on the individual alone, rather than familial, societal, and otherwise shared aspects of disorder. Again, the standard manuals for diagnosis and treatment are not sufficient to address the concerns of critics of GMH. They are in fact counterproductive by advancing a concept of mental disorder that rules out the way in which mental disorders are at least partly socially constructed.

Psychiatry is rationalistic in the sense that both diagnosis and treatment are limited to the language of empirical science. It is also rationalistic insofar as mental disorder is linked to status of the patient's own rationality—another important mark of autonomy. If a mental disorder disrupts a person's ability to make rational choices, then mental disorder is associated, if not equated, with irrationality. If a person's autonomy depends on being able to make rational choices about their own treatment (the very criterion of autonomy present in mainstream bioethics), then those afflicted with mental disorders lack autonomy. But rationality, too, is a normative concept that carries certain assumptions about what standards of rationality count most.

In her work on mental disorders, philosopher Lisa Bortolotti argues that irrationality is neither necessary nor sufficient for diagnosis of a mental disorder. It is not sufficient since many instances of irrationality (e.g., beliefs that a person maintains contrary to counterevidence, such as racist beliefs), are not typically considered pathologies (Bortolotti 2015, 73). Nor is it necessary, given evidence that depressed persons make more accurate predictions as opposed to the more optimistic person (Bortolotti 2015, 74). This is relevant to the problems facing GMH for several reasons. First, if the person diagnosed with a mental disorder is not by definition irrational, then the patient is also not necessarily lacking agency and autonomy. Second, and more importantly, the practitioner is just as prone to irrationality as the patient, so proper treatment not only requires attending to the patient, but to one's own biases.

Thus far, it looks as though GMH and mainstream bioethics are moving on separate but parallel tracks. Both fields see the need to revise their fundamental principles in light of culturally specific practices without lapsing into relativism. In advocating for a "social bioethics," Nelson and Williams suggest that bioethics involve itself in the mental health field to learn its aims and practices. But given the specific problems associated with psychiatry's conception of mental disorder, looking to beliefs and practices of psychiatry for guidance will reveal only the same sorts of problems that beset bioethics in the first place, namely, prioritization of an individualistic conception of autonomy and the dilemma of colonialization and moral relativism. Where, then, might bioethics look for guidance?

ACCOUNTING FOR EPISTEMIC INJUSTICE IN GLOBAL MENTAL HEALTH

The threat of medical colonialization is not just an ethical problem, but also an epistemological problem. The values and concepts endorsed by the GMH movement can conflict with the beliefs and knowledge systems of the populations they treat. In failing to take seriously those knowledge systems either by ignoring them, overriding them, or "translating them" into psychiatric concepts, GMH is effectively committing what philosopher Miranda Fricker terms "epistemic injustice" (Fricker 2007). Framing the problems facing GMH in terms of epistemic injustice illuminates the specific harm that is caused when these problems go unacknowledged. This framework also provides substantive guidelines for avoiding harm that complement the guidelines for ethical cross-cultural mental health advocacy.

Epistemic injustice in general occurs when "someone is wronged specifically in her capacity as a knower" (Fricker 2007, 20). Fricker identifies two forms of epistemic injustice: testimonial injustice and hermeneutical injustice. Testimonial injustice occurs when a person does not take a speaker seriously, owing to a prejudice or negative stereotype that person has regarding the speaker's social identity (Fricker 2007, 28). The example Fricker gives is of an African American person not being believed by the police when reporting a crime against her due to the police officer's prejudice toward African Americans. This is easily applicable to persons suffering from mental disorders: their community and care providers do not grant them credibility due to prejudices about their identity as a mental patient. A physician ignoring a patient's subjective experience and looking only to objective, empirical evidence for a diagnosis is one such example.[6]

An important aspect of this type of injustice is that it is *systematic*. That is, the prejudice consists in a false or distorted belief about a person's membership in a group that is endemic to the society in which one lives, particularly the web of beliefs, practices, and attitudes that perpetuate negative stereotypes. In the psychiatrist's case, the web of beliefs consists in the discipline-specific conception of mental disorder, which may very well harbor prejudices about the value of a patient's own input. In Fricker's example, the particular instance of testimonial injustice occurs among members of one society.

In a cross-cultural context, things are somewhat more complicated, for there can be two systems of prejudice at work, that of psychiatry's biases about a patient's agency and rationality and the beliefs of the local culture in which the afflicted person lives that cause the person to be isolated or even institutionalized. In addition, a person's credibility could be deflated not just because of negative stereotypes about mental disorders but also about that person's race, gender, or ethnicity. GMH must contend with all of these potential biases.

Hermeneutical injustice "occurs at a prior stage, when a gap in collective interpretive resources puts someone at an unfair disadvantage when it comes to making sense of their social experiences" (Fricker 2007, 1). Fricker gives several examples, but most germane is her example of a woman who is disadvantaged because she, and society at large, lack the concept of postpartum depression. Fricker relates Susan Brownmiller's report of a woman who blamed herself (and was blamed by her husband) for her feelings of worthlessness, lack of energy, and poor concentration after childbirth until she learned about postpartum depression. Only then did she recognize that her condition was not simply a personal failure (Fricker 2007, 149). Fricker's example may oversimplify matters given the problems already identified for the values and beliefs of psychiatry.

While psychiatric categories can help make sense of one's experience in ways more beneficial than society's tendency toward moral blame, it can still hinder full credibility if it still relies on the psychiatric conception of mental disorder as hyponarrative, individualistic, empirically based, and irrational. This itself can be a misguided or insufficient hermeneutical resource for making sense of a person's disorder. In the context of cross-cultural psychiatry, where the patient's subjective experience is embedded in norms of her culture, the "gap" in hermeneutical resources can exist between patient and psychiatrist or others within the patient's own society. This gap is precisely the source of the dilemma between medical paternalism and moral relativism: GMH is caught between imposing negative prejudices encoded in psychiatric values and giving way to potentially negative prejudices of a local culture.

Being subject to epistemic injustice opens the door for a variety of other injustices, such as the sorts of harms that are typically identified by critics of GMH that result from not taking the afflicted person seriously (e.g., misdiagnosis, stigmatization, and further decline of health). But the fundamental harm of epistemic injustice is that it undermines its victim's very *identity* as a human being: "[t]o be wronged in one's capacity as a knower is to be wronged in a capacity essential to human value. . . . [O]ne suffers an intrinsic injustice" (Fricker 2007, 44). Systematically having one's capacity as a knower undermined erodes confidence in oneself, one's ability to know oneself and the world, and one's courage in standing up for one's beliefs (Fricker 2007, 49).

In other words, being subject to epistemic injustice undermines a person's agency and autonomy. It also shows that autonomy and agency are fundamentally relational.[7] A person's self-determination depends on their self-confidence which, in turn, depends on the level of credibility they are afforded as a knower *by others*. This harm is more fundamental than Gbadgesin's autonomy-based principle of human flourishing. Flourishing depends on the hermeneutical situation: if a society lacks the proper resources to make sense of their experience, no amount of self-determination or freedom is going to overcome that.

Identifying the nature and harm of epistemic injustice also reveals ways to correct for it and develop the virtue of epistemic justice. Fricker (2007) argues that "responsibility requires a distinctly *reflexive* critical social awareness" (91). The hearer must not only attend to what the speaker is saying but also attend to her own moments of cognitive dissonance, where her prejudice conflicts with what she is actually experiencing with the speaker. This should prompt reflection on whether prejudice has influenced her attitude toward the speaker.

The practice of epistemic justice in GMH therefore requires care providers to reflect on the impact that interactions with members of local cultures have on her own beliefs and revise accordingly. Recent work on addressing epistemic injustice in psychiatry applies this line of thought more generally, and in doing so it echoes many of the suggestions made by advocates of a culturally sensitive approach to GMH. Crichton et al. (2017), for instance, suggest that psychiatric training include rounds "which allow health professionals to focus on the existential, ethical, and personal aspects of a medical case" (67). Kurs and Grinshpoon (2018), too, advocate prioritizing the voice of the patient as well as sensitivity to the social and environmental factors that influence the patient's affliction (340). It is not enough, however, to understand another culture and incorporate that into one's perspective. Gathering evidence of another's status as a knower is half of the work, to be sure. But doing this alone sounds a lot like GMH's reductive exercise of translating or reducing cultural idioms to their underlying pathology.

This does little to solve the problems inherent in psychiatric concepts of mental disorders. For that, there needs to be reflection on whether conflicts between the two reveal prejudices in the collective hermeneutical resources of psychiatry. The *DSM* and *ICD* do not offer guidance for navigating the existential, ethical, and personal aspects of a person's experience of a disorder, much less reconcile them with its psychiatric conception. In fact, these manuals may resist such efforts. To get beyond this, guidance is needed from philosophy.[8]

Epistemic injustice is a valuable framework for avoiding the twin horns of paternalism and moral relativism facing GMH. Gbadgesin's principle of flourishing is meant to resolve this dilemma by offering a principle that could determine the moral value of beliefs and practices across cultures. But as I point out above, it relies on an individualistic notion of autonomy, when the harm of epistemic injustice that the principle should identify is more fundamental. Autonomy is possible only if the individual is not subject to epistemic injustices that affect her identity and self-worth.

Because of this, autonomy is also relational. Respecting autonomy is not simply a matter of counseling someone on their diagnosis and allowing her to decide what treatments to undergo, given the gap in hermeneutical resources of psychiatry. It is a collaborative effort between the care provider and patient to engage in reflection about potential prejudices that conflict with the lived experience of the patient.

While epistemic injustice helps overcome a dilemma facing GMH, it is not a failsafe solution given the unique complexities of providing mental health services in a variety of diverse contexts. For one thing, accounting for prejudices in the care provider may not be sufficient, given that the patient may be subject to additional prejudices from her community. Nevertheless, psychiatry alone is not sufficient to address these prejudices, which underscores the need for bioethics to fill the gap, particularly a bioethics that draws from rich philosophical resources such as epistemic injustice. Epistemic justice is both an intellectual and moral virtue (Fricker 2007, 120). As such, it is not an act- or duty-based moral theory but one that is grounded in a person's disposition. As I mentioned at the start, GMH relies on "task sharing" or training nonspecialists as primary care providers. This training cannot come from psychiatry alone, nor can it come in the form of guidelines or rules that satisfy a duty-based ethics.

The challenge, then, is especially great if there is a need to develop or identify affective dispositions, as well as cognitive ones. In many ways, the problem facing GMH recalls the ancient quarrel between medicine and philosophy, each with its own claim to human flourishing. It also recalls Socrates's point in Plato's *Gorgias* that, while medicine may know how to heal, it is up to the moral expert to determine when and why.

REFERENCES

American Psychiatric Association. 1994. *Diagnostic and Statistical Manual of Mental Disorders.* 4th ed. Washington, DC: American Psychiatric Association.

Bemme, D., and N. D'Souza. 2012. "Global Mental Health and Its Discontents." *Somatosphere.* Published July 23, 2012, http://somatosphere.net/2012/07/global-mental-health-and-its-discontents .html.

Bortolotti, Lisa. 2015. *Irrationality.* Cambridge: Polity.

Boyle, Philip J., and Daniel Callahan. 1995. *What Price Mental Health? The Ethics and Politics of Setting Priorities.* Washington DC: Georgetown University Press.

Brison, Susan J. 2002. *Aftermath: Violence and the Remaking of a Self.* Princeton, NJ: Princeton University Press.

Callahan, Daniel. 1999. "The Hastings Center and the Early Years of Bioethics." *Kennedy Institute for Ethics* 9, no. 1: 53–71.

Chang, R. 2015. "Value Pluralism." In *International Encyclopedia of the Social and Behavioral Sciences*, Volume 25, 2nd ed., edited by James Wright, 21–26. New York: Elsevier.

Cohen, Alex, Vikram Patel, and Harry Minas. 2014. "A Brief History of Global Mental Health." In *Global Mental Health: Principles and Practice*, edited by Vikram Patel, Harry Minas, Alex Cohen, and Martin J. Prince, 3–26. New York: Oxford University Press.

Crichton, Paul, Havi Carel, and Ian Kidd. 2017. "Epistemic Injustice in Psychiatry." *British Journal of Psychiatry Bulletin* 41: 65–70.

Fernando, Suman. 2010. *Mental Health, Race, and Culture*. London: Palgrave.

Fulford, K. M. W. 2003. "Mental Illness." In *Encyclopedia of Bioethics*, Volume 3, 3rd ed., edited by Stephen G. Post, PAGES. New York: Macmillan.

Fricker, Miranda. 2007. *Epistemic Injustice: Power and the Ethics of Knowing*. New York: Oxford University Press.

Gavey, Nicola. 2005. *Just Sex? The Cultural Scaffolding of Rape*. New York: Routledge.

Gbadgesin, Segun. 2012. "Culture and Bioethics." In *A Companion to Bioethics*, 2nd ed., edited by Helga Kuhse and Peter Singer, 24–35. Oxford: Wiley-Blackwell.

Kirmayer, Laurence J., and Leslie Swartz. 2014. "Culture and Global Mental Health." In *Global Mental Health: Principles and Practice*, edited by Vikram Patel, Harry Minas, Alex Cohen, and Martin J. Prince, 41–62. New York: Oxford University Press.

Kurs, Rena, and Alexander Grinshpoon. 2018. "Vulnerability of Individuals with Mental Disorders to Epistemic Injustice in Both Clinical and Social Domains." *Ethics & Behavior* 28, no. 4: 336–46.

Mills, China. 2014. *Decolonizing Global Mental Health*. New York: Routledge.

Nelson, Janet. 2003. "Bioethics and the Marginalization of Mental Illness." *Journal of the Society of Christian Ethics* 23, no. 2: 179–97.

Patel, Vikram. 2006. "Beyond Evidence: The Moral Case for International Mental Health. *American Journal of Psychiatry* 163, no. 9: 1312–15.

Patel, Vikram. 2010. "Global Mental Health: A New Global Health Field Comes of Age." *Journal of the American Medical Association* 303, no. 19: 1976.

Patel, Vikram. 2012. "Global Mental Health: From Science to Action." *Harvard Review of Psychiatry* 20, no. 1.

Sadler, John Z. 2005. *Values in Psychiatric Diagnosis*. Oxford: Oxford University Press.

Shay, Jonathan. 1995. *Achilles in Vietnam: Combat Trauma and the Undoing of Character*. New York: Simon & Schuster.

Szaz, Thomas. 1961. *The Myth of Mental Illness*. London: Harper.

Summerfield, Derek. 2008. "How Scientifically Valid Is the Knowledge Base of Global Mental Health?" *British Medical Journal* 336: 992–94.

Williams, Arthur R. 2016. "Opportunities in Reform: Bioethics and Mental Health Ethics." *Bioethics* 30, no. 4: 221–26.

World Health Organization. 1992. *The ICD-10 Classification of Mental and Behavioural Disorders: Clinical Descriptions and Diagnostic Guidelines*. Geneva: World Health Organization.

World Health Organization. 2001. *World Health Report 2001: Mental Health: New Understanding, New Hope*. Geneva: World Health Organization.

NOTES

1. "WHO Mental Health Gap Action Programme (mhGAP)," World Health Organization, accessed October 25, 2019, https://www.who.int/mental_health/mhgap/en/; see also Cohen et al. (2014), 15.

2. For instance, the most widely used text in bioethics, *The Principles of Biomedical Ethics*, by Beauchamp and Childress (5th edition, 2001), makes only cursory mentions of mental illness and "mental

retardation." Some recent papers addressing this neglect are Janet R. Nelson (2003) and A. R. Williams (2016).

3. The impetus toward community-based outpatient care had already been made by the federal government through the National Mental Health Act of 1946, but the proliferation of especially cruel treatments, such as electroshock therapy and lobotomies, returned the spotlight to mental asylums.

4. This is explicit in Patel et al. (2006, 1312), where he argues that the scientific basis of diagnosis being settled, it is "unethical to deny effective, acceptable, and affordable treatment."

5. WHO *World Health Report* references the *ICD-10*, which uses the phrase "clinically recognizable." The newest version, the *ICD-11* (2018), uses the phrase "clinically significant." The phrase was moved later in the definition for the most recent version of the *DSM* (*DSM-V*, 2013).

6. Crichton et al. (2017); Kurs and Grinshpoon (2018).

7. On identity as fundamentally relational, see Brison 2002.

8. Kurs and Grinshpoon (2018) suggest that patients be involved in the revision process of the *DSM*, which has the potential to address problems within psychiatric nosology (341), but without the guidance of philosophical analysis of mind/body, ethics, and related areas, psychiatry does not have the resources to address these problems.

3

Long-Term Care for Elderly People Globally

A Feminist Perspective

Rosemarie Tong

ABSTRACT

Global aging will increase the need for long-term care (LTC) worldwide. Social critics have raised serious questions about whether it is primarily the responsibility of governments, individuals, or families to provide for the requirements of elderly people. In this chapter, I speculate that families will more and more be asked to care for their elderly members. From a feminist point of view, this situation would be less worrisome if, contrary to fact, most countries were not tempted to turn to women to meet their need for more unpaid family caregivers. Asking women to leave the paid workforce to do unpaid family care work may weaken women's recent economic and social gains and jeopardize their physical and psychological health status. Therefore, I propose another solution to the family care problem, namely, a thorough deconstruction of ingrained notions about who should do paid work (men) and who should provide unpaid care work (women).

INTRODUCTION: THE GLOBAL PHENOMENON OF AGING

Aging is a global phenomenon. People are living longer in both developed and developing countries. Worldwide, approximately 531 million people were age 65 or older in 2010. This number will swell to 1.5 billion in 2050 (Kochhar 2014, 1), when, in the United States, the population of people older than 65 will surpass that of people younger than 15 (Kochhar 2014, 3). Also by 2050, the majority of people in Japan, South Korea, and Germany are likely to be older than 65 (Weisman 2060, A01). Moreover, many developing countries are aging at a faster rate than developed countries. It took the United States 69 years to increase the size of its over-age 65 population from 7 to 14 percent (Department of State 2007, 15), but Singapore accomplished this same feat in only 19 years (Department of State 2007, 7).

The primary reason for global aging are twofold. First, fertility rates are decreasing in most developing countries, as well as most developed countries. Up to 1965, the global fertility rate was five children per woman, but since then the global fertility rate has halved to 2.5 children per woman (Brilliant Maps 2015, 3). Given that the ideal replacement level is 2.0 children per woman, particularly striking is Singapore's replacement rate where it is just 0.8 percent (Brilliant Maps 2015, 3). Nearly all of Europe (except France, Ireland, and Turkey), three of the four BRIC countries (China, Russia, and Brazil), and all of Japan, Canada, and Australia are also below replacement level (Brilliant Maps 2015, 3). It is theorized that low replacement levels are largely due to strides in women's "empowerment" (Roser 2017, 10).

Among the factors said to lower people's interests, especially women's interest, in having a large number of children are (1) better education, especially education for women; (2) women's increased participation in the paid workforce; (3) lower child mortality rate; (4) decreased need for child labor in most nonagrarian countries; (5) increased prosperity in many developing, as well as developed countries (the richer people are, the more choices they have, including the choice to remain child free); (6) declining religiosity in many countries that previously espoused a biblical "be-fruitful-and-multiply" ethos; and (7) growing availability of family planning counseling and contraceptive services (Roser 2017, 10–32).

The other primary cause of global aging is the simple fact that people are living longer in many developing countries, as well as most developed countries. Between 1960 and 2000, life expectancy at birth grew from 50.4 to 71 in East Asia (Shrestha 2000, 207), from 56.8 to 70.4 in Latin American and the Caribbean (Shrestha 2000, 207), and from 69.7 to 76.9 in the United States (Arias 2002, 33). Especially noteworthy is that by 2030, South Korean women and men are expected to live to slightly more than ages 90 and age 84, respectively (Senthilingam 2017).

On the face of it, increased life expectancy and lower fertility rates would seem to be an occasion for global celebration (Kinsella and Phillips 2005, 1–42). But when human beings fail to produce enough children at the very same time they begin to live far longer lives than before, a crisis situation can be produced relatively rapidly. First, there is the most obvious problem: How do young people support elderly people, if the number of elderly people significantly exceeds the number of young people?

For example, in 2010 there were 100 US working age people for every 49 dependents (people younger than 15 and older than 65) (Kochhar 2014, 5). By 2015, that same number of US workers will need to support 66 dependents (Kochhar 2014, 5). Moreover, also by 2050, in the seven most developed countries, there will be only two workers for every one retiree in need of support (Department of State 2007, 3), and in Japan only 100 working age people for every 96 dependents (Angel 2018, 19–23).

Throughout the world, there will be a "great-grandparent boom" (Department of State 2007, 11). Working age people will find themselves simultaneously responsible for supporting more than one generation of elderly people. In China, this state of affairs is termed the "four-two-one" problem. As the first cohort of China's now-abandoned one-child policy reach adulthood, they may find themselves singly responsible for both their parents' and grandparents' LTC (Green 2014). There has even been alarmist talk in China about the "eight-four-two-one" problem: one adult Chinese child responsible for the LTC of two elderly parents, four elderly grandparents, and eight elderly great-grandparents (Liu 2008, 29).

Second, the costs of caring for large numbers of elderly people are probably greater than the costs of caring for large numbers of young people. Increasingly, chronic diseases such as diabetes, hypertension, coronary heart disease, arthritis, and dementia account for a higher percentage of the overall global disease burden (National Institute on Aging 2011, 13–15). According to the Global Burden of Disease Project, in 2008, noncommunicable diseases accounted for an estimated 86 percent of disease in high-income countries, 65 percent in middle-income countries, and a "surprising" 37 percent in low-income countries (National Institute on Aging 2011, 1). In India, where the battle against death from diarrhea, malaria, pneumonia, and other infectious diseases continues, stroke, coronary heart disease, and lung disease are the three top killers of people (World Life Expectancy 2015). Moreover, people in developing countries constitute two-thirds or more of dementia sufferers worldwide (Alzheimer's Disease International 2010).

Third, and related to the growing population of elderly people with costly chronic diseases, is the fact that, worldwide, there are not nearly enough health care workers, let alone health-care workers who specialize in geriatrics. In 2012, for example, there were only 7,356 geriatricians in the United States, and there was only about one geriatric psychiatrist for every 23,000 elderly people, a number that is going to increase to one geriatric psychiatrist for every 43,000 elderly people in 2030 (Chernof and Warshawsky 2013, 19).

Moreover, by 2020, the number of available US skilled nurses will simply be insufficient to tend to the needs of elderly US people, a reality exacerbated by a very high turnover rate for homecare workers (44 to 46 percent) and certified nurse assistants (48 percent), the workers who do the bulk of hands-on US eldercare (Chernof and Warshawsky 2013, 19–20). Among the factors explaining this turnover rate are low wages, poor employment benefits, lack of promotion opportunities, inadequate training, negative public image, lack of respect, and little direct involvement in patient-care decisions (Maun 2007).

Not surprisingly, high-income developed countries have sought to secure extra healthcare workers from low-income developing countries where hard labor is typically compensated with low wages. In a 2010 study, Martha Hill found that in the United States and United Kingdom there were about 1,000 nurses per 100,000 people, while there were only 20 nurses per 100,000 people in poor countries like Chad, Gambia, and Uganda (Hill 2010). The situation was particularly bad in Chad, where there is less than one physician for every 20,000 people and just four hospital beds for every 10,000 people. Because of increased healthcare needs and a "noticeable reduction in the number of healthcare workers due to HIV/AIDS related deaths" (Tankwanchi et al. 2015), Chad will need 300 percent more healthcare workers over the next few years. This statistic is especially worrisome given the large number of physicians and nurses who emigrate from low-income sub-Saharan African countries to high-income developed countries (Tankwanchi et al. 2015).

GOVERNMENT AS PRIMARY LTC PROVIDER

Given the state of affairs sketched above, people may think their respective governments should have the primary responsibility for providing individuals with LTC, but as it turns out an increasing number of governments are seeking to privatize healthcare services. In Russia, state-sponsored healthcare services are on the verge of collapse due to Russian's poor economy, low birth rate, and corruption among healthcare workers (Ostrousky 2005), and in China and India, ever burgeoning populations make government-funded healthcare services ever elusive (Lum 2012, 563–69). Moreover, many European countries, including some of those that had been lauded for the healthcare benefits they provide to citizens (Walker 2000, 83), now question whether their public programs can be sustained as their populations gray. Retrenchments in LTC are noticeable in Belgium, France, Greece, Italy, Portugal, Luxembourg, Germany, Netherlands, and the United Kingdom (Walker 2000, 83). Still, the Nordic countries resist the privatization of long-term healthcare insurance and/or services. For example, Norway and

Denmark remain especially committed to providing public-subsidized LTC to their citizens for two reasons: (1) their populations remain willing to pay very high taxes for social welfare programs (Blackman 2001, 185–88), and (2) their populations are decidedly opposed to marginalizing care work (Williams 2000, 57–58). Indeed, the Danish state "is based on the explicit principle of social inclusion for both older people and women of working age who are relieved of any duty to provide unpaid care work" (Blackman 2001, 184).

Other countries that have inaugurated or continue to subsidize LTC for their citizens are Japan and Israel. In 1996, the Japanese Ministry of Health and Welfare proposed and subsequently passed a publicly subsidized LTC bill for all of its elderly people (Hong and Liu 2000, 221). In 1988, Israel made LTC care in one's home a legal right (Schmid 2005, 191). Israel provides for two levels of benefits: (1) a 100 percent disability allowance for citizens who are highly dependent on help from others to carry out some activities of daily living and (2) up to a 150 percent disability allowance for citizens who are completely dependent on others to carry out most activities of daily living (Schmid 2005, 192). Eligibility is means tested, but not in the stringent ways it is tested in the United States, for example.

The United States is conspicuous among developed countries for not providing much in the way of long-term, government-subsidized LTC services. Established in 1965 the Medicare program provides US people over the age of 65 with only limited in-patient hospital costs, out-patient hospital costs, physicians' fees, medical supplies, surgical services, diagnostic tests, and prescription drug benefits. Contrary to many Americans' general belief, Medicare does not provide for any more than 100 days of care in a skilled nursing home following an at least three-day hospital stay. Moreover, the services must be related to acute healthcare needs, and the recipient must be "expected to recover" (Eisenberg 2017, 3–4). Because Medicaid does not provide funds to assist elderly US people with activities of daily living (ADLs), such as toileting, bathing, dressing, getting in and out of bed, money managing, meal preparing, shopping, and housecleaning, elderly US people who need this type of help must pay for it themselves from savings, private LTC insurance, or assistance from charities or by qualifying for the US Medicaid program (Paying for Senior Care 2018).

Established in 1964, the Medicaid program is the "default" program for LTC in the United States. It covers "functionally elligi[ble]" individuals (unable to perform at least one of six ADLs on their own) who are also very poor (without assets exceeding around $2,000 excluding a care and home). If the individual is married to someone who is living in the community, the spouse can keep roughly $120,000 in assets plus a home and car (Eisenberg 2017, 4–5). Because poverty is the entry condition for the Medicaid program, some elderly US people try to hide their assets in protected investments and/or transfer them to family members or even friends ahead of time, making themselves look like indigent people. These people are acting illegally if not also immorally, says Binstock, because they "take advantage of a program for the poor without actually being poor themselves" (Binstock 1998, 10). Therefore, if the US government determines "that you have given away or transferred your assets within the five years of the date you are applying (two and a half in California), you will be ineligible for Medicaid benefits for a period of time" (Eisenberg 2017, 5). While the asset maximum for Medicaid sounds very low, Janet Grant, regional vice president for the Great Plains Region at Aetna Medicaid says, "almost everyone has depleted their funds after a couple of years of long-term care" (Eisenberg 2017, 4, 5). The average rate in 2012 for a private room was $4,466 to $9,375 per month in a skilled nursing home and $2,414 to $5,713 per month in an assisted living residence (Consumer Reports Money Advisor 2012, 3).

Slowly the US population, like populations throughout the world, is being educated about the high cost of LTC and the fact that governments may lack sufficient funds to pay for not only it but also other traditional benefits. Specifically, the US government may require US workers to labor until they are 70 instead of 65 before receiving the first one of their Social Security checks. It is estimated that this change in Social Security alone would cut public debt by $6.2 trillion by 2085 (Fabian 2011).

In addition to the United States, many European countries and the United Kingdom have similar plans to reduce social security benefits to offset rising LTC costs. In particular, in Italy, "historically one of the most generous welfare states," men's retirement age will be raised from 62 and 60 for women to ages 69 and 70, respectively, by 2050. Even more noteworthy is the fact that Greece will raise its retirement age for men from 55 to 67 (Brown 2012). Both of these countries claim that they simply cannot fund their people's retirement years as generously as they traditionally have.

The belief that individuals should finance their own LTC is growing not only in Western countries but also in Eastern countries (Tao et al. 2007; Chan and Pang, 2007; Zhai and Qiu, 2007; Borsaubin et al. 2007; and Engelhardt 2007). For example, a sample study of Hong Kong families, healthcare professionals, and healthcare administrators showed support for the view that individuals should either save funds for their own LTC voluntarily or be required by the government to do so (Chan and Pang 2007, 422). In a similar study conducted in Beijing, there was also support for compulsory saving for LTC (Zhai and Qui 2007, 442). Moreover, Singapore already requires individuals to save for their own LTC needs (Engelhardt 2007, 520). But requiring people to work longer to finance their own LTC needs is reasonable only if the people in question are relatively healthy. Similarly, requiring people to save money for their own LTC needs is reasonable only if they can do so without jeopardizing their ability to meet their other basic needs such as food, clothing, and shelter.

So, too, it may not be reasonable to expect elderly people to purchase their own private LTC insurance. Such policies are expensive, especially if people hold them 20 years or more and never need to make a claim on them (Chernof and Warshawsky 2013, 26–29). In 2015, between seven and nine million Americans had a private LTC insurance policy, approximately 8 percent of the age 45 and older US population (Logeland 2015). That percentage has not increased appreciably in recent years despite the increase in numbers of elderly US people. Slow growth in the number of LTC insurance policyholders is not surprising given not only the high cost of LTC insurance (for example, in New York a 70-year-old person might pay between $2,650 and $9,900 a year) but also because LTC insurance companies frequently hike their rates (130 percent in some cases) (LaPonsie 2016), deny claims, and, even worse, simply go out of business (Kristof 2009). According to Howard Gleckman, in 2015, sales of new LTC insurance policies fell by 75 percent as compared to sales in 2005, and 90 percent of the carriers that were offering LTC insurance in 2005 had stopped selling them by 2015 (Gleckman 2015).

FAMILIES AS PRIMARY LTC PROVIDERS

Given that many individuals may neither be able to work into their 70s and 80s nor able to save enough funds from their low pay to meet their own LTC needs, governments are increasingly asking and, in some instances, requiring families to financially assist them (Parker and Dickerson 2001, 247). Families all over the world already do a lot of eldercare. The United

States is a case in point, where the value of family caregiving exceeds the total value of all paid long-term services and support. Does there come a point in time when it becomes simply unfair to ask family caregivers to provide for their elderly members? With respect to this sensitive issue, US bioethicist Daniel Callahan had this to say over 25 years ago when the burden of eldercare was much lower:

> [I]t is an old and hard moral question to know what we should make of demands for self-sacrifice. Most moral rules have common sense and practicality to commend them. Murder, lying, and theft ordinarily have tangibly bad consequences for those who commit such acts. Even our self-interest commends us to avoid them. Matters are otherwise when we are morally asked to give up our lives, or personal hopes, for the sake of another. Only under special circumstances can that seem to make any sense of all from the viewpoint of self-interest, even of the most benign sort. It is not for nothing that almost all Western moralities have been careful to distinguish between duty and supererogation. They all recognize that everyone cannot be a saint or a selfless paragon of altruism. The notion that we might as a matter of social policy burden families with the heroic duty of caring for the chronically ill or those in need of a course of rehabilitation that may fail and render them chronically ill or disabled ought at least to raise a red flag of warning. (Callahan 1991, 157–58)

To be sure, questioning young people's obligations to elderly people is disconcerting. If people worldwide believe that parents have the primary responsibility to care for their young children, then, why should there be any question about whether adult children should have the primary responsibility to care for their elderly parents? Why should children who take care of an elderly parent view themselves as "heroes" or "saints" rather than persons simply discharging a duty? Why should children, as in contemporary China, be legally and not simply morally required "to provide for the emotional and physical needs of their parents, which includes visiting them often or facing fines and potential jail time"? (Russo 2013).

In addressing these questions it is important to stress that although all cultures explain children's obligations to elderly parents in terms of some duty or affection for them, some cultures emphasize duty and others emphasize affection. For example, in those Asian countries with a still intact Confucian tradition, all children, but especially the oldest son, still believe it is their moral duty to take care of their elderly parents (Li 1994, 71–72).

Because parents give life to their children and take care of them until they are adults, children reason that they owe their parents a debt of gratitude. Therefore, not to take care of one's elderly parents in their years of need is shameful and enough to warrant society's condemnation (Hong and Liu, 2000, 165–82; Liu 2000, 183–99; Koyano 2000, 200–23; Hi and Chou, 2000, 224–48; Lee et al. 2000, 269–96; Wong 2000, 297–21; Yu et al. 2000, 322–38).

The need to reciprocate one's parents for the gift of life and more is felt by most adult children in the West, although the emphasis seems to be on affection rather than duty. In fact, in a now classic article, philosopher Jane English (1991) has claimed that affection, not duty, is the primary basis for adult children's obligations to parents. She comments that:

> Although I agree that there are many things that children *ought* to do for their parents, I will argue that it is inappropriate and misleading to describe them as things "owed." I will maintain that parents' voluntary sacrifices, rather than creating "debts" to be "repaid," tend to create love or "friendship." The duties of grown children are those of friends, and result from love between them and their parents, rather than being things owed in repayment for the parents' earlier sacrifices. . . . Seen in this light, parental requests for children to write home, visit, and offer them a reasonable amount of emotional and financial support in life's crises are well founded, so long as a friendship still exists. (147, 152–53)

But whether filial obligation is based mostly on duty or mostly on affection, worrisome issues still remain. For example, who has the responsibility to care for individuals who have no children or who are totally estranged from the children they do have? In modern societies, about 20 percent of women do not give birth, and this percentage is growing more rapidly than previously expected (Department of State 2007, 16). In addition, many women and men are childless because they lose their children to disease, war, or other violence. Childless single men and women are particularly vulnerable in their old age if they are poor (Lee et al. 2000, 292). Still another issue is simply that as the world ages, young people's well-being and their children's well-being are being mortgaged to provide for elderly people's well-being. In the United States, for example, a recent American Association of Retired People study "projected a dramatic decline over the next 20 years in the caregiver support ratio: from 7 potential care-givers for every person in the high-risk years of 80-plus in 2010 to 4 for every person 80-plus in 2030" (Chernof and Warshawsky 2013, 19–20).

Is it fair that an only child should have to shoulder the entire burden of caring for one or two elderly parents, whereas a child with siblings can share this duty? Similarly, is it fair for siblings to expect whichever one of them feels most obligated to help their parents to do so? Why should the most generous sibling be burdened in ways that his or her ungenerous siblings escape? Finally, is it fair to ask children in their 60s who have looked forward to their retire-ment as a responsibility-free time to become the primary caregivers for their elderly parents? (Montgomery, Borgatta, and Borgatta 2000, 33–35).

Emphasizing that caring for one's elderly parents can be burdensome is troubling. Yet it is not necessarily wrong for adult children to have reservations about being primarily responsible for their parents' LTC. Economist Carroll Estes has stressed that women in particular should think carefully before leaving their paid jobs to care for a family member. Importantly, she notes that elderly US women are not nearly as well off as elderly US men because US benefits for the elderly are gender biased against women in at least three ways. Specifically, Estes (2006) observes that:

1. Retirement income is linked to waged labor, which is itself gendered;
2. Nonwaged reproductive labor, performed predominantly by women, is not recognized or counted under state policy as labor; and
3. Retirement policy is based on a model of family status as married with male breadwin-ner (and with marital status as permanent rather than transient) (88–89).

Because of these three factors, says Estes, state policy "sustains the subordination of women by imposing a normative and preferential view of a particular family form with a male bread-winner and a dependent wife that is inherently disadvantageous to the majority of older women (the majority of whom are not married, especially among women of color and the very old." In sum, elderly US women are often poorer than elderly US men largely because they have not worked long enough in the paid workforce, instead devoting their energies to unpaid family work (Estes 2006, 89).

Caregiving does not only take a disproportionate toll on women as compared to men; it takes a toll on them health-wise. According to the Family Caregiver Alliance in the United States, "[t]he impacts of . . . women's intensive caregiving can be substantial" (Family Caregiver Alliance 2015). Various studies have found that "hallmarks" of women's caregiving experience include "a higher level of hostility and a great decline in happiness for caregivers of a family member; greater increase in systems of depression; less personal mastery and less self-acceptance; less high caregiving-related stress" (Marks et al. 2002). In addition, a 2003 study found that 26 percent of female caregivers reported fair to poor health compared to 12 percent of women generally (Australian Bureau of Statistics 2004). This is not to say that being a caregiver has no positive effects. Often women caregivers report that they feel "more purpose in life than their noncaregiving women peers" (Marks et al. 2002, 657–61). But this advantage does not negate the negative toll of eldercare on women, especially minority and low-income female caregivers. One telling study found "that the caregiving time burden falls most heavily on lower-income women: 52 percent of women caregivers with incomes at or below the national median of $35,000 spend 20+ house each week providing care" (The Commonwealth Fund 1999).

CONCLUSION

As the world's population ages, new arrangements will need to be made between governments, individuals, and families to meet elderly people's LTC requirements. No matter how the responsibilities for elderly people's LTC are allocated, however, families will continue to be called on for major help.

To be sure, many elderly people will not need much in the way of family-provided LTC. They will remain healthy enough to care for themselves (Choi and Dinse 1998, 159) or wealthy enough to hire nonfamilial caregivers (Rosen 2007, 13). Moreover, a good measure of elderly people will find government-provided LTC benefits sufficient to meet their needs. But there will still be millions of elderly people who will look to their families or family-like persons (close friends, charitable individuals/groups, people who share the same plight) for help to meet their LTC needs, and many societies will automatically call on women to provide this help. For example, after decades of sex-selecting males for their one and only child, a practice that has resulted in a dramatic sex-ratio imbalance of 119.6 males for every 100 females in China (Hudson and Boer 2008, 186), the Chinese are now starting to sex select for girls (Liu 2008, 28).

Apparently, many young Chinese couples believe that daughters are more likely than sons to minister to them in their old age. Moreover, some elderly Chinese couples that do not have a daughter or are childless are trying to acquire "a daughter" through a process akin to adoption. Advertisements for "daughters" now appear in Chinese newspapers, some of them promising ample reward to the women who answer them (Liu 2008, 29).

Clearly, unless developed and developing countries explode the gender system that captures their collective imaginations, they will run the risk of not having enough caregivers to meet their needs. The challenges of global aging present a unique opportunity to weaken the two norms that uphold the world's gender systems, namely, the ideal worker norm, theorized by Joan Williams (Williams 2000, 1), and the ideal care worker norm, alternately celebrated and criticized by feminist care ethicists (Gilligan 1982; Held 2006; Kittay 1999; Noddings 1984).

Williams (2000) reasons that "domesticity" is a rigid gender system that separates market work from family work and then structures market work "around the ideal of a worker who works full time and overtime and takes little or no time off for childbearing or child rearing." As Williams sees it, "though the ideal worker norm does not define all jobs today, it defines the good ones; full-time blue-collar jobs in the working-class context, and high-level executive and professional jobs for the middle class and above" (Williams 2000, 1). Structured in this way, market work has no patience for caregivers who are distracted by family work. Workers who put their families above their work commitments are punished with marginalization in the workforce. But this state of affairs has negative consequences for caregivers. Their marginalization disqualifies them from the rewards of market work, including not only "responsibility and authority" but also the extra money they need to care for themselves and others. The only way to change this inequitable state of affairs, argues Williams, is to make the workplace conform to the family rather than the family to the workplace. The ideal worker would then become someone who has time for both family and work and is able to care because of the way the workplace is structured.

US women continue to be the ones who worsen their social, economic, and physical/psychological health to meet their elderly relatives LTC needs (The Swaddle Team 2018). Countries that are really serious about gender equity realize that the only way not to marginalize care work is not to twick but to destroy both the ideal care worker norm and the ideal worker norm. These countries do not aim to pull women out of the paid workforce so men can stay in it. Instead, they not simply permit but also require men to take time off for family matters. For example, in Iceland, both women and men get three months' post-childbirth leave at 80 percent of their salary plus another three months they can split anyway they want. Neither the man nor the woman can transfer their three months' paternity or maternity leave to each other. Weller (2016) says "the government wants to ensure both parents can work and that kids get to spend time with both."

Significantly, most workplace family-care leave and benefit policies still emphasize childcare leaves. But, in the future, they will probably have to emphasize eldercare leaves just as much, if not more. This shift in emphasis from childcare to eldercare may, in my estimation, present new opportunities for society to view men as just as able as women to deliver care. Because women give birth to children, they were assigned the duty to rear them (Tong 2009, 85–86). But there is no equivalent "natural" reason for women to care for elderly people, and so the rationale for men not caring for elderly people is not as plausible as the rationale for men not taking caring of infants and children. Thus, men as well as women should be equally obligated to be caregivers for elderly people.

To be sure, most men did not actually do the care work assigned to them. Their wives, sisters, and daughters did it for them. Consider Japan where daughters-in-law did the brunt of eldercare, even though their husbands were officially in charge of taking care of their aged parents (Care of the Elderly 2016). But in the face of a burgeoning aging population, now may be the ideal time to ask men to develop their caregiving skills. There are too many elderly people with too many needs. Women cannot be expected to meet all of the world's increasing caregiving needs. Men will have to help women care for elderly people or elderly people will need to fend for themselves.

Men have started to care for children more than in the past (Yogman and Garfield 2016). There is simply no compelling reason they cannot also care for elderly family members' needs (Belkin 2008). To be sure, eldercare may be particularly frightening for men. The bodies of elderly people speak of diminishment, disintegration, and death—threats to the autonomous self who charts the course of *his* destiny. They speak of nature, materiality, and that which cannot be controlled but must instead be accepted. But it is precisely by coming to terms with the reality of enfleshment that men could join with women to overcome the dichotomies that are at the root of job segregation and gender inequity. Vulnerability is our common fate as human beings. We need to construct our workplaces and families in ways that acknowledge our dependence on each other. In order for us to be properly autonomous, men as well as women need to do care work. Only then will women's old age be as good as men's (Dodds 2007, 500–10).

REFERENCES

Agich, G. J. (2007). Reflections on the function of dignity in the context of caring for old people. *The Journal of Medicine and Philosophy* 32(5), 483–94.

Alzheimer's Disease International. (2010). *World Alzheimer's Report.* Retrieved on April 9, 2018 from http://www.alz.co.uk/research/files/WorldAlzheimerReportpdf.

Angel, J. L. (2018). Aging policy in a majority-minority nation. *Public Policy & Aging People* 28(1), 19–23. Retrieved on April 6, 2018 from https://doi.org/10.1093/ppar/pry005.

Arias, E. (2002). National vital statistics reports: United States life tables, 2000. *National Center for Health Statistics* 51(3), 33.

Binstock, R. H. (1998). The financing and organization of long-term care. In L. C. Walker, E. H. Bradley, and T. Wetle (eds.), *Public and private responsibilities in long-term care.* Baltimore: Johns Hopkins University Press.

Blackman, T. (2001). Conclusion: Issues and solutions. In T. Blackman, S. Brodhurst, and J. Convey, (eds.), *Social care and social exclusion.* New York: Palgrave Publishers.

Borsaubin, E. V., Chu, A., and Catalano, J. M. (2007). Perceptions of long-term care, autonomy, and dignity, by residents, family, and care-givers: The Huston experience. *The Journal of Medicine and Philosophy* 32(5), 447–64.

Brilliant Maps. (2015). The astounding drop in global fertility rates between 1970 and 2014. Retrieved on April 2, 2008 from https://brilliantmaps.com/fertility-rates/.

Brown, E. N. (2012). The takeaway: 14 countries raising retirement age. *The American Association for Retired People (AARP).* Bulletin Today.

Callahan, D. (1991). Families as caregivers: The Limits of Morality. In N. S. Jecker (ed.), *Aging and ethics: Philosophical problems in gerontology.* Totowa, NJ: Humana.

Chan, H. M., and Pang, S. (2007). Long-term care: dignity, autonomy, family integrity, and social sustainability: The Hong Kong experience. *The Journal of Medicine and Philosophy* 32(5), 401–24.

Chernof, B., and Warshawsky, M. (2013). *Commission on long-term care:* Report to the Congress, 1–58.

China Population Association. (2010). Are "four-two-one" families really a problem? (in Chinese). Retrieved on April 7, 2018, from the original article on 2011-07-07.

Consumer Reports Money Advisor. (2012). Long-term-care insurance: insurers of funding to boost premiums or stop selling policies, 3. Retrieved on April 13, 2018, from https://www.consumers-reports.org/cro/2012/081/long-terminsurance/index.htm.

Department of State and the Department of Health and Human Services, National Institute on Aging, National Institutes of Health. (2007). *Why population aging matters: A global perspective.* US Department of State.

Eisenberg, Richard. (2017). "Medicare, Medicaid, and long-term care: your questions answered." *Forbes.* Retrieved on April 12 from https://www.forbes.com/sites//2017/ 11/21/medicare-medicaid-and-long-term-care-2017/11/21/medicare-medicaid-and-long-term-care-your-questions-answered/a3e22d17699.

Engelhardt, H. T. Jr. (2007). Long-term care: The family, post-modernity, and conflicting moral life-worlds. *The Journal of Medicine and Philosophy* 32(5), 519–36.

English, J. (1991). What do grown children owe their parents? In N. S. Jecker (ed.), *Aging and ethics: philosophical problems in gerontology.* Totowa, NJ: Humana.

Estes, C. (2006). Critical feminist perspectives, aging, and social policy. In J. Baars, D. Dannefer, C. Phillipson, and A. Walker (eds.), *Aging, globalization and inequality: the new critical gerontology.* Amityville, NY: Baywood Publishing Co., Inc.

Fabian, Jordan. (2011). GOP senators: Raise retirement age to 70. Retrieved on April 14, 2018, from https://thehill.com/blogs/blog-briefing-room/news/155715-gop-senators-raise-retirement-age-to-70.

Family Caregiver Alliance. (2015). Women and caregiving: Facts and figures. https://www.caregiver.org/women-and-caregiving-facts-and-figures.

Fran, R. (2007). Which care? whose responsibility? and why family? A Confucian account of long-term care for the elderly. *The Journal of Medicine and Philosophy* 32(5), 495–518.

Fields, S. (2008, June 19). Death, be not proud. *The Washington Times*, A17.

Gilligan, C. (1982). *In a different voice.* Boston: Harvard University Press.

Gleckman, Howard. (2015). The long-term care insurance industry ponders its future. Retrieved on April 13, 2018, from https://www.forbes.com/sites/howardgleckman/2015/04/09/the-long-term -care-insurance-industry-ponders-its-future-seven-trends-to-watch/#4d6d88dcf6fe.

Green, Denis. (2014). Elderly care—coping with the 4:2:1 problem. *China Outlook.*

Held, V. (2006). *The ethics of care: Personal, political and global.* New York: Oxford University Press.

Hill, Martha. (2010). Nursing shortage knows no boundaries. *The Baltimore Sun*, September 13, 2010.

Hong, Y., and Liu, W. T. (2000). The social psychological perspective of elderly care. In W. T. Liu and H. Kendig (eds.), *Who should care for the elderly?* Singapore: Singapore University Press.

Hudson, V. M., and Boer, A. D. (2008). China's security, China's demographics: Aging, masculinization, and fertility policy. *Brown Journal of World Affairs* 14(2), Spring/Summer 2008, 185–200.

Kinsella, K., and Phillips, D. R. (2005). Global aging: the challenge of success. *Population Bulletin* 6(1), 1–42.

Kittay, E. F. (1999). *Love's labor: Essays on women, equality, and dependency.* New York: Routledge.

Kochhar, R. (2014). 10 projections for the global population in 2050. *Pew Research Center.* Retrieved on April 1, 2018, from https://www.pewresearch.org/fact-tank/2014/02/03/10-projections-for-the -global-population-in-2050/.

Kristof, Kathy. (2009). Long-term-care insurance: 4 biggest risks to avoid. Retrieved on April 15, 2018, from https://www.cbsnews.com/news/long-term-care-insurance-4-biggest-risks-to-avoid.

LaPonsie, Maryalene. (2016, March 10). The high cost of long-term care insurance (and what to use instead). *US News & World Report.* Retrieved on April 14, 2018, from https://money.usnews.com/ money/personal-finance/family-finance/articles/the-high-cost-of-long-term-care-insurance-and-what -to-use-instead.

Lee, R. L., Lee, J., Yu, E. S. H., Sun, S., and Liu, W. T. (2000). Living arrangements and elderly care: The case of Hong Kong. In W. T. Liu and H. Kendig (eds.), *Who should care for the elderly?* Singapore: Singapore University Press.

Li, C. (1994). The Confucian concept of Jen and the feminist ethics of care: A comparative study. *Hypatia* 9(1), 70–89.

Liu, M. (2008, March 17). Playing with the old blood rules. *Newsweek*, 27–29.

Liu, W. T. (2000). Values and caregiving burden: The significance of filial piety in elder care. In W. T. Liu and H. Kendig (eds.), *Who should care for the elderly?* Singapore: Singapore University Press.

Logeland, Denise. (2015). Can long-term care insurance work for more people? *Forbes.* Retrieved on April 26, 2018, from https://www.forbes.com/sites/nextavenue/2015/12/03/can-long-term-care -insurance-work-for-more-people/#3f5573ea3b35.

Lum, Terry. (2012). Long-term care in Asia. *Journal of Gerontological Social Work* 55(7), 563–69.

Marks, N., Lambert, James David, and Choi, Heejong. (2002). Transitions to caregiving, gender, and psychological well-being: A prospective U.S. national study. *Journal of Marriage and Family* 64(3), 657–67.

Mason, Barry. (2004). World health report: Life expectancy falls in poorest countries. *World Socialist Web Site.* Retrieved on April 11, 2018, from https://www.wsws.org/en/articles/2004/01/whor-j12.html.

Maun, Clint. (2007). Turnover rates and statistics in long-term care and hospitals. Retrieved on April 10, 2018, from http://clintmaun.com/index.php5?cID=265.

Montgomery, R. J. V., Borgatta, E. F., and Borgatta, M. L. (2000). Societal and family change in the burden of care. In W. T. Liu and H. Kendig (eds.), *Who should care for the elderly?* Singapore: Singapore University Press.

National Institute on Aging and World Health Organization. (2011). Global health and aging. https:// www.who.int/ageing/publications/global_health.pdf.

Noddings, N. (1984). *Caring: A feminine approach to ethics and moral education.* Berkeley: University of California Press.

Ostrousky, Arkady. (2005). Bribery in Russia up tenfold to $316 bn in four years. *Financial Times.*

Parker, M., and Dickerson, D. (2001). Resource allocation. In M. Parker and D. Dickerson (eds.), *The Cambridge medical ethics workbook: case studies commentaries and activities.* Cambridge, UK: Cambridge University Press.

Paying for Senior Care. (2018). How to pay for nursing home care/convalescence care. Retrieved on May 15, 2018, from https://www.payingforseniorcare.com/longtermcare/paying-for-nursing-homes.html.

Rosen, R. (2007). The care crisis. *Nation* 284(10), 11–16.

Roser, Max. (2017). Fertility rate. *Our World in Data.* Retrieved on April 3, 2018, from https://our worldindata.org/fertility-rate.

Russo, F. (2013). Caring for parents: Should there be a law? *Time,* July 22, 2013.

Schmid, H. (2005). The Israeli long-term care insurance law: Selected issues in providing home care services to the frail elderly. *Health and Social Care in the Community* 13(3), 191–200.

Schmid, R. E. (2008). Health care system not ready for Boomers, report says. *SFGate.* Retrieved July 1, 2008, https://www.sfgate.com/business/article/Health-care-system-not-ready-for-Boomers-report -3217790.php.

Senthilingam, Meera. (2017). South Korea will take lead in life expectancy by 2030, study predicts. CNN.

Shrestha, Laura B. (2000). Population aging in developing countries. *Health Affairs* 19(3), 207.

Tankwanchi, A. B. S., Vermund, S., and Perkins, D. (2015). Monitoring sub-Saharan African physician migration and recruitment post-adoption of the WHO code of practice: temporal and geographic patterns in the United States. Retrieved on April 27, 2018, from https://doi.org/10.1371/journal. pone.0124734.

Tao, J., & Wah, L. (2007). Dignity in long-term care for older persons: A Confucian perspective. *The Journal of Medicine and Philosophy* 32(5), 465–82.

Tao, J., Wah, L., Chan, H. M., and Fan, R. (2007). Exploring the bioethics of long-term care. *The Journal of Medicine of Philosophy* 32(5), 395–400.

The Commonwealth Fund. (1999). Informal caregivers (Fact Sheet). https://www.commonwealthfund. org/sites/default/files/documents/___media_files_publications_data_brief_1999_may_informal_ caregiving_caregiving_fact_sheet_pdf.pdf

The Economist. (2017). The Economist: longevity in rich countries. *Kyiv Post.* Retrieved on April 4, 2018, from https://www.kyivpost.com/world/economist-longevity-rich-countries.html.

The Swaddle Team. (2018). The key to being a couple with equitable, dual careers. Retrieved on April 29, 2018, from https://theswaddle.com/couple-equitable-dual-careers-long-term-planning/.

Tong, R. (2009). *Feminist thought: A more comprehensive introduction.* 3rd edition. Boulder, CO: Westview.

Walker, A. (2000). Sharing long-term care between the family and the state—a European perspective. In W. T. Liu and H. Kendig, (eds.), *Who should care for the elderly?* Singapore: Singapore University Press.

Williams, J. (2000). *Unbending gender: Why family and work conflict and what to do about it.* New York: Oxford University Press.

World Life Expectancy. (2015). World health review: China vs. India. Retrieved on April 8, 2018, from https://www.worldlifeexpectancy.com/world-health-review/china-vs-india.

Yogman, M., and Garfield, C. F. (2016). Fathers' roles in the care of development of their children: The role of pediatricians. Retrieved on April 30, 2018, from https://pediatrics.aappublications.org/ content/138/1/e20161128.

Zhai, X., and Qiu, R. Z. (2007). Perceptions of long-term care, autonomy, and dignity, by residents, family, and caregivers: The Beijing experience. *The Journal of Medicine and Philosophy* 32(5), 425–46.

4

The Human Rights Dimensions of Virginity Restoration Surgery[1]

Alison Dundes Renteln

ABSTRACT

This chapter considers the ethical issues that arise when women seek revirgination surgeries to avoid "honour"-related violence. The preoccupation with virginity in many societies exerts tremendous pressure on women to be, or at least appear to be "pure" on their wedding nights. Sometimes the cultural imperative is so serious that women fear for their lives. Although many consider this social control so objectionable that women should feel compelled to undergo these procedures that they would ban the surgeries, the question is whether the principle of autonomy should empower women to seek what ever type of medical treatment they wish, particularly if their lives are at stake. While in an ideal world hymenoplasties would be unnecessary, surgeons' refusal to perform this surgery arguably violates women's human rights.

"A woman's honor is like a match, it can only be lit once."[2]

INTRODUCTION

Although health is often treated as a neutral concept that can be analyzed in objective terms, in reality cultural context shapes the interpretation of what constitute beneficial medical practices.[3] Women may sometimes find themselves at the mercy of medical professionals who question their motivations for seeking surgical procedures. This is particularly the case regarding "elective" surgery not deemed necessary by "cosmopolitan" medicine. One such operation is hymenoplasty (also known as hymenorrhaphy), a type of reconstructive or cosmetic procedure to repair a woman's hymen (the thin membrane that stretches across the vagina). While a number of activities can cause the hymen to break, it is most commonly ruptured when a girl or woman has sexual intercourse for the first time. A ruptured hymen is, therefore, often presumed to be evidence of past sexual activity, and for a variety of reasons some women want to avoid that presumption.

Taking the hymenoplasty debate as a starting point, in this chapter I consider whether physicians should have the power to refuse women access to surgery based on their possibly misguided concern for their patients' presumed lack of autonomy or the presumption that they suffer from "false consciousness."[4] Denying adult women access to elective procedures in the name of women's rights or on the basis of other justifications raises serious questions about whether they enjoy genuine autonomy in liberal democracies.

The anatomical status of unmarried girls is a concern across the globe. According to customary law in many societies, their condition affects family honor because premarital sex is often thought to bring shame on the family.[5] Sexual activity before marriage may be dangerous for women in countries with strict codes of sexual morality, and the problem is exacerbated when women from these societies move to countries with more sexual freedom. Differing moral codes concerning sexual conduct inevitably complicate the lives of young women who move from Islamic polities to European countries.[6]

Many have to maneuver in new social worlds where more liberal attitudes toward sexual activity exist, while at the same time having to adhere to the more conservative rules of their families and communities. To function as required in both realms, some women ask surgeons to repair their hymens in order to conceal their past sexual activities.[7] While the question of whether a type of sexual behavior alters virginity may appear to be relatively trivial, for these women it can be a matter of life and death.[8] They fear that if they do not appear to be virgins on their wedding night, they may become victims of honor killings.[9]

In this context, one asks whether women seeking hymen reconstruction should be legally guaranteed access to this surgical procedure, despite the well-intentioned objections of surgeons, especially when denial of "revirgination" could result in death. In deciding how to formulate public policy regarding hymenoplasty, one should take into account the serious qualms doctors have about performing this surgery, including the commonly expressed view that hymen reconstruction perpetuates sexist attitudes toward women.[10] For surgeons, the basic question is whether performing a hymenoplasty is consistent with domestic law and international human rights standards; for women seeking the surgery, the question is whether the denial of the surgery violates their fundamental human rights.

In what follows, I assess the debate about hymen restoration. This study of a controversial surgical practice, complicated by cultural conflicts regarding its necessity, affords insight into biases inherent in the medical profession.[11] The analysis of this operation requires consideration of the motivations of those seeking it, as well as a brief assessment of the social value of virginity. Most importantly, this study demonstrates the necessity of having a realistic understanding of the consequences of defloration for women in particular cultural communities.

THE CULTURAL SIGNIFICANCE OF VIRGINITY

In some societies women are expected to be virgins when they marry;[12] this is ostensibly to ensure the paternity of future offspring.[13] Although this expectation of virginity on the wedding night was prevalent in European countries and North America in the not-so-distant past, it has ceased to play as crucial a role since the mid-twentieth century and the advent of the sexual revolution.[14] Virginity continues to be an important requirement for individuals in some communities, including Islamic societies.[15] A study of South Asian women in Ontario, for instance, emphasizes the importance of the norm of virginity in the context of explaining the cultural motivation for domestic violence.[16]

Although many assume there is a single understanding of "virginity," its meaning has changed over time and varies in different parts of the world. Scholarship about the historical significance of virginity usually associates it with an intact hymen.[17] For the purposes of this analysis, that definition is the relevant one, although it should be noted that relying on the hymen as the indicator of virginity is misleading. Not only can the appearance of an intact hymen can vary considerably[18] but, as mentioned above, its rupture can occur for reasons other than sex.

Moreover, the breaking of the hymen does not always result in bleeding. Indeed, studies indicate that only half of women observed blood during their first sexual experience.[19] This matters because traditionally, in societies in which the virginity of the bride had to be demonstrated, the presence of blood on the sheets was crucial. It is also erroneous to presume that virginity is necessarily related to what 'Westerners' might call chastity or purity. For instance, an ethnographic study of the sexual experience of young adults in Morocco noted that while young women accept the proposition that they should be virgins when they marry, they enjoy sexual intimacy without vaginal penetration.[20] The pressure to find alternative ways to have sexual experience without risking the loss of virginity, as understood in the community, has also intensified because the age of marriage has risen.

As virginity plays a significant role in marriage negotiations, families in many countries have been known to require virginity testing of their daughters. This practice has been strongly condemned by human rights organizations such as Human Rights Watch because it is regarded as an affront to women's dignity.[21] Moreover, as virginity testing is often compelled as a prerequisite to a forced marriage, it is considered even more reprehensible.[22]

In some societies rituals are performed to celebrate the virginal status of girls. For instance, regions in South Africa such as the province of KwaZulu Natal have experienced a revival of *umhlanga*—a Zulu reed dance ceremony celebrating virginity—despite vociferous protests against virginity testing.[23] To take part in *umhlanga*, girls must be "certified" virgins. Although some fear the certification may put girls at risk because it may attract men who want a virgin in order to avoid contracting AIDS, others contend that the virginity testing is actually beneficial because it protects young girls. So, despite trenchant criticisms of virginity testing,[24] some commentators defend the practice because it is accepted by the communities.[25]

While many people assume that there is no longer a preoccupation with virginity in modern societies in the twenty-first century, wedding customs in modern societies reflect the continuing importance of this "virtue," even though it is conveyed in symbolic terms. For instance, at American weddings the bride typically wears a white gown that ostensibly signifies her pure state. Before she departs for her honeymoon, it is customary for the bride to throw her bouquet, which symbolically represents her "defloration." Another wedding ritual that arguably reflects the cultural value attached to virginity is the breaking of glass. For example, at Jewish weddings after the bride and groom drink out of the same glass, the groom breaks it under his foot.[26] While it is unlikely that those participating in such rituals are deliberately perpetuating sexist or misogynistic attitudes requiring the purity of women at the time of marriage, they nevertheless they reinforce these societal understandings.

THE DEMAND FOR HYMENOPLASTY

One should not conflate virginity testing of young girls with the quite distinct debate about adult women requesting hymen restoration surgery to avoid honor-related violence.[27] An adult woman's decision to undergo a reconstructive surgery that does not involve any serious risk of physical harm has nothing to do with the question of the best interests of the child nor does it necessarily involve duress.

In Europe and North America women have been requesting hymenoplasty for the past few decades.[28] According to one study, "hymenoplasty has proliferated in various parts of Europe,"[29] and the American Society of Plastic Surgeons says vaginal surgery, including hymenoplasty, is one of the industry's fastest-growing segments.

The increase in demand for "revirgination" surgeries in European countries and North America may be a consequence of increased migration, the reality that young women are caught between two cultures, and the fact that they marry at a later age. Underlying it all, however, is women's need to avoid honour-related violence or at least allay their fears that it might occur.

As hymen repair seems to be occurring more frequently, the medical profession is addressing the question of its legitimacy with a sense of urgency.[30] The pressure on surgeons to perform hymenoplasties led to an intense discussion about the ethical challenges they face: on one hand, is the possibility that performing the surgery simply reinforces gender inequities in certain cultural milieus; on the other hand, is women's fear that they will be subjected to honour-related violence and even death if the procedure is not performed.

Such ethical dilemmas regarding hymen restoration surgery are not limited to liberal Western countries. In Iran, for example, where hymenoplasty is illegal and doctors can be prosecuted for performing it, Ahmadi remarks that some doctors nevertheless went to great lengths to do the surgery in order to protect women from honor-related violence:

> The physicians seemed to assume the moral burden of protecting these women's welfare, suggesting they would have felt morally culpable if something were to happen to them, when knowing that performing a simple medical procedure may have prevented reprisal. Perceiving the risk of not performing hymenoplasty as too great, the physicians respect the autonomy of those requesting . . . the surgery.[31]

Social science supports the claim that adult women in Europe also seek hymen repair because they fear they will be victims of honor-related violence if they are discovered not to be virgins on their wedding night.[32] Research is available on the plight of young Muslim women in Spain, Sweden, and the Netherlands.[33] In light of past research on the importance of marriage traditions to immigrants, enforcement of norms regarding sexual morality may take on a special significance for migrants to ensure the maintenance of cultural identity.[34] Scholars contend that young women caught between Islamic and European norms concerning "sexuality, virginity and marriage exposes these young women to very specific and severe forms of acculturative stress."[35] They also point out that keeping secrets from their families may result in "feelings of guilt and anxiety."[36]

Medical professionals, however, tend to handle questions of the proper nature of surgeries without adequate consideration of the consequences for their female patients, revealing the paternalism of medicine. Rather than allowing medical elites to decide a question on their own that affects the well-being of many women, it would be preferable to weigh the arguments for and against hymenoplasty.

OBJECTIONS TO HYMENOPLASTY

The primary argument against hymen restoration is that it perpetuates sexist attitudes toward women. In essence, surgeons performing the procedure would be reinforcing the patriarchal notion that women must be virgins, or at least must appear to be, on their wedding night. Even though women are the ones requesting the surgery, its performance has the effect of undermining the dignity of women. Professor Jacques Lansac, president of the National College of Gynaecologists and Obstetricians of France, comments: "The surgery is an attack on women's dignity . . . [and] liberty."[37]

This argument is reminiscent of the position taken by the Human Rights Committee when it rejected the contention by Manuel Wackenheim, a man with dwarfism, that he had the right to employment in dwarf-tossing competitions.[38] France banned the contests because they allegedly undermined the dignity of persons with disabilities. According to this line of argument, a paternalistic approach to human rights is justifiable because the state has an obligation to protect the dignity of members of a group even if particular individuals fail to appreciate how their choices and actions undermine their own self-interest.[39]

A second objection is the "virginity fraud" involved. As the purpose of the surgery is to deceive a future husband about the status of his wife's hymen and thereby create the illusion of virginity, some surgeons find the fraud involved objectionable; they regard their involvement as a form of complicity in the deceit.[40] According to this line of argument, they owe a duty not only to the woman who is the patient, but also to the husband and family.[41] This deceit is not new; for centuries women have used a number of circumvention techniques to fool their grooms on their wedding nights.[42] One trick was to ensure that the groom was sufficiently inebriated that he would not notice the difference in the bride's condition.

Techniques discussed in the literature include having midwives repair the broken hymen with needle and thread and animal membrane;[43] using a vial (or sponge or capsule) of animal's blood and surreptitiously spreading it in the appropriate place; concealing a small blade in the wedding dress to make a small cut; and substituting already bloodied sheets. Another more contemporary option is the use of kits available online; some produced in China cost as little as $30. They involve the insertion of red substance that mimics blood. A company in Germany, VirginiaCare, also claims to sell artificial hymens that are basically pouches of bovine blood.[44]

But it is the relatively new use of surgery that implicates the medical profession in the wedding night schemes and may partly explain their reluctance to perform the surgery.[45] The fact that some physicians have conscientious objections to performing the procedure should not constitute a reason for disallowing the surgery altogether, provided another surgeon can be found to operate.

A number of professional associations have taken a position opposing the surgery on the grounds that "refusal to do a hymenoplasty represented the best practice and current standard of medical care."[46] Physicians opposed to the surgery referred to a policy statement from the American College of Obstetrics and Gynaecology, "Vaginal Rejuvenation and Cosmetic Vaginal Procedures," which officially discouraged the procedure "because of a paucity of information about their safety and efficacy."[47]

The mostly consistent rejection of hymenoplasty by medical professional organizations—including the Royal College of Obstetricians and Gynaecologists and the National College of Obstetricians and Gynaecologists of France—reflects a genuine desire to undermine the patriarchal ideology that women must be virgins at the time of marriage.[48] The policy of the U.K.-based Royal College of Obstetricians and Gynaecologists states explicitly that cultural or religious norms which place women in positions of vulnerability or subservience are unacceptable. This includes cultures in which women fear for their safety if it is discovered that their hymen is perforated. . . .

   While the Standards Board supports the concept of patient and professional autonomy, it believes that any decision to provide cosmetic genital surgery should be based entirely on clinical grounds.[49]

While this position of trying to reject patriarchal logic by refusing to perform hymen repair is not without merit, it is an approach that may prove short-sighted if it winds up sacrificing the very individuals that the policy is designed to save.

   Principles of biomedical ethics also enter into the debate. The key principle is non-maleficence, or do no harm. Some doctors consider the procedure unjustifiable because the women are not "sick," the procedure is not "medically necessary," and it appears to be a type of harm or mutilation.[50] Although hymenoplasty is usually a minor surgery lasting 30–45 minutes, performed under either local or general anesthesia, it does involve some risk, as do all surgical procedures.[51] The recovery may take four to six weeks, although innovations may reduce that.[52] As a matter of principle, there is a question as to whether doctors are required to perform surgeries that may be regarded as "self-mutilation" or "self-harm" when there is no medical reason for it.[53] On this basis, surgeons might decline to operate.

   Moreover, if the women who were their patients are attacked or killed and family members are prosecuted, the physicians worry that they might be required to testify in court, which may be another disincentive to performing the surgery. Even more worrisome may be the possibility that the doctors themselves could be subject to retaliation if the family members discover that they have performed the surgery. The experience of doctors running abortion clinics in the United States surely demonstrates the possibility that communities can show their extreme displeasure when they disagree with a specific type of surgery.

   Another major concern of surgeons is the legal status of the practice. As various countries have enacted laws that ban genital surgeries, medical personnel have expressed concern about the legally ambiguous status of the procedure.[54] They contend that European laws that ban female genital mutilation (FGM) are broad in scope and appear to apply to genital cosmetic surgery and hymen repair. Although there may not yet exist a definitive interpretation of relevant statutes, the vagaries of the laws may also discourage surgeons from operating.

   The high profile prosecution of a physician in the United Kingdom suggests that this concern is not unfounded.[55] The doctor delivered a baby to a woman who had undergone female genital cutting in her homeland of Somalia. After the delivery, he stitched the area to repair tearing she had experienced during labor. To his surprise, he was prosecuted under the national law prohibiting surgery of the female genitalia. This charge was absurd insofar as the law was designed to prevent *removal* of parts of the female anatomy of little girls who lack legal capacity to consent; it was not intended to prevent surgeons from performing reconstructive surgery on consenting adult women. Fortunately, the doctor was acquitted.[56]

   This case indicates that legal officials may see fit to prosecute doctors for "revirgination" under statutes that do not clearly distinguish among different types of surgeries. That surgeons must operate in the shadow of the vague laws may, in fact, discourage them from providing reconstructive surgery that adult women urgently request and actually need.

ARGUMENTS IN FAVOR OF ALLOWING HYMENOPLASTY

The Principle of Patient Autonomy

The most significant argument in favor of hymen repair is the autonomy interest of women. Simply put, women as patients should have the ability to decide what types of surgical procedures they wish to have, whether they are medically necessary or not. That patients who are in control of their mental faculties and have legal capacity should make decisions about surgery is hardly controversial. Patient autonomy, while admittedly not an absolute principle that should be limited in extreme cases of self-harm, is a well-established principle in medical ethics.

Even if one does not subscribe to full autonomy and supports the prohibition of some procedures, women should at least be able to have reconstructive surgery. The hymenoplasty debate emerged following heated public discussion of female genital mutilation, a surgery that has been designated as a criminal offense in many jurisdictions because it is considered a form of mutilation.[57] Yet it is unclear why some types of operations are condemned as "mutilation" while others are accepted as elective procedures. Although many people in modern societies condone the pervasive trend toward "flesh wounds,"[58] FGM has usually been condemned as an extreme form of violence against women.

A new double standard has emerged, which becomes particularly evident when one considers that certain types of genital surgeries are treated as permissible, while hymenoplasties to avoid "honor"-related violence are not. In "Western" societies adult women are increasingly opting for genital surgeries for aesthetic reasons,[59] giving rise to a new field called "cosmetogynecology." According to the American Society for Aesthetic Plastic Surgery, 400 girls 18 and younger had labiaplasty in 2015—an 80 percent increase over the previous year—and a 2013 British report noted a fivefold increase over ten years.[60] These cosmetic genital surgeries have as of yet not been subject to regulation, nor have they generated much public debate about their legitimacy. This constitutes selective enforcement of laws that apply to female genitalia.

It is worth emphasizing here the major difference between FGM and hymenoplasty. Unlike female genital cutting, which involves the permanent removal of parts of the body, hymen restoration is a reconstructive surgery. Also, whereas female genital cutting is generally performed on very young girls, those seeking hymenoplasties are predominantly adult women. While some might question their judgement, it seems perfectly reasonable for the women to request the surgery when they face a credible threat of honor-related violence. Given that the surgery is restorative and requested by adults, women should be entitled to have it performed.

HUMAN RIGHTS AS A BASIS FOR HYMENOPLASTY

Not only does the principle of patient autonomy supports the argument in favor of hymenoplasty; the framework of human rights law also offers some basis for requiring that states ensure the availability of the procedure. A growing body of literature and global policies support the proposition that there is a right to health.[61] Even without such an explicit right, women arguably have a right of access to health care and medical services under existing instruments, particularly the international Covenant on Economic, Social and Cultural Rights. Article 12 stipulates that there is a human right to the highest attainable standard of health. This provision has been elaborated in General Comment Number 14 (2000), which calls for paying attention to women's right to health in particular.[62]

Although the right to health is considered a well-established human right, whether it applies to the right to surgery is not an entirely settled question. While some scholars regard it only as an "emerging" norm, others support an expansive interpretation of the right to health that includes a right to essential surgery.[63] This logic is convincing: if the International Covenant of Economic, Social, and Cultural Rights guarantees a right to the highest attainable standard of health, then this right should be construed as encompassing the right to surgery.

If such a right to surgery is accepted, there would have to be further debate about whether hymenoplasty constitutes an essential surgery. It stands to reason that this relatively innocuous procedure should be covered as essential surgery if it can spare women from violence or death. In addition, the fact that women live in fear of honor-related violence serves as a mental health argument in favour of interpreting the surgery as essential.

Another relevant human right is the right to culture. Here the argument is that women may choose to remain a part of their cultural communities despite certain oppressive, patri-archal practices, and this choice is protected by international human rights law.[64] The right to culture guarantees the right to participate in the cultural life of the community, even if the relevant moral code is inconsistent with views of external observers. Hence, women should be guaranteed access to the surgery so they can continue to take part in the major activities of their communities. Although it may seem peculiar that deceit should be authorized as part of cultural rights, it may be a necessary means by which participation can be maintained.

The right to bodily integrity is another argument women could invoke in support of access to hymenoplasty. Although usually employed as part of campaigns against surgeries such as male circumcision and FGM, there is no reason why bodily integrity must necessarily be interpreted as *prohibiting* certain forms of surgery. After traumatic and disfiguring injuries, some people might argue that they have a right to reconstructive surgery in order to *restore* their bodily integrity. In a similar vein, women can justifiably argue that they want to restore the hymen because they consider it essential for their understanding of bodily integrity and their sense of well-being.

Feminists take differing positions on the propriety of this surgery. While some oppose it because it reflects patriarchal values, others champion it as an expression of autonomy. Although it would be preferable to live in a world that no longer valued virginity and used it as a cruel means of social control, the question is whether adult women should have the right to a reconstructive procedure in the interim.

WEIGHING THE ARGUMENTS

In the previous sections I considered arguments for and against hymenoplasty. Ultimately I conclude that women should have the right to undergo the procedure if they choose to do so.[65] Patient autonomy is important and should be recognized in legal systems as a general matter and certainly with regard to reconstructive surgery. If autonomous decision-making is to be protected, then the autonomy of physicians should be protected as well. If surgeons have objections to the surgery, whether based on feminist principles, a judgement that it is medi-cally unnecessary, or other grounds, they ought to have the right to decline to do so.

The law as it is currently designed in some jurisdictions may not afford protection to doctors who perform the surgery. The fact that adult women elect to have the procedure may be insufficient to protect doctors again prosecution: the statutes may stipulate either that culture cannot justify the performance of the surgery or that consent is not a defence when the operation represents a form of mutilation.

Recognizing these risks, what policy changes should be implemented? For surgeons willing to perform hymen reconstruction, the question is whether the laws ought to be modified to address the ambiguous status of this procedure. That would at least avoid the worry that the surgery constituted a crime. For those who do not wish to perform the hymenoplasty, the code of medical ethics should permit an opt-out policy.

Questions also arise about whether doctors who do not wish to perform the procedure should be ethically required to refer women to other doctors or to other sources of counseling.[66] When young women migrate to new lands from countries that require virginity at the time of marriage, they often lack the mentoring of older women about how to handle their precarious situation. As a consequence, some medical professionals have suggested that counseling young immigrant women about possible alternatives to hymenoplasty might reduce the number of requests for this type of surgery.[67] According to one scholar, in the absence of mentors, surgeons in the Netherlands who declined to perform the surgery recommended use of the circumvention techniques mentioned earlier in the chapter.[68] Establishing more extensive counselling programmes with absolutely strict confidentiality could yield real benefits for both the young women and surgeons.

AUTONOMY IN THE MEDICAL CONTEXT

In the field of biomedical ethics, the principle of autonomy is ordinarily of paramount importance. This means in practical terms that patients should be treated with dignity and that they are entitled to decide whether or not to accept medical treatment. Leading texts emphasize that as long as patients possess legal capacity and are informed of the potential risks of medical procedures, they should be able to make their own decisions about taking drugs, having surgeries, or making changes to their lifestyles.[69] With respect to surgical ethics, the conventional wisdom is that patients should be able to choose whether or not to undergo surgeries, even if the procedures are not medically necessary. Autonomy also requires that medical professionals operate in the best interests of their patients.[70]

Interestingly, recent studies of hymenoplasty regard the decision to undergo the surgery as an act of resistance. It demonstrates that women recognize the constraints of their social environment and cleverly find means to function within that reality. Those who conduct ethnographic research increasingly highlight the "empowering" nature of the decision to "medicalize" the procedure. One study concludes with the nuanced argument that "that women seeking HR [hymen reconstruction] are both victims and agents: they cannot realistically hope to be completely free of coercive patriarchal attempts to control their bodies, but they may resist such attempts by seeking HR."[71] Nevertheless, it is still possible that by acting in this manner they reinforce patriarchal norms that demand "purity" of women.[72] Future research will reveal whether this procedure serves the interests of women or not.

CONCLUSION

In an ideal world there would be no double standard regarding premarital sex for men and women, and women would not need to deceive their husbands. Until such time as women enjoy the same liberties as men, they will have to maneuver within patriarchal systems. As they strive to circumvent the sexist customs that limit their activities, the medical profession must reconsider its ill-conceived policies recommending that surgeons refuse to provide the "revirgination." Even if one wishes that women did not have to resort to surgery to avoid serious threats to their well-being, in democratic systems the possibility of requesting reconstructive surgery should be available to them.

The empowerment of patients should mean that they can choose to have elective surgeries whether physicians are eager to perform them or not. Surgeons' refusal to operate on women seeking hymenoplasty who believe it is necessary to save their lives clearly interferes with their autonomous decision-making. They should consider the possible consequences for their patients. Whether the state is obligated to fund the surgeries is another matter, but the absence of government financing would most likely result in the further victimization of poor women if they cannot obtain hymenoplasties.

While many types of cosmetic and reconstructive surgery could be condemned as reflecting self-hatred on the part of women,[73] only some types of surgical procedures seem to attract widespread condemnation. Despite the possible negative aspects of allowing hymenoplasty, it is ultimately better to empower women to make their own health care decisions. Instead of assuming that the choice to undergo the knife reflects a lack of agency, a feminist reconsideration could regard this choice as one that is strangely empowering.

NOTES

1. This essay was previously published in Marie-Claire Foblets, Michele Graziadei, and Alison Dundes Renteln (Eds.) *Personal Autonomy in Plural Societies: A Principle and Its Paradoxes*. Routledge, 2018, pp. 206–20. Reprinted with permission.

2. K Shaheen, "Hymenoplasty: Why Do Women Get Virginity Back?" *The Daily Star* (Beirut, 8 October 2013) <www.dailystar.com.lb/News/Lebanon-News/2013/Oct-08/233897-hymenplasty-why -do-women-get-virginity-back.ashx> accessed 24 April 2017.

3. CO Airhihenbuwa, *Health and Culture: Beyond the Western Paradigm* (Sage 1995); S Johnsdotter and B Essén, "Genitals and Ethnicity: The Politics of Genital Modifications" (2010) 18 Reproductive Health Matters 29.

4. Some see this rather as a form of "relational autonomy," whereby individuals willingly allow their choices and decision-making to be constrained by their social settings. See J Nedelsky, *Law's Relations: A Relational Theory of Self, Autonomy, and Law* (Oxford University Press 2011); in Foblets et al. (Eds.) see also Deveaux (Ch. 5), Johnson (Ch. 15), Benda-Beckmann (Ch. 16), and Ali and Kazmi (Ch. 19).

5. FH Stewart, *Honor* (University of Chicago Press 1994); A Agarwal, *Crimes of Honor: An International Human Rights Perspective on Violence against Women in South Asia* (PhD Dissertation, University of Southern California 2008). Fatima Mernissi asserts that "The concepts of honour and virginity locate the prestige of a man between the legs of a woman. It is not by subjugating nature or by conquering mountains and rivers that a man secures his status, but by controlling the women related to him by blood or by marriage, and forbidding them any contact with male strangers." F Mernissi, "Virginity and Patriarchy" (1982) 5 *Women's Studies International Forum* 183. See also R Husseini, *Murder in the Name of Honour: The True Story of One Woman's Heroic Fight Against an Unbelievable Crime* (Oneworld Publications 2009) 83.

6. A Steigrad, 'Muslim Women in France Regain Virginity in Clinics' (*Reuters*, 3 April 2007) <www.reuters.com/article/us-muslimwomen-europe-virginity-idUSL2532025120070430> accessed 24 April 2017; S Meichtry and M Colchester, 'Secular, Muslim Culture Clash Ensnares French Doctors. Hymenoplasty Spotlights Debate Over Repression' *Wall Street Journal* (New York, 10 June 2008) A11;

E Sciolino and S Mekhennet, "In Europe, Debate Over Islam and Virginity" *New York Times* (New York, 11 June 2008) <www.nytimes.com/2008/06/11/world/europe/11virgin.html> accessed 24 April 2017; "More Women Becoming Virgins Again with Hymen Replacement Operations on the NHS" *Daily Mail* (London, 30 July 2010) <www.dailymail.co.uk/news/article-1298684/Surge-virginity-repair-operations -NHS.html> accessed 24 April 2017.

7. The status of this tissue is of such monumental significance that women in some societies worry about participating in athletic activities such as cycling, which can, in rare cases, result in the rupture of the hymen.

8. N Shalhoub-Kevorkian, "Imposition of Virginity Testing: A Life-Saver or a License to Kill" (2005) 60 Social Science & Medicine 1187, 1190.

9. TT Pham, *Moroccan Immigrant Women in Spain: Honor and Marriage* (Lexington Books 2014) 113.

10. G Heinrichs, "Is Hymenoplasty Anti-Feminist?" (2015) 26 *Journal of Clinical Ethics* 158.

11. Among important considerations of this practice, see, e.g., A Longmans et al., "Ethical Dilemma: Should Doctors Reconstruct the Vaginal Introitus of Adolescent Girls to Mimic the Virginal State?" (1998) 361 *British Medical Journal* 459; RJ Cook and BM Dickens, "Hymen Reconstruction: Ethical and Legal Issues" (2009) 107 *International Journal of Gynecology and Obstetrics* 266.

12. There is a double standard in that there is no such expectation for men.

13. D Holtzman and N Kulish, "Nevermore: The Hymen and the Loss of Virginity" (1996) 44 (suppl) *Journal of the American Psychoanalytic Association* 303; H Blank, *Virgin: The Untouched History* (Bloomsbury 2007); TT Dao Jensen, "Visions of Virginity in the Abstinence-Only Curriculum" (PhD Dissertation, Arizona State University 2008). For rules governing how to evaluate paternity in light of the length of gestation, see I Ghanem, *Islamic Medical Jurisprudence* (Arthur Probsthain 1982) 30. DNA tests would provide a reliable method instead.

14. Evidence of continuing concern with virginity is reflected in U.S. practices such as abstinence and virginity pledges and the 'true love waits' movement. Controversies over "slut walks" suggest that there continues to be a preoccupation with virginity in the United States; see A North, "Should 'Slut' Be Re-tired?," *New York Times* (New York, 3 February 2015) <https://op-talk.blogs.nytimes.com/2015/02/03/ should-slut-be-retired/?_r=0> accessed 24 April 2017. A sensational televised story of a few young women auctioning off their virginity for hundreds of thousands of dollars to pay for their college educa-tion and help support their families also suggests its enduring value in North America; see AB Wang, "'It's my decision.' This Woman Is Auctioning Off Her Virginity to Help Her Family" *The Washington Post* (Washington, 25 October 2016) <www.washingtonpost.com/news/wonk/wp/2016/10/25/its-my -decision-this-woman-is-auctioning-off-her-virginity-to-help-her-family/?utm_term=.6c1caa84dc6d> accessed 24 April 2017.

15. BR van Moorst et al. contend that virginity is important in the religious ethics of many groups; see "Backgrounds of women applying for hymen reconstruction, the effects of counselling on myths and misunderstandings about virginity, and the results of hymen reconstruction" (2012) 17 *The European Journal of Contraception and Reproductive Health Care* 93, 94. It also is used metaphorically to signify a lack of (business) experience, as with Richard Branson's Virgin Atlantic airlines, and high quality, as with extra virgin olive oil. For a famous essay analysing the trauma associated with the loss of virginity, see S Freud, "The Virginity Taboo" in S. Whiteside (tr), *The Psychology of Love* (Penguin Classics 2006 [1918]) 262.

16. S Hunjan and S Towson, "'Virginity is Everything': Sexuality in the Context of Intimate Partner Violence in the South Asian Community" in SD Dasgupta (ed), *Body Violence: Intimate Violence against South Asian Women in America* (Rutgers University Press 2007) 53, 59. See also Husseini (n 4) 83: "So much of the problem of violence against women in general, and specifically in so-called honor crimes, revolves around the hymen—the proof of virginity; a literal seal of virtue. It represents the 'honour' of the girl and, more importantly, of her family."

17. J-J Amy provides a definition: "*Virginity* could be defined as the *absence of any prior sexual inter-course with penetration of the vagina that caused an identifiable lesion of the hymen.*" J-J Amy, "Certificates

of Virginity and Reconstruction of the Hymen" (2008) 12 European Journal of Contraception and Re-productive Health Care 111; see also D Pollack, "Virginity Testing: International Law and Social Work Perspectives" (2008) 51 International Social Work 262–267; J Awwad et al., "Attitudes of Lebanese University Students Towards Surgical Hymen Reconstruction" (2013) 42 Archives of Sexual Behavior 1627. In Christianity some struggle to explain the status of the Virgin Mary because although conceived through the Immaculate Conception, baby Jesus arrived through vaginal birth; see M Mayblin, "People Like Us: Intimacy, Distance, and the Gender of Saints" (2014) 55 (suppl 10) *Current Anthropology* S 271.

18. Amy (n 16).

19. This fact is widely known (see, e.g., Pham [n 8] 100). Nevertheless, it seems not to have obviated the need for women to produce blood on their wedding night.

20. F Bakass, M Ferrand, and the ECAF team, "Sexual Debut in Rabat: New 'Arrangements' between the Sexes" (2013) 68 Population F 37. Surprisingly, this empirical study makes no reference to hymeno-plasty. Likewise, a study of Lebanon also mentioned that "more than half of Lebanese female university students approved premarital sexual contact without vaginal penetration." The researcher concludes: "This finding underpins the fact that sexual taboos seem to relate more to the physical state of virginity than to the virtue of chastity." See Awwad et al. (n 16) 1633.

21. Human Rights Watch, see <www.hrw.org/news/2014/12/01/un-who-condemns-virginity-tests> accessed 24 April 2017.

22. Parents sometimes take their minor daughters to doctors for testing and possible hymen restora-tion, if necessary, before marrying them off. L Kopelman, "Make Her a Virgin Again: When Medical Disputes about Minors are Cultural Clashes" (2013) 39 *Journal of Medicine and Philosophy* 8.

23. L Vincent, "Virginity Testing in South Africa: Re-Traditioning the Postcolony" (2006) 8 *Culture, Health & Sexuality* 17. For a comparative analysis of testing in Brazil and South Africa, see LB Brown, "Abject Bodies: The Politics of the Vagina in Brazil and South Africa" (2009) 56 Theoria 1.

24. For oppressive use of virginity tests, see, e.g., K Engelhart, "Brides Forced to Take Tests for Vir-ginity" *Maclean's* (Toronto, 27 July 2009) <www.macleans.ca/news/world/brides-forced-to-take-tests-for -virginity/> accessed 24 April 2017.

25. While Vincent concedes that some may object to the testing as a violation of the privacy rights of girls, her article (n 22) questions why it is treated differently from male circumcision under the Chil-dren's Rights Bill. For a defence of the testing as beneficial to girls, see A Wickström, "Virginity Testing as a Local Public Health Initiative: A 'Preventive Ritual' More than a 'Diagnostic Measure'" (2010) 16 *Journal of the Royal Anthropological Institute* 532.

26. For the association between unbroken glass and virginity, see A Dundes, "The Psychoanalytic Study of Folklore" in A Dundes, *Parsing Through Customs: Essays by a Freudian Folklorist* (University of Wisconsin Press 1987) 32. It is probably no coincidence that the barrier to women's success in the workplace is usually called the "glass ceiling."

27. Although it is difficult to know whether the restoration surgery succeeds in protecting women from honor-related violence, there is some evidence in this direction. In Egypt hymen restoration was considered responsible for reducing the rate or honor killings by 80 per cent. See P Kandela, "Egypt's Trade in Hymen Repair" (1996) 347 *Lancet* 1615; M O'Connor, "Reconstructing the Hymen: Mutila-tion or Restoration?" (2008) 16 *Journal of Law and Medicine* 164.

28. MHJ Bekker et al., "Reconstructing Hymens or Constructing Sexual Inequality? Service Provi-sion to Islamic Young Women Coping with the Demand to be a Virgin" (1996) 6 *Journal of Community & Applied Social Psychology* 329; A Chozick, "Virgin Territory: U.S. Women Seek a Second First Time. Hymen Surgery Is on the Rise and Drawing Criticism" *Wall Street Journal* (New York, 15 December 2005) A1.

29. Pham (n 8) 106; B Crumley, "The Dilemma of 'Virginity' Restoration" *Time* (New York, 13 July 2008) <http://content.time.com/time/world/article/0,8599,1822297,00.html> accessed 24 April 2017.

30. L Seng Khoo and V Senna-Fernandes, "Hymenoplasty and Virginity—An Issue of Socio-Cultural Morality and Medical Ethics" (2015/2016) 3 *PMFA News* 1.

31. A Ahmadi, "Ethical Issues in Hymenoplasty: Views from Tehran's Physicians" (2014) 40 *Journal of Medical Ethics* 430.

32. See Steigrad (n 5).

33. See especially B Essén, A Blomkvist, L Helström, and S Johnsdotter, "The experience and responses of Swedish health professionals to patients requesting virginity restoration (hymen repair)" (2010) 18 *Reproductive Health Matters* 38; see also S Ayuandini, "How Variability in Hymenoplasty Recommendations Leads to Contrasting Rates of Surgery in the Netherlands" (2017) 19 *Culture, Health, & Sexuality*; Pham (n 8); Bekker et al. (n 27).

34. F Strijbosch, "The concept of the Pela and Its Social Significance in the Community of Immigrant Moluccans in The Netherlands" (1985) 17 *Journal of Legal Pluralism* 177.

35. Ibid 331.

36. Ibid 333.

37. Steigrad (n 5). A judgment in Lille where a judge annulled a marriage because a woman had lied about being a virgin sparked great controversy.

38. *Wackenheim v France*, Communication No 854/1999: France, 26/07/2002, CCPR/C/75/D/854/1999 (Jurisprudence).

39. For a thoughtful consideration of this decision, see E Stamatopoulou, *Cultural Rights in International Law* (Martinus Nijhoff 2007) 118.

40. Insofar as all cosmetic surgery involves deceit, taken to its logical extreme this argument would require rejection of all such procedures. P de Lora, "Is Multiculturalism Bad for Health Care? The Case for Re-Virgination" (2015) *Theoretical Medicine and Bioethics* 141, 154.

41. DD Raphael, "Commentary: The Ethical Issue is Deceit" (1998) 316 *British Medical Journal* 460.

42. C Addison, "Enlightenment and Virginity" (2010) 2 *Inkanyiso: Journal of Humanities and Social Sciences* 71, 77; "Virginity for Sale" (*Marie Claire*, 20 January 2010) <www.marieclaire.com/politics/a3809/fake-hymens-for-sale/> accessed 24 April 2017; see also R Evelth, "Artificial Hymens Have Come a Long Way Since Blood-Filled Fish Bladders" *Smithsonian* (Washington, 12 August 2013) <www.smithsonianmag.com/smart-news/artificial-hymens-have-come-a-long-way-since-blood-filled-fish-bladders-27752278/> accessed 24 April 2017.

43. This is according to a former director of the Kinsey Institute for Research in *Sex, Gender, and Reproduction*, quoted in Chozick (n 27).

44. R Gert, "Women Simulate Virginity with Artificial Hymens. German Company Sells Easy-to-Use Product Ensuring Blood on Wedding Sheets" (*The Times of Israel*, 18 December 2015) <http://www.timesofisrael.com/women-simulate-virginity-with-artificial-hymens/> accessed 24 April 2017.

45. People were concerned about fake or "falsified" virginity in earlier centuries. Tassie Gwilliam provides an interesting analysis comparing faked virginity to counterfeit money, implying that the fraud devalues virginity just as "fake money devalues coinage." It also suggests women's bodies are comparable to commodities for exchange. Male authors have written at length in novels about virginity fraud or counterfeit maidenhead; see T Gwilliam, "Counterfeit Maidenheads in the Eighteenth Century" (1996) 6 *Journal of the History of Sexuality* 518. In an influential essay, Fatima Mernissi refers to the phenomenon as "artificial virginity" (n 4).

46. Kopelman (n 21) 10.

47. Despite the declared "paucity of information," the committee that issued the policy warned that the surgery "could cause scarring, pain, altered sensation, and sexual dysfunction"; see Kopelman (n 21) 10.

48. See Royal College of Obstetricians and Gynaecologists, Statement No. 6, "Hymenoplasty and Labial Surgery" (July 2009) 1–3 and a subsequent position paper. This document lists the organizations in other countries such as France, New Zealand, Malaysia opposed to hymenoplasty. But see the Swedish National Board of Health and Welfare's Ethical Committee's Protocol No. 43 (19 March 2004) (discussed in Essén et al. [n 32] 42–43) which allows the surgery if a woman's life is in danger.

49. See Royal College of Obstetricians and Gynaecologists, Statement No. 6, "Hymenoplasty and Labial Surgery" (July 2009) 1–3.

50. For a discussion of whether consent should be treated as a defense to self-harm, see AD Renteln, "Cutting Edge Debates: A Cross-Cultural Consideration of Surgery" in W Teays et al. (eds), *Global Bioethics and Human Rights: Contemporary Issues* (Rowman & Littlefield 2014) 220, and DJ Baker, *The Right Not to Be Criminalized: Demarcating Criminal Law's Authority* (Ashgate 2011).

51. Amy (n 16) 112; Steigrad (n 5).

52. D Shaw and BM Dickens, "A New Surgical Technique of Hymenoplasty: A Solution, but for Which Problem" (2015) 130 *International Journal of Gynecology and Obstetrics* 1.

53. For a discussion of the ethics of amputation for individuals who want to have certain body parts removed when there is no medical necessity, see D Patrone, "Disfigured Anatomies and Imperfect Analogies: Body Integrity Identity Disorder and the Supposed Right to Self-Demanded Amputation of Healthy Body Parts" (2009) 35 *Journal of Medical Ethics* 541. This topic is beyond the scope of this analysis, and has little bearing on my argument inasmuch as the operation central here is *reconstructive* surgery.

54. O'Connor (n 26) 16.

55. S Laville, "First FGM Prosecution: How the Case Came to Court" *The Guardian* (London, 14 February 2015) <www.theguardian.com/society/2015/feb/04/first-female-genital-mutilation-prosecution-dhanuson-dharmasena-fgm> accessed 24 April 2017.

56. S Laville, "Doctor Found Not Guilty of FGM on Patient at London Hospital" *The Guardian* (London, 4 February 2015) <www.theguardian.com/society/2015/feb/04/doctor-not-guilty-fgm-dhanuson-dharmasena> accessed 24 April 2017.

57. See, e.g., M Mabilia, "FGM or FGMo? Cross-Cultural Dialogue in an Italian Minefield" (2013) 29 Anthropology Today 17.

58. See, e.g., V Blum, *Flesh Wounds: The Culture of Cosmetic Surgery* (University of California Press 2005).

59. Johnsdotter and Essén (n 2); BJ Hill, *Supra-Natural: Genderventions and Genitalia* (PhD Dissertation, Indiana University 2013) 101.

60. RC Rabin, "A Baffling Trend in Surgery: More Teenage Girls are Seeking Cosmetic Changes to Genitalia" *New York Times* (New York, 26 April 2016) D4.

61. BCA Toebes, *The Right to Health as a Human Right in International Law* (Intersentia/Hart 1999). Toebes discusses women's health issues but makes no mention of hymenoplasty.

62. See <www.refworld.org/pdfid/4538838d0.pdf> accessed 24 April 2017.

63. See, e.g., KA McQueen et al., "Essential Surgery: Integral to the Right to Health" (2010) 12 Health and Human Rights 137; Renteln (n 49).

64. LL Veazey, *A Woman's Right to Culture; Toward Gendered Cultural Rights* (Quid Pro, LLC 2015).

65. For an argument in favor, see de Lora (n 39) 141.

66. S Bastami, "When Bleeding Is Vital: Surgically Ensuring the 'Virginal' State" (2015) 26 *Journal of Clinical Ethics* 154. In the U.S. a survey of 1,000 physicians showed they were divided over the question of referral.

67. S Ayuandini, "Finger Pricks and Blood Vials: How Doctors Medicalize 'Cultural' Solutions to Demedicalize the 'Broken' Hymen in the Netherlands" (2017) 177 *Social Science & Medicine* 61, 64.

68. Ibid.

69. R Young, "Informed Consent and Patient Autonomy" in H Kuhse and P Singer (eds), *A Companion to Bioethics* (2nd ed, Wiley-Blackwell 2009) 530; TL Beauchamp and JF Childress, *Principles of Biomedical Ethics* (6th ed, Oxford University Press 2009) 99.

70. A McLean, *Autonomy, Informed Consent and Medical Law: A Relational Challenge* (Cambridge University Press 2009).

71. V Wild et al., "Hymen Reconstruction as Pragmatic Empowerment? Results of a Qualitative Study from Tunisia" (2015) 147 *Social Science & Medicine* 54, 60.

72. M Kaivanara, "Virginity Dilemma: Re-Creating Virginity Through Hymenoplasty in Iran" (2016) 18 *Culture, Health & Sexuality* 71, 81.

73. V Pitts-Taylor, "Becoming/Being a Cosmetic Surgery Patient" (2009) 10 *Studies in Gender and Sexuality* 119.

5

Immigration Detention and the Right to Health Care

Rita Manning

ABSTRACT

There are now over 1.1 million people overseen by Immigration and Customs Enforcement (ICE), with about 33,000 detained in jails and federal detention centers around the United States at any particular time. The average detention time is two months, but some are detained for much longer periods. Since its inception, 121 deaths and countless cases of medical neglect have occurred. Given its secrecy and lack of oversight, it is not clear how many of these deaths are the result of inadequate medical care. ICE is a branch of a government agency in a democratic country, thus citizens have an obligation to ensure that it operates in conformity with the fundamental principles of justice on which this nation was founded. ICE is a young and rapidly growing bureaucracy with little oversight. It operates using a mix of federal, state, local and private centers, many of which are penal institutions. It has a history of abuse, and even when in conformity with its penal standards, it inflicts additional harm onto vulnerable people, especially asylum seekers and parents of minor children. It thus requires constant vigilance and concern. Our immigration policies and detention practices are deeply troubling, but until we elect to reform them, we have a special obligation to the vulnerable populations that we house in ICE detention.

INTRODUCTION

Francisco Castaneda came to the United States when he was ten years old, a refugee from the civil war in El Salvador. His mother died before she could apply for refugee status for the family, and Francisco ended up in ICE detention following his arrest for minor drug charges. Francisco repeatedly requested medical attention for a lesion on his penis, but was repeatedly denied care until the settlement of an ACLU lawsuit on his behalf. He subsequently died of penile cancer in 2008, at the age of 35 (Mooty 2010).

Victoria Arellano, a transgender woman from Mexico with AIDS, was detained in 2007. During detention, she was given her AIDS medication on a very random schedule. Despite repeated requests for help, and symptoms ranging from nausea, vomiting blood, and fever,

ICE denied her medical care until a week before her death. She died from pneumonia and meningitis at the age of 23 (Papst 2009).

These cases are truly horrifying, and given its secrecy, and lack of accountability and oversight, it is not clear how many of the one hundred and twenty one deaths that have occurred to date in ICE detention are equally the result of grossly inadequate medical care (ICE detainee deaths). In what follows, I will describe the problem in more detail and argue that ICE has a moral obligation to offer adequate medical care to all its detainees.

GLOBAL BACKGROUND

There are approximately 191 million displaced persons in the world. Of that number, about 17 million are designated by the UN High Commission on Refugees as refugees and stateless persons, with an additional 16 million person internally displaced (UN High Commission on Refugees). In the United States, there are approximately 11.2 million undocumented persons (Passel and Taylor 2010). Just under 50,000 of that number are asylum seekers (UN High Commission on Refugees). While undocumented persons do have some limited rights to health care in the United States, in practice their access to health care is extremely limited. *Plyer v. Doe* (1982) ruled that undocumented people were persons under the Fourteenth Amendment whose fundamental rights, including, presumably some rights to health care, were thereby protected.

The 1986 Emergency Medical Treatment and Active Labor Act (EMTALA) mandates that all persons are entitled to receive emergency medical care until their condition is stabilized, but the 1996 Personal Responsibility and Work Opportunity Reconciliation Act (PRWORA) restricted most federal public benefits, including health care, for all classes of immigrants, legal and undocumented. One could argue that all persons have a right to health care, but here I will make a more modest claim, that those undocumented persons who are held in immigration detention are entitled to appropriate health care. Since many medical conditions may be a natural consequence of the current ICE detention practices, this may turn out to be a far-ranging critique.

There are now over 1.1 million people overseen by ICE, with about 33,000 detained in jails and federal detention centers around the country at any particular time (Schriro 2009). The average detention time is two months, but some are detained for much longer periods. Some detainees from the Mariel boat lift from Cuba were detained for thirty years until the Supreme Court ordered their release (*Clark v. Martinez* 2005).

But the United States is not alone in detaining undocumented persons. This practice also occurs in Austria, Canada, Finland, Germany, Mexico, Netherlands, the United Kingdom, Japan, France, Italy, Greece, Spain, and Australia (Global Detention Project). While I think that a similar argument could be made for access to health care in all these countries, I will confine my remarks to immigration detention in the United States. Before I begin my argument, a bit of background is in order.

US IMMIGRATION DETENTION POLICIES

The United States began detaining immigrants at Ellis Island in 1852, but this practice was largely discarded until the 1996 Illegal Immigration Reform and Immigrant Responsibility Act. Among its provisions are the following:

1. Most criminal offenses are grounds for mandatory, permanent deportation and this provision applies even to offenses committed before the enactment of this legislation.
2. Mandatory detention is the norm for those in deportation proceedings.
3. The elimination of the right to federal review of INS (The Homeland Security Act of 2002 replaced INS with Immigration and Customs Enforcement, ICE; United States Citizenship and Immigration Services; and Bureau of Customs and Border Protection) decisions,
4. Expedited removal procedures that allow INS (now ICE) employees broad discretion to deny admission, even to asylum seekers.
5. Evidence not available to immigrants or their lawyers can be used in deportation proceedings.

The 1996 Antiterrorism and Effective Death Penalty Act allows states to collaborate with Homeland Security in enforcing illegal immigration via 287(g) agreements. Florida was the first state to enter into a 287(g) agreement, which it did in 2002, and currently there are sixty-nine agencies in twenty-four states with 287(g) agreements (ICE factsheet).

While ICE's emphasis on deporting immigrant "criminals" suggests that these are the only persons in ICE detention, this is far from the case. The categories of persons in ICE detention include asylum seekers; undocumented persons who are not asylum seekers, but who are not accused of any crime; undocumented persons who are accused of trivial offenses, including identity theft or felonious reentry; undocumented persons accused of serious offenses; and legal permanent residents who have committed a deportable offense. Until 2009, ICE also detained the children of undocumented adults, most of whom were American citizens. The practice of detaining "unaccompanied alien children" ended in 2003 with the transfer of these children to the Office of Refugee Resettlement.

ICE currently houses detainees in at least sixty-nine detention facilities (ICE detention reform). This is a constantly shifting number because ICE operates three different kinds of centers: Service Processing Centers (SPCs) that are run by ICE, Contract Detention Facilities (CDFs) that are run by private prison companies like Corrections Corporation of America and GEO, and centers run under contract with state or local government correctional agencies.

Various concerns have been raised about these detention centers: they are often distant from the detainee's place of residence making legal representation very difficult. In the prisons and jails that lease space to ICE, detainees are treated, in most respects, like prisoners, regardless of their status. Because correctional space is committed to other uses, detainees are transferred often and with little notice, making it difficult to find detainees. (ICE recently included a detainee locator device on its website.) Even when detainees can be located and are at a facility that allows the possibility of visitation, it is difficult and limited.

All detention centers require visitors to possess valid government issued identification, and many family members of detained persons may not have such documents. Various other restrictions are put on visitation with some centers mandating that all visits be noncontact and limited to 30 minutes (ICE visitation).

CONCERNS ABOUT ICE HEALTH CARE

Finally, a number of very serious concerns have been raised about the lack of adequate health care in ICE detention facilities (Priest and Goldstein 2008; Keller 2003; Guzman 2009). Homer D. Venters, an attending physician at the Bellevue/NYU Program for Survivors of

Torture, in New York City, said that "after adjusting for average length of detention, the data show that the mortality rate increased 29% between 2006 and 2007, from 27 to 34 per 100 000 detention-years" (AMA 2008).

First, though ICE adopted standards for the provision of health care in 2008, these standards were developed for penal institutions and are thus inappropriate for civil detention (Pabst 2009). Second, there are no clear provisions for enforcing the standards—and the number of serious complaints continue to arise. These range from suicide (Goldstein and Priest 2008) and lack of treatment for mental illness (Tillman 2009) to the denial of abortion services for a detainee who was raped (Walden 2009) to preventable deaths (Ferrell 2008; Florida Immigration Advocacy Center 2009). Concerns about the lack of translators and health care staff indifference and incompetence have also been raised (Mooty 2010).

ICE recently agreed to provide immigration detainees at two of its facilities with "constitutionally adequate levels of medical and mental health care" as part of an agreement to settle an American Civil Liberties Union lawsuit (*Woods v. Morton* Settlement). While this is clearly a step in the right direction, the limit of the agreement to two sites, and ICE's history of intransigence on this issue suggest that continued vigilance and oversight is warranted. Kelsey Pabst summarizes the reports of ICE Inspector General for the years 2004–6 and notes that despite the serious violations, as of 2008, ICE had not even responded to the report (Pabst 2009).

I begin by distinguishing three categories of medical conditions, one of which imposes a different sort of moral obligation. The first is preexisting conditions, the second those that occur in detention but which have no causal connection to the conditions of detention, and the third are conditions that have a causal relationship to detention. All of the arguments I shall give for our obligation to provide adequate health care to detainees apply to all three categories of detainees, but the last category of detainees provides an especially compelling case. Here, we are obligated to mitigate the harm that is created by the detention practices that the United States chooses to employ.

Many detainees will enter detention with preexisting conditions. This is not surprising since this is a very vulnerable population. Most left their home countries for economic reasons and their immigration status makes it very difficult to obtain care in the United States. The federal Emergency Medical Treatment and Active Labor Act (EMTALA) requires that hospitals treat and stabilize patients who present with emergencies, but at the same time there are no requirements to offer long term or curative care.

In addition, the Personal Responsibility and Work Opportunity Reconciliation Act (PRWORA) restricts most federal public benefits, including medical care, for all classes of immigrants, legal and undocumented. Many hospitals are currently dealing with this conflict by repatriating undocumented patients, often without their fully informed consent (Johnson 2009; Bresa 2010; Babu and Wolpin 2010). It is reasonable to suppose that part of the reason why some people enter detention with preexisting conditions is because of the restrictions on access to health care that are enshrined in federal law.

The second category includes those that occur in detention but which have no causal connection to the conditions of detention. The final category is conditions that are either exacerbated or caused by the detention itself. Foremost among these are mental health problems.

MENTAL HEALTH ISSUES IN ICE DETENTION

The psychological effects of detention are profound and long lasting. Coffee et al. describe some of the mental health problems directly attributable to detention: isolation and fractured relationships, demoralization and depression, and changes in view of self (Coffey et al. 2010). When the detainee is an asylum seeker, these problems are magnified through the lens of their previous mistreatment. Cutler cites problems in this population ranging from "anxiety to features of depressive illness, and features of post-traumatic stress to more serious conditions such as self-harm and suicide attempts" (Cutler 2005). These problems are especially serious for mothers. As one immigration attorney described it,

> It seems to me that there are so many unique issues with [detained] women. It's a higher psychological toll to be separated from their children. It gets to the point where you cannot even communicate with your client at all [because they are so distraught]. With men, there's definitely an impact, but with women it takes over their entire being. Anybody who works with women detainees who have been transferred away from children will tell you it's so much more emotionally taxing for them. (Rabin 2009)

While ICE claims to be continually upgrading its health care, as of May 2011, the only "reforms" they cite in the area of mental health are convening one workshop and a "full day mental health roundtable" (ICE detention reform).

COLLATERAL DAMAGE

The effect of ICE detention extends well beyond the detainee. Communities are undermined by the absence of contributing members. The fear of ICE detection encourages people to stay away from community activities and to endure abusive living and working conditions (Ray 2006; Kim 2009). The children of detained parents will often have the parent detained at a distant location, and in the worst case, the child will lose the parent through deportation. If the child is among the approximately 4 million US-born children with at least one noncitizen parent, and 79 percent of the children with undocumented parents were born in the United States (Passel and Taylor 2010), she may well face a devastating choice: to remain in the United States without the parent or move to a unfamiliar country, with prospects that are likely to be exceedingly poor (Rome 2010).

Since the experience of having one's parent detained in a prison like facility to which one has little access is very similar to the experience of having one's parent incarcerated for a criminal offense in a correctional institution, one would expect that long term effects on children of parents detained by ICE would be roughly similar to those experienced by children of incarcerated parents. These consequences include severe and trauma-related stress: depression and difficulty forming attachments, difficulty sleeping and concentrating; withdrawing emotionally; cognitive delays; difficulty developing trust, autonomy, initiative, productivity, and achieving identity (Miller 2006).

ARGUMENTS FOR OBLIGATION TO DETAINEES: PUBLIC HEALTH

There are a number of arguments for the obligation to provide health services to detainees, and many of these arguments parallel the arguments offered in support of medical care for immigrants generally. The first is public health. Some of the detainees will later be released and they may pose a threat to themselves or others if their health concerns are not addressed.

One of the problems with this argument is that it does not go far enough. One could address this concern by offering services only to those that have a high probability of release into the United States, or to those who have a medical condition that would pose a public health hazard. Of course defenders of this argument point out that one doesn't know who will constitute a public health hazard until they have been medically assessed. The CDC (2005) discussion of the prevalence of asymptomatic tuberculosis is instructive here.

JUSTICE

The question of justice most often comes up in bioethics in the context of the allocation of health care. The relevant issue for this paper is whether and when persons are entitled to a minimum standard of health care. Rawls's (1999) principle of equal opportunity is often appealed to in this context. He argues that, in a fair bargaining situation, all persons would agree that everyone is entitled to equal opportunity. Meaningful equal opportunity requires, among other things, a right to a least a minimum standard of health care.

Defenders of a right to health care, such as Norman Daniels, argue that failure to respect this right is fundamentally unjust (Daniels 1998). This injustice is compounded when we note that people in ICE detention are unable to access health care on their own. Thus, even if one were persuaded that the right to health care is merely a negative right—one which requires only that others refrain from interfering with a person's act of securing health care—one would have to grant that the conditions of detention must either allow health care providers access to their detainee patients, or, if security requires limiting outside access, that health care be provided by ICE.

Critics might allege that a right to health care is something that society need only respect for its members and that persons in ICE detention are at best future members. But most defenders of the equal right to health care would base such a right on membership, not in any particular political community, but in the human community. Thus, the denial of health care violates a fundamental human right.

Defenders of a right to health care would argue that failure to provide at least a minimum standard of health care is fundamentally unjust (Daniels 1998). This injustice is compounded when we note that people in ICE detention are unable to access health care on their own. Thus, even if one were persuaded that the right to health care is merely a negative right—one which requires only that others refrain from interfering with a person's act of securing health care—one would have to grant that the conditions of detention must either allow health care providers access to their detainee patients, or, if security requires limiting outside access, that health care be provided by ICE.

Critics might allege that a right to health care is something that society need only respect for its members and that persons in ICE detention are at best future members. But most defenders of the equal right to health care would base such a right on membership, not in any particular political community, but in the human community. Thus, the denial of health care violates a fundamental human right.

PROFESSIONAL RESPONSIBILITY

The third argument appeals to the professional responsibility of detention medical staff. They may be ICE employees or contractors, but I would argue that even in this conflict of dual loyalties, their professional responsibility is primarily as health care practitioners. We can appeal here to four principles generally recognized in health care ethics: autonomy, justice, beneficence, and nonmaleficence. I think it is fairly obvious that denying appropriate health care to detainees runs afoul of some of these principles. Presumably no rational person would choose to have their health issues ignored. Beneficence points in the direction of offering care, and nonmaleficence deems cooperation of health care practitioners in detention practices which exacerbate health problems as professionally irresponsible. This provides another reason for thinking that the dual loyalty conflict must be settled in favor of the detainee patient.

STATE COERCION

The next argument is that state coercion is a sufficient condition for having certain basic rights. These rights include the right to participate in the government in some fashion. Michael Walzer argues that "the processes of self-determination through which a democratic state shapes its internal life, must be open, and equally open, to all those men and women who live within its territory, work in the local economy, and are subject to local law" (Walzer 1984). Following Henry Shue (1996), I would argue that this fundamental political right cannot be meaningfully exercised unless one's basic subsistence rights are also provided for.

The Supreme Court made a similar argument in *Plyer v. Doe* where they claimed that undocumented children were persons under the Fourteenth Amendment and thus entitled to protection of their basic rights. One might respond here that no one is coerced into illegally migrating into the United States. I have two responses. The first is that there is indeed an element of coercion here and I will return to this in the discussion of the US role in causing migration. Second, once a person is in ICE detention, they are subject to substantial state coercion and thus should have some protections against the excessive use of state power. This leads into the next argument.

CRUEL AND UNUSUAL PUNISHMENT

The next argument applies specifically in the case of ICE detention. The Supreme Court has ruled that the denial of health care to incarcerated persons constitutes impermissible cruel and unusual punishment (*Brown v. Plata* 2011). As Justice Kennedy writes in *Plata*,

> As a consequence of their own actions, prisoners may be deprived of rights that are fundamental to liberty. Yet the law and the Constitution demand recognition of certain other rights. Prisoners retain the essence of human dignity inherent in all persons. Respect for that dignity animates the Eighth Amendment prohibition against cruel and unusual punishment. . . . To incarcerate, society takes from prisoners the means to provide for their own needs. . . . A prison that deprives prisoners of basic sustenance, including adequate medical care, is incompatible with the concept of human dignity and has no place in civilized society.

One might argue here that immigration detention is not identical to criminal incarceration and thus that *Plata* does not apply. However, in *Youngsberg v. Romero* (1982) the Supreme Court held that persons who are involuntarily committed are entitled to better treatment than convicted criminals "whose conditions of confinement are designed to punish." Thus I would argue that ICE detainees, who are subject to administrative and not criminal proceedings, are constitutionally entitled to adequate medical care.

DUE PROCESS

Detainees are detained during the processing of their various immigration pleas and while awaiting arrangements to be deported. During this process, they are constitutionally entitled to due process (*Demore v. Kim* 2003). Here we can appeal again to Shue's argument that basic political rights depend for their exercise on basic subsistence rights. It is very difficult, and sometimes impossible to assert one's rights in any immigration process if one's basic health needs are not met.

FAMILY MEMBERSHIP

Family reunification has been a criterion for immigration since the Immigration Act of 1965. The underlying principle here is that strong family ties are important, both for individuals and for a flourishing national culture. This principle should apply to all families. The difficulty of reentering the United States has resulted in an undocumented population that is increasingly made up of families with minor children (Passel 2006). There are approximately 4 million US-born children with at least one noncitizen parent, and 79 percent of the children with undocumented parents were born in the United States (Passel and Taylor 2010).

Given these statistics, it is reasonable to assume that a high percentage of people in ICE detention are the parents, siblings, or other relatives of US citizens. This provides a general argument for loosening immigration restrictions on such persons. If such persons are morally entitled to consideration for entry on family grounds, presumably their treatment in detention should reflect their status as members, to some extent, of our society, and this status can ground the obligation to provide adequate health care to them.

COLLATERAL DAMAGE

If ICE detention imposes collateral damage on the innocent children of detainees, and if there is an acceptable alternative to detention, then we have a reason for supposing that we have an obligation to mitigate the harm. One simple way to do this it to move away from detention—at least for parents of minor children. There is good reason to think that alternatives to detention will not only mitigate some of the harms caused by detention, but will be an effective and cost saving alternative to detention. A program run by the Vera Institute showed an appearance rate of over 90 percent for undocumented immigrants enrolled in its alternative nondetention program (Root 2000).

If the collateral damage undermines the detainee's ability to assert her rights in immigration proceedings, as it seems to do in the case of mothers, then we have an additional reason to adopt alternatives to detention. If this solution is not politically feasible, we are not thereby absolved of all obligation toward detainee parents. One way we can discharge some of our obligation is to offer them the appropriate health services to mitigate the harm that they are suffering in virtue of this collateral damage.

RECIPROCITY

James Dwyer argues that, "Most undocumented workers do the jobs that citizens often eschew. They do difficult and disagreeable jobs at low wages . . . they have the worst jobs and work in the worst conditions," and that such work is a "social construction" that forms the basis of our obligation to provide health care (Dwyer 2004).

I would add that in addition to doing this work, undocumented workers pay taxes and receive few comparable benefits in return. They pay Social Security taxes under fake numbers that, according the Social Security Administration, add about $50 billion dollars annually to the system (Porter 2005). In addition, they pay sales taxes, and some are homeowners who also pay property taxes. At the same time they are prohibited by the 1996 Personal Responsibility and Work Opportunity Reconciliation Act from collecting most public benefits.

US ROLE IN CAUSING HEALTH PROBLEMS AND/OR IN CAUSING MIGRATION

Many theorists have argued that the political and economic policies of the global North are direct causes of migration. Thomas Pogge offers a global analysis and critique: "The existing global institutional order is neither natural nor God-given, but shaped and upheld by the more powerful governments and by other actors they control (such as the EU, NATO, UN, WTO, OECD, World Bank, and IMF)."

At least the more privileged and influential citizens of the more powerful and approximately democratic countries bear then a collective responsibility for their governments' role in designing and imposing this global order and for their governments' failure to reform it toward greater human-rights fulfillment." (Pogge 2008). Whether or not one is convinced of such a global thesis, other theorists offer more local, empirically based accounts. David Bacon, for example, offers a detailed look at how US policies created, and continue to create, tremendous pressures for Mexican illegal migration to the United States (Bacon 2008). I will not debate this issue here, but if these theorists are correct, then we have reason to assert a negative duty to stop the policies that created the problem and a positive duty of reparation to mitigate the harm that we have caused.

Whether or not one is convinced that US policies are causally implicated in undocumented immigration, there is no doubt that some detention practices are directly implicated in harm to detainees. The denial of care that results in unnecessary death or impaired function is a clear example. The prison like detention conditions that detainees are subjected to, especially asylum seekers who are fleeing state torture, are a direct cause of subsequent mental health problems and exacerbations of such problems (Robjant, Robbins, and Senior 2009). In these cases, the only question is whether the duty of reparation should apply only to those directly wronged or to the larger class of detainees. I would argue that since ICE makes no real attempt to sort out asylum seekers and other vulnerable people from other less vulnerable detainees, it has an affirmative duty to provide appropriate health care for all detainees.

ARGUMENTS AGAINST THE OBLIGATION TO DETAINEES: DETERRENCE

Brietta Clark discusses some of the standard objections to providing health care to undocumented immigrants in general, and these arguments apply to detainees as well (Clark 2008). First she discusses the deterrence argument, that restricting such benefits would act as a deterrent to illegal immigration and that providing them would act as an incentive to such immigration.

Her response to this argument is that it is employment, not health care, which is the primary motivator for illegal immigration. Given the restrictions on health benefits for immigrants required by PRWORA, and the fact that by 2008, twenty-eight states had also restricted health care benefits for immigrants (Matthew 2010), it is very difficult to believe that undocumented immigrants come to the United States in search of publically subsidized health care.

LIMITED HEALTH CARE RESOURCES

The next argument she turns to is that we must restrict health care benefits because our health care resources are very limited. Her response is that health care is not an individual but a public good and that restricting it has overall bad consequences. Presumably one might point to public health here. James Dwyer offers an additional response to this objection. He argues that we need not choose between health care for citizens and the undocumented. There are many other possible tradeoffs. Secondly he points out that health care is a basic need and, as such, it is inappropriate to distribute it by appeal to a principle of desert.

DENIAL OF BENEFITS IS APPROPRIATE PUNISHMENT FOR LAWBREAKING

The final argument Clark considers is that benefit restrictions are justified as punishment for violations of the social contract. She has two responses here. The first is that not all excluded immigrants are undocumented—the five year waiting period for Medicaid applies to legal immigrants as well. This first response seems to exclude persons in ICE detention, but I would argue that it does not. Recall the categories of persons in ICE detention: asylum seekers; undocumented persons who are not asylum seekers, but who are not accused of any crime; undocumented persons who are accused of trivial offenses, including identity theft or felonious reentry; undocumented persons accused of serious offenses; and legal permanent residents (LPRs) who have committed a deportable offense. Asylum seekers, in particular, are clearly not in violation of any social contract. Presenting oneself for asylum is within the rules of national and international law.

We can make a similar case for LPRs who are detained for committing a deportable offense. First, even if the offense occurred after the 1996 Illegal Immigration Reform and Immigrant Responsibility Act, I would argue that deportation is grossly disproportionate to most of the offenses that are currently classed as deportable offenses (DUI, for example). Second, the law allows for the deportation of LPRs for offenses which occurred in the past, even before the act became law.

The second response Clark gives is that while criminal sanctions might be seen as appropriate for violations of immigration law, this does not imply that denial of health care should be part of the punishment. Indeed, the Supreme Court has explicitly stated this position in *Plata*—denial of health care is a violation of the Eighth Amendment ban against cruel and unusual punishment.

RIGHT TO EXCLUDE AND RIGHT NOT TO TREAT

Some theorists have argued that legitimate states have a prima facie right to exclude immigrants from their territory (Wellman 2008). If undocumented persons have no right to be in the country, then it might seem to follow that they have no rights to benefits available to legitimate members of the state. But I would argue that even if we accepted this position, such persons would still have a right against harm. Imagine that someone enters my property without my permission. Surely I would not be justified in shooting the intruder. I would argue that the case is similar for detainees. The denial of needed medical services for someone who is otherwise unable to procure them in virtue of being detained is a harm, as is the unnecessary infliction of psychological distress on already vulnerable persons, such as asylum seekers. I think there is actually a much stronger case to be made for the obligation to provide health care for all, but the appeal to a right against harm suffices to show that persons who are detained by ICE have at least the right to be protected from the denial of medical services.

INSUFFICIENT RECIPROCITY

Some would argue that undocumented immigrants take more resources than they provide and thus are not entitled to services based on a principle of reciprocity. "They are taking our jobs" is one way this concern is raised. I think there is something right about this objection, but I don't think it accurately fixes the source of the problem. Richard Trumka (2010), AFL-CIO president, states the problem very succinctly: "Too many U.S. employers actually like the current state of the immigration system—a system where immigrants are both plentiful and undocumented—afraid and available."

Too many employers like a system where our borders are closed and open at the same time—closed enough to turn immigrants into second-class citizens, open enough to ensure an endless supply of socially and legally powerless cheap labor. In *Hoffman Plastics* (2002) the Supreme Court ruled that undocumented workers were not entitled to back pay, even if their various employment claims were sustained, since they were not legally available for work. This decision provides a perverse incentive to hire undocumented workers—no matter what you do to them they cannot be compensated with back pay in any lawsuit against you (Manning 2010). It is thus likely that having a class of exploitable workers does result in fewer jobs for American workers along with depressing wages in the unskilled sector. But the fault here is with employers and the Court, not with the undocumented workers.

A related objection is that immigrants don't pay enough in taxes to cover all the public benefits they use. This objection rests on an empirical claim about how much undocumented immigrants pay in taxes versus what they use in services. But even if we granted that the balance tilts in favor of the use of services, this is not the end of the story. We can appeal to James Dwyer's response to this objection here. This objection sees society as a private business venture where one benefits on the basis of what one invests, and, as Dwyer (2004) writes, "The business model is not an adequate model for thinking about voting, legal defense, library services, minimum wages, occupational safety and many other social benefits" (37).

EVEN IF UNITED STATES IS CAUSALLY IMPLICATED IN MIGRATION, THE BEST WAY TO FIX THE PROBLEM IS IN HOME COUNTRIES

I turn now to the final argument: that even if we accepted all the justifications for providing health care, and the causal role that wealthy countries play in creating migratory pressures, encouraging undocumented immigration is the wrong approach because it exacerbates the problem by encouraging the youngest most productive workers to emigrate, leaving their home countries even worse off than they already are. While I am convinced that a more comprehensive, global solution is ultimately in order, this simply does not absolve us of our obligation to those who are already within our borders, and especially those within our detention facilities.

CONCLUSION

ICE is a branch of a government agency in a democratic country, thus the citizens on whose behalf it allegedly operates have an obligation to ensure that it operates in conformity with the fundamental principles of justice on which this nation was founded. ICE is a young and rapidly growing bureaucracy with little oversight. It operates using a mix of federal, state, local and private centers, many of which are penal institutions. It has a history of serious abuse, and even when it operates in conformity with its penal standards, it inflicts additional harm onto vulnerable people, especially asylum seekers and parents of minor children. It thus requires our constant vigilance and concern. Our immigration policies and detention practices are deeply troubling, but until we elect to reform them, we have a special obligation to the vulnerable populations that we house in ICE detention. Minimally, that includes being attentive to their medical needs.

REFERENCES

American Medical Association. (2008). *JAMA*, 300(2).

Bacon, D. (2008). *Illegal People*. Boston: Beacon Press.

Babu, Maya A. and Wolpin, Joseph B. (2010). Undocumented immigrants, healthcare access, and medical repatriation after serious medical illness. *American Health Lawyers Association, Journal of Health & Life Sciences Law*, 3(3), 83–101.

Bresa, Lindita. (2010). Uninsured, illegal, and in need of long-term care: the repatriation of undocumented immigrants by U.S. hospitals. *Seton Hall Law Review*, 1663–96.

Brown v. Plata, 563 U.S. 678, 687 (2011).

Centers for Disease Control and Prevention (CDC). (2005). Trends in Tuberculosis. Retrieved August 2, 2012, from http://www..gov/mmwr/preview/mmwrhtml/mm5511a3.htm.

Clark v. Martinez, 543 U.S. 371 (2005).

Clark, Brietta R. (2008). The immigrant health care narrative and what it tells us about the U.S. health care system. *Loyola University Chicago School of Law, Beazley Institute for Health Law and Policy, Annals of Health Law*, 17, 229–78.

Coffey, Guy J., Kaplan, Ida, Sampson, Robyn C., and Tucci, Maria Montagna. (2010). The meaning and mental health consequences of long-term immigration detention for people seeking asylum. *Social Science & Medicine*, 70, 2070–79.

Cutler, Sarah. (2005). Fit to be detained? Challenging the detention of asylum seekers and migrants with health needs. Report by *BID (Bail for Immigration Detainees)*, based on the findings of a report by *Médecins Sans Frontières*.

Daniels, Norman. (1998). Is there a right to health care and, if so, what does it encompass? *A Companion to Bioethics,* eds. Kuhse and Singer. Oxford, UK: Blackwell Publishers, 316–25.

Demore v. Kim, 538 U.S. 510, 553 (2003).

Dwyer, James. (2004). Illegal immigrants, health care, and social responsibility, *The Hastings Center Report*, Jan/Feb, 35–40.

Ferrell, J. (2008, May 10). Map: a closer look at 83 deaths. *Washington Post*, http://www.washingtonpost .com/wp-srv/nation/specials/immigration/map.html.

Goldstein, A., and Priest, D. (2008, May 13). Five detainees who took their lives," *Washington Post*, http://www.washingtonpost.com/wp-dyn/content/article/2008/05/12/AR2008051202694.html.

Guzman, Esther Morales. (2009). Imprisonment, deportation, and family separation: my American nightmare. *Social Justice* 36(2), 106–109.

Global Detention Project, http://www.globaldetentionproject.org/home.html.

Hoffman Plastics Compounds, Inc. v. NLRB3, 535 U.S. 137 (2002).

ICE detainee deaths, http://www.ice.gov/doclib/foia/reports/detaineedeaths2003-present.pdf.

ICE detention reform, http://www.ice.gov/detention-reform/detention-reform.htm.

ICE factsheet, http://www.ice.gov/news/library/factsheets/287g.html.

ICE visitation, http://www.ice.gov/doclib/dro/facilities/pdf/etowaal.pdf.

Johnson, Kit. (2009). Patients without borders: extralegal deportation by hospitals. *University of Cincinnati Law Review*, Winter, 78, 657–97.

Keller, Allen S. (2003). The impact of detention on the health of asylum seekers. *Journal of Ambulatory Care Management*, 26(4), 383–85.

Kim, Kathleen. (2009). Civil rights and the low-wage worker: The trafficked worker as private attorney general: a model for enforcing the civil rights of undocumented workers. *The University of Chicago Legal Forum*, 247–310.

Manning, Margaret. (2010). A mockery of the American dream: How to prevent employers from exploiting immigration status and escaping Title VII liability post-*Hoffman* (unpublished).

Matthew, Dayna Bowen. (2010). Race and healthcare in America: The social psychology of limiting healthcare benefits for undocumented immigrants - moving beyond race, class, and nativism. *Houston Journal of Health Law & Policy*, Spring, 10, 201–26.

Miller, Keva M. (2006). The impact of parental incarceration on children: An emerging need for effective interventions. *Child and Adolescent Social Work Journal*, 23(4), 472–86.

Mooty, Brianna M. (2010). Solving the medical crisis for immigration detainees: Is the proposed detainee basic medical care act of 2008 the answer? *Law and Inequality: A Journal of Theory and Practice*, 28, 223–53.

Papst, Kelsey E. (2009). Protecting the voiceless: ensuring ICE's compliance with standards that protect immigration detainees. *McGeorge Law Review*, 40, 261–89.

Passel, Jeffrey. (2006). The size and characteristics of the unauthorized migrant population in the U.S.: Estimates based on the March 2005 Current Population Survey. Washington, DC: Pew Hispanic Center.

Passel, Jeffrey, and Taylor, Paul. (2010). Unauthorized immigrants and their U.S. born children. Washington, DC: Pew Hispanic Center.

Plyer v. Doe, 457 U.S. 202 (1982).

Pogge, T. (2008). *World poverty and human rights*. Cambridge, UK: Polity Press.

Porter, E. (2005, April 5). Illegal immigrants are bolstering Social Security with billions. *New York Times*, http://www.nytimes.com/2005/04/05/business/05immigration.html.

Priest, D., and Goldstein, A. (2008, May 11–14). Careless detention: System of neglect, *Washington Post*, http://www.washingtonpost.com/carelessdetention.

Rabin, Nina. (2009). Unseen prisoners: Women in immigration detention facilities in Arizona. *Georgetown Immigration Law Journal*, Summer, 23, 31–32.

Ray, Mohar. (2006). Undocumented Asian American workers and state wage laws in the aftermath of Hoffman Plastic Compounds. *Asian American Law Journal*, 13, 91–114.

Robjant, Katy, Robbins, Ian, and Senior, Victoria. (2009). Psychological distress amongst immigration detainees: A cross-sectional questionnaire study. *British Journal of Clinical Psychology*, 48, 275–86.

Rome, Sunny Harris. (2010). Promoting family integrity: The Child Citizen Protection Act and its implications for public child welfare. *Journal of Public Child Welfare*, 4(3), 245–62.

Saucedo, Leticia. (2006). The employer preference for the subservient worker and the making of the brown collar workplace. *Ohio State Law Journal,* 67, 964–66.

Schriro, Dora. (2009). Immigration and Customs Enforcement: Rethinking civil detention and supervision, *Arizona Attorney,* 45, 26–27.

Shue, H. (1996). *Basic rights.* Princeton: Princeton University Press.

Tillman, Laura. (2009, February 19). America's immigration gulags overflowing with mentally ill prisoners, *Brownsville Herald,* http://www.alternet.org/story/127451/.

Trumka, Richard. (2010, June 18). Remarks at the City Club of Cleveland, http://www.aflcio.org/media center/prsptm/sp06182010.cfm.

UN High Commission on Refugees, http://www.unhcr.org/4cd91dc29.html.

Walden, Alexandria. (2009). Abortion rights for ICE detainees: Evaluating constitutional challenges to restrictions on the right to abortion for women in ICE detention. *University of San Francisco Law Review,* 43, 979–1012.

Walzer, M. (1984). *Spheres of justice.* New York: Basic Books, 1984, 60.

Wellman, Christopher Heath. (2008). Immigration and freedom of association. *Ethics* 119, 109–41.

Woods v. Morton, http://www.aclu.org/files/assets/2010-12-16-WoodsvMorton-SettlementAgreement .pdf.

Youngsberg v. Romeo, 457 U.S. 307 (1982).

6

Solitary Confinement[1]

Wanda Teays

ABSTRACT

In this chapter I discuss what many consider the worst form of torture, solitary confinement. A disaster in terms of a method of rehabilitation (as intended by the Quakers who put it to use years ago), solitary confinement has brought about any number of harms and no apparent benefits. The days of the Quakers thinking solitary confinement purifies the soul are long gone. In its place is we find a practice that causes both mental and physical suffering with long-term damage. We will look at five cases to get a sense of the potential harm of solitary. They include a lawyer, a detainee, two hostages, three prisoners, and three men on Death Row. The picture that they present is truly alarming. Each of these cases indicates why solitary confinement should be banned or restricted to a matter of hours if absolutely necessary. We then look at the examples of countries that have made changes and, within the U.S., the actions of Rick Raemisch, the Colorado prisons director who put an end to long-term solitary in his state.

When forces are beyond your control, there's not a lot you can do.

—Albert Woodfox

It's an awful thing solitary. . . . It crushes your spirit and weakens your resistance more effectively than any other form of mistreatment.

—Sen. John McCain

There is torture of mind as well as body; the will is as much affected by fear as by force. And there comes a point where this court should not be ignorant as judges of what we know as men.

—Justice Felix Frankfurter

INTRODUCTION

It is no mistake on Nel Noddings' part to consider isolation a manifestation of evil. The utter cruelty of confining another person to a cell, cage, or box boggles the mind. That it can go on for years or even decades is unimaginable. Where was the outcry when Zacarias Moussaoui was sentenced to life in prison in solitary confinement with no possibility of parole for his role in the attacks on 9/11?

The fantasy of the Quakers who thought solitary confinement would purify the soul and be an effective form of rehabilitation has been shown to be groundless. That it has continued to the present day and is commonly used in prisons and detention centers indicates how misguided is this policy and how urgent is the need to put an end to it.

Let's assume for the moment that there could be therapeutic benefits to a short period of isolation. If that were the case, we would need to clarify what they are and whether they outweigh the long-term risks. The practice needs to be assessed by medical professionals to fully grasp the potential harms and consider the alternatives.

Cyrus Ahalt and Brie Williams (2016) are right on track in raising this concern: "Aside from conducting some important studies that have linked even relatively brief isolation to worsening mental health, the medical community has been largely absent from the national debate over solitary confinement. That absence is conspicuous."

It's conspicuous and it needs to change. This is particularly so, given the rampant misuse of the practice. We see this with the number of minor infractions that result in "segregation" (= solitary).

THE MISUSE OF SOLITARY

Joshua Manson cites examples from a United Nations' report.

> In both the U.S. immigration and detention and federal prison systems, for example, people can be held in solitary confinement for the sole reason that they will be released, removed, or transferred within 24 hours. Also under U.S. federal law, people can be held in solitary confinement if they are HIV-positive and there is "reliable evidence" that they may "pose a health risk" to others.
>
> In California, people may be subject to isolation just because they are "a relative or associate of a staff member." In Pennsylvania, people may be subject to solitary confinement, against their will and consent, because they are "at a high risk of sexual victimization" if there exists no "alternative means of separation from the likely abuser." Also in Pennsylvania, people may be subject to solitary confinement simply because "there is no other appropriate bed space." (Manson 2016)

And so on. You don't have to be a danger to others to end up in solitary confinement, contrary to what we might think. This is particularly disturbing in light of the potential harms of being placed in solitary for even short periods. It can cause long-lasting trauma, mental suffering, and psychological harm.

Solitary can also heighten the risk of suicide. We see this, for example, with the case of Jack Letts. A British Canadian man who went off to Syria to join ISIS, Letts was captured and held in prison by Kurdish authorities. He ended up in solitary.

He told the [Canadian] consular official that he had attempted suicide after his first month in solitary confinement but was found in time by his Kurdish guards. "I started to go insane and talk to myself and I thought dying was better than my mother seeing me insane," Letts said. "So I tried to hang myself." He has since been allowed to live in a cell with other prisoners (Brewster 2018).

Jack Letts's reaction to solitary matches the experience of one after another after another. We can see this in the following five cases—the use of solitary on a lawyer, a detainee, two hostages, three prisoners, and three on Death Row. Each case paints a bleak picture of the use of solitary confinement.

First Case: Lawyer Xie Yanyi

Xie Yanyi had spent much of his career in China representing clients in sensitive legal cases involving victims of official corruption, police violence, or religious persecution. John Sudworth (2017) of the BBC reports on China's "war on law":

> The crackdown on China's already beleaguered human rights field began in mid 2015, halfway through Xi Jinping's first term. Now, anointed in office for a second term by the Communist Party Congress that ended this week, it stands as one of his most gloomy legacies. In total, more than 300 lawyers, legal assistants and activists have been brought in for questioning, with more than two dozen pursued as formal investigations.

Xie Yanyi, one of those arrested, said he didn't see sunlight for six months and that he was kept in a stress position and crouched on a low stool from 6:00 in the morning until 10:00 at night. He elaborates:

> After 15 days like this, [he said], his legs went numb and he had difficulty urinating. At times he was denied food and was beaten. . . . But harder to bear was the time spent in solitary confinement, he asserts. "I was kept alone in a small room and saw no daylight for half a year. I had nothing to read, nothing to do but to sit on that low stool." In his view, "People could go mad in that situation. I was isolated from the world. This is torture—the isolation is more painful than being beaten." (Sudworth 2017)

Second Case: Detainee Jose Padilla

Detainee and American citizen Jose Padilla was held over three years in solitary confinement. The conditions were harsh: his windows were blacked out; there was no clock or calendar and only a steel platform to sleep on (no mattress) before having access to legal counsel (Sontag 2006).

Two psychiatrists and a psychologist who conducted examinations of Padilla contend that both his extended detention in solitary and interrogation left him with severe mental disabilities. All three say he may never recover. In their opinion, "Padilla's ordeal in the brig was so psychologically unsettling that it has left him terrorized. Any reminder of the ordeal through questions by his lawyers or others triggers a recurrence of the disorganizing terror Padilla experienced" (Richey 2007).

Third Case: Hostages Terry Anderson and Frank Reed

Journalist Terry Anderson was covering Lebanon's civil war of 1975–90 when he was kidnapped along with other foreigners. He was released in 1991 after being held prisoner in an underground dungeon for six-and-a-half years (History.com 2009).

Fellow hostage Frank Reed, an American private-school director, was held in solitary confinement for four months before being put in with Anderson. Surgeon and public health commentator Atul Gawande reports on Reed's condition: "By then, Reed had become severely withdrawn. He lay motionless for hours facing a wall, semi-catatonic. He could not follow the guards' simplest instructions. Released after three and a half years, Reed ultimately required admission to a psychiatric hospital" (2016).

Anderson didn't fare so well either:

> After a few months without regular social contact . . . he started to lose his mind. He talked to himself. He paced back and forth compulsively, shuffling along the same six-foot path for hours on end. Soon, he was having panic attacks, screaming for help. He hallucinated that the colors on the walls were changing. He became enraged by routine noises—the sound of doors opening as the guards made their hourly checks, the sounds of inmates in nearby cells. After a year or so, he was hearing voices on the television talking directly to him. He put the television under his bed, and rarely took it out again. (Gawande 2009)

Fourth Case: Prisoners Robert King, Herman Wallace, and Albert Woodfox, AKA "The Angola Three"

The three Black Panther-activists were convicted in the early 1970s of a prison guard's murder (they claimed they were framed). Each spent decades in solitary—King 29 years, Wallace 41 years, and Woodfox 43 years, the longest in US history. King commented on the conditions:

> The cells were pretty bare, and they were maybe about . . . 3 feet wide and about 6 feet long. It was almost like it was in a tomb, and there was a slab of concrete that you slept on. You ate three meals a day—you had two slices of bread each meal. During the wintertime, you froze, and during summertime, you were overheated. But in any event, you were starved. (Kennedy 2016)

Wallace died three days after his release in 2013. In a February 2016 interview with *The Guardian (UK)*, Woodfox remarked on the brutality of solitary:

> Some of the guys found the pressure so great that they just laid down in a fetal position and stopped communicating with anybody. I've seen other guys who just want to talk and make noise, guys who want to scream. Breaking up manifests itself in any number of ways in individuals." (Pilkington 2016)

As for himself, Woodfox observed that,

> The panic attacks started with sweating. You sweat and you can't stop. You become soaking wet—you are asleep in your bunk and everything is soaking wet. Then when the claustrophobia starts it feels like the atmosphere is pressing down on you. That was hard. I used to talk to myself to convince myself I was strong enough to survive, just to hold on to my sanity until the feeling went away. (Pilkington 2016)

Fifth Case: Death Row Convicts Marcus Hamilton, Winthrop Eaton, and Michael Perry

Convicted of first-degree murder in Louisiana and sentenced to death, all three men have been in solitary confinement for over 25 years. They aren't the only ones: according to Liam Stack (2017), 71 prisoners sentenced to death in Louisiana are being held in solitary confinement at the Angola state penitentiary.

They spend 23 hours a day in windowless concrete cells that measure 8 by 10 feet. They are allowed to leave the cell for one hour each day to shower, make phone calls or walk along the tiered walkway beside their cells. Three times a week, they can use that hour to go outside to sit in a small outdoor cage. (Stack 2017)

Evidently "a lot, if not most" of the states that have the death penalty house their Death Row inmates in solitary confinement, according to Betsy Ginsberg, the director of the civil rights clinic at the Benjamin N. Cardozo School of Law (Stack 2017).

The damaging effects of prolonged solitary confinement on the mental and physical health of prisoners have been well established, as Stack points out. Social psychologist Craig Haney notes that even those with no history of mental illness were engaged in a "constant, ongoing struggle to maintain their sanity." In addition, "These conditions predictably can impair the psychological functioning of the prisoners who are subjected to them," he [observed]. "For some prisoners, these impairments can be permanent and life-threatening" (Stack 2017).

OVERVIEW OF ISSUES

On any given day, approximately 80,000 prisoners are being held in solitary confinement in the United States alone. That's not all. According to the Bureau of Justice Statistics, over the course of a year, nearly 1 in 5 (= 20 percent) U.S. prisoners spent time in solitary confinement. This adds up to 400,000 people who are incarcerated are also in solitary during a given year (Ahalt and Williams 2016). With such staggering numbers, much more needs to be done to justify this practice.

Others convey similar sentiments and raise important concerns. For instance, it's not only prisoners who are subjected to solitary confinement. Immigrants in detention facilities are also at risk.

John V. Kelly, US Department of Homeland Security Acting Inspector General points out that, "Staff did not always treat detainees respectfully and professionally, and some facilities may have misused segregation" (Sacchetti 2017). He cites the example of a detainee reported being locked down for multiple days for sharing coffee with another detainee (Office of Inspector General, Homeland Security 2017). This is clearly an overreaction to a minor offense.

THE HARMS OF SOLITARY

Misuse is one concern. So are the extreme conditions and the resulting psychological effects. Social scientist Craig Haney undertook a two-year study of inmates who were subjected to prolonged use of solitary confinement at Pelican Bay prison in California. He states that,

Sealed for years in a hermetic environment—one inmate likened the prison's solitary confinement unit to "a weapons lab or a place for human experiments"—prisoners recounted struggling daily to maintain their sanity.

They spoke of longing to catch sight of a tree or a bird. Many responded to their isolation by shutting down their emotions and withdrawing even further, shunning even the meager human conversation and company they were afforded. (Goode 2015)

Haney, said that, after months or years of complete isolation, many prisoners begin to lose the ability to initiate behavior of any kind. In extreme cases, "prisoners may literally stop behaving," thus becoming "essentially catatonic" (Gawande 2016).

In addition, almost 90 percent of these prisoners had difficulties with "irrational anger," as Terry Anderson notes about his own experience. In contrast, only 3 percent of the general population are said to suffer extreme anger. Not surprising, Haney claims that many prisoners in solitary become consumed with revenge fantasies.

This is a far cry from the rehabilitation that Quakers sought in turning to solitary confinement. Rather than a time to cool off, solitary seems more likely to bring emotions to the boiling point. Just look at some of the harms that have been documented.

Atul Gawande (2016) reports that studies show diffuse slowing of brain waves after a week or more of solitary confinement. He cites the 1992 case of fifty-seven prisoners of war whose EEGs showed brain abnormalities months after a six-month detention in Yugoslavia. Such evidence indicates solitary confinement has both physical as well as psychological harms.

ABUSIVE AND AGGRESSIVE FORMS OF SOLITARY

If things aren't bad enough when people are confined to 8 x 10' cells, there have been even more alarming cases. A macabre turn of events has been the use of boxes (for example with Abu Zubaydah) to cram suspected terrorists into. Yes, boxes. Presumably this is to encourage them to be more forthcoming, as if subjecting them to such miserable conditions would inspire them to divulge useful information. The result is that their confinement is more physically taxing than the use of rooms or prison cells.

Such an extreme has been accepted if not sanctioned at the highest level. In fact, psychologist masterminds Drs. Mitchell and Jessen recommended using such "aggressive techniques" as part of the interrogation process on so-called high-value captives. This included detainees Abu Zubaydah and Mohamed Ben Soud being placed in wooden boxes with holes poked in them to allow air flow (Fink and Risen 2017). They were then forced into crouched positions, unable to stand up or move about. The Senate Intelligence Committee Report details Zubaydah's confinement to a box:

> He spent a total of 266 hours (11 days, two hours) in the large (coffin size) confinement box and 29 hours in a small confinement box, which had a width of 21 inches, a depth of 2.5 feet, and a height of 2.5 feet. . . . According to the daily cables . . . Abu frequently "cried," "begged," "pleaded," and "whimpered," but continued to deny that he had any additional information. (2014, 52–53)

To add to the pressure, then US District Attorney Jay Bybee authorized via a memo the use of insects placed in the box to exploit the victim's phobias and fears. The memo permitted Zubaydah to be kept in a dark, confined space small enough to restrict his movement (*CNN* 2009).

> In addition, putting a [so-called] harmless insect into the box with Zubaydah, who "appears to have a fear of insects," and telling him it is a stinging insect would be allowed, as long as Zubaydah was informed the insect's sting would not be fatal or cause severe pain. "If, however, you were to place the insect in the box without informing him that you are doing so . . . you should not affirmatively lead him to believe that any insect is present which has a sting that could produce severe pain or suffering or even cause his death," the memo said. (CNN 2009)

DESCRIPTIONS AND DENIALS

The five cases of solitary confinement are disturbing enough when looking at the individuals affected, not to mention those like Abu Zubaydah and Ben Soud, who were crammed into boxes. It is also important to consider the scope of the use of solitary and how it can be obscured or hidden by the way it is described. We see this in the following mixture of linguistic manipulation and denial:

> "The Bureau [of Prisons] does not recognize the term solitary confinement. Therefore, the Bureau does not have a definition or reference to provide," the BOP told investigators with the DOJ [Department of Justice] Office of the Inspector General.
>
> One former BOP official told investigators that "solitary confinement does not exist" within the federal prisons system. But the inspector general's office said the Bureau of Prisons is just arguing semantics. (Reilly 2017)

Moreover, as law professor Joseph Margulies points out, there is no upper bound on holding a detainee in solitary confinement or being subjected to interrogations (2006, 107). To get a sense of the enormity of the problem in the US, look at the numbers reported in July 2017 by the US Department of Justice on the Federal Bureau of Prisons:

> As of June 2016, of the 148,227 sentenced inmates in the BOP's [Federal Bureau of Prisons'] 122 institutions, 9,749 inmates (7 percent) were housed in its three largest forms of Restricted Housing (RHU). . . . Although the BOP states that it does not practice solitary confinement, or even recognize the term, we found inmates, including those with mental illness, who were housed in single-cell confinement for long periods of time, isolated from other inmates and with limited human contact.
>
> Although the BOP generally imposes a minimum amount of time that inmates must spend in RHUs, it does not limit the maximum amount of time . . . As a result, inmates, including those with mental illness, may spend years and even decades in RHUs. (Office of the Inspector General, DOJ 2017)

THE USE OF EUPHEMISMS

One of the ways that solitary confinement was made more palatable was through distorting language. Whitewashing it with euphemisms like "disciplinary segregation," "administrative segregation" or "Segregated Housing Units (SHU)" does not alter the fact that such isolation is harmful and its extensive use alarming. With such labeling, they can avoid admitting that they practice solitary confinement. To what advantage? Colin Dayan asserts, "Since prison officials claim that these units are non-punitive, they are difficult to fight" (2007, 54).

The *Washington Post* editorial board (2017) responded to the Department of Justice report by declaring solitary confinement to be torture. "Restrictive housing placement is the bureau's preferred terminology," they stated, "but the report released last week made clear that is a semantic dodge." *The Post* pointed out that:

> Among those forced to languish alone were inmates with serious mental illness, some of whom were isolated for more than five years. A number of state prison systems have taken steps to limit or end their use of solitary confinement because of mounting evidence of its detrimental effects.

The Inspector General cited research that isolation can cause anxiety, depression, anger, paranoia and psychosis among prisoners. "You have no contact, you don't speak to anybody, and it's a form of torture on some level," a psychologist at one prison told investigators.

WHERE IS THE OUTRAGE?

Given this is the case, it is puzzling how little outcry there is among medical personnel and the general public. The solution? *The Post* (2017) calls it:

> Ending such barbarity is not only morally correct but also has practical benefits in improving public safety. Prisoners subjected to solitary confinement have difficulty reentering society and are more likely to re-offend.

Colin Dayan observes that solitary confinement was once considered the most severe deprivation and now its use is normalized (2007, 54). However, change is finally afoot. We see this in the practice of solitary confinement being banned in the state of Colorado. Rick Raemisch, the executive director of the Colorado Department of Corrections, explains:

> Long-term solitary was supposed to be rehabilitative, but it did not have that effect. Studies have found that inmates who have spent time in solitary confinement are more likely to reoffend than those who have not. Data shows that prisoners in solitary account for about half of all prison suicides; self-harm is also more common in solitary units than in less-restrictive ones.
>
> One social psychologist even found that the degree of loneliness experienced by people in solitary is matched only by that of terminal cancer patients. In addition, solitary confinement was intended to be a last resort for those who were too violent to be in a prison's general population. But then we gradually included inmates who disrupted the efficient running of an institution. In other words, inmates could be placed in solitary for almost any reason, and they were. (Raemisch 2017)

WORKING FOR CHANGE

Raemisch came to see that major changes were in order. He noted how he benefited from listening to the perspectives of others. This came about in 2015 when he assisted the State Department with other United Nations countries in modernizing international standards for the treatment of prisoners—known as the Nelson Mandela Rules. It was decided, Raemisch (2017) reports, that keeping someone for more than 15 days in solitary was torture.

This conclusion was echoed in a report of the Human Rights Clinic at the University of Texas School of Law. "Its authors concluded," reports Jacey Fortin, "that solitary confinement in Texas violates international human rights standards and amounts to a form of torture" (2017). The bottom line is that:

> We agree that if somebody commits a crime, they should receive a punishment. . . . But we say, at the same time, that once you impose a punishment on a person, you need to keep treating that person with humanity and with dignity. (Fortin 2017)

Raemisch would concur. As he puts it, "There now is enough data to convince me that long-term isolation manufactures and aggravates mental illness. It has not solved any problems; at best it has maintained them. That's why, in September, Colorado ended the practice" (2017).

This decision is significant; others should follow their example. We need to recognize that its widespread use in the U.S. doesn't make it right. Many other countries are in the same boat in the use and misuse of solitary.

In an October 17, 2016 UN Special Rapporteur on Torture, Juan E. Méndez, presented a report to the General Assembly detailing and comparing solitary confinement practices around the world. He declared that solitary confinement may amount to cruel, inhuman, or degrading treatment and in some cases torture, and may thus, under certain conditions, be prohibited under international law.

In that 2011 report, Méndez further called for a categorical ban on subjecting juveniles and people with mental illness to solitary confinement, and to end the practice of prolonged and indefinite solitary confinement. (Solitary Watch 2016)

In contrast, Norway is at the other end of the spectrum in its use of solitary confinement. As Ahalt and Williams (2016) indicate, Norwegian leaders realized that the old model simply did not work, that it did more harm than good and the time had come for its replacement. Norway's approach stands as a dramatic contrast with the systemic overuse of solitary.

WHAT ROLE CAN DOCTORS PLAY?

Doctors have a role to play in this. The Norwegian model is worth serious consideration. Ahalt and Williams (2016) offer their recommendation—one it behooves health professionals to take. "We believe the health professions have a responsibility to work with criminal justice policymakers to assess the risk of health-related harm underlying correctional practices such as solitary confinement. Fortunately, a compelling model for such a partnership exists." This they saw practiced at a Norwegian maximum security prison. It housed 250 men, many serving long sentences for violent crimes.

We asked the warden how many prisoners were being held in isolation and were surprised to hear his answer: one. That morning, a prisoner had trashed his cell. Guards, using motivational interviewing strategies, tried unsuccessfully to defuse the situation. The man was now cooling off in isolation under the close supervision of a health care team." As soon as he calms down," the warden told us, "he will return to the general population." We asked how long that might take." Tonight?" the warden guessed. "Tomorrow, certainly." (Ahalt and Williams 2016)

In comparison:

In a U.S. prison of the same size, we would expect to find 25 prisoners in solitary, and roughly half of them would be confined for more than a month. But here there was only one serving less than 1 day, with enhanced attention rather than minimal human contact.

The Norwegian criminal justice leaders we spoke with told us that 20 years ago their correctional system resembled ours: overcrowded and violent, with frequent use of solitary confinement. Then, motivated by prison riots, Norwegian leaders undertook broad reform. (Ahalt and Williams 2016)

Norway is not alone casting a critical eye on solitary in trying to make changes with this outdated and harmful model. What is going on in Britain also deserves our attention. Jean Casella (2015) of Solitary Watch reports on controls that have been put in place:

Britain has a long history of using solitary confinement. In 1842, it mimicked the United States in opening a prison, . . . devoted to isolating prisoners so they could contemplate their sins. The practice was largely abandoned on both sides of the Atlantic once it became clear that solitary led to madness, not penitence. Prison isolation was revived in the late 20th Century, but never on the scale seen in the United States.

Today, a series of rules allow the short-term use of solitary confinement, but are meant to check its overuse and abuse. Prison governors (wardens) may place individuals in what are officially called "care and separation" units to preserve the "good order and discipline" of the prison. But after 72 hours, their continued segregation requires the approval of not only the governor, but—as confirmed in a recent court decision—the Cabinet Secretary for Justice. With the necessary approvals, terms in solitary can stretch longer, but must be reviewed and renewed every 14 days.

With the additional oversight and a high-level approvals process, the abuse of solitary confinement should be curtailed. Moreover, this model allows for more transparency and thus has less likelihood of misuse.

CONCLUSION

There is little doubt that solitary confinement is cruel and unusual punishment and, for any extended period, is a form of torture. It has virtually no value as an instrument of rehabilitation. That it is not been banned or subject to strict limitations in terms of use and duration is simply deplorable.

Both Norway and Britain have moved to a different model of addressing behavioral or other issues that made solitary seem a legitimate option. We need to give close attention to the approaches they have taken and consider the range of alternatives to solitary.

Although it seems unreasonable to have oversight by a governor, a director of justice or the like, an oversight committee could be employed to help end the abuses taking place with solitary confinement.

One option might be to use a review board such as a bioethics committee or a variation drawing upon medical professionals, clergy, and members of the community. In other words, we need more transparency about what is taking place and more controls on what is being done.

REFERENCES

Ahalt, Cyrus, and Brie Williams. 2016, May 5. "Reforming Solitary-Confinement Policy—Heeding a Presidential Call to Action," New England Journal of Medicine; 374:1704-1706. http://www.stopsoli taryforkids.org/wp-content/uploads/2016/05/NEJM-Solitary-May-2016-p1601399.pdf. Retrieved 5 June 2018.

Brewster, Murray. 2018, February 8. Alleged ISIS Operative 'Jihadi Jack' Begs Canada to Let Him Come Here, CBC News, http://www.cbc.ca/news/politics/jihadi-jack-isis-consular-1.4526882. Retrieved 5 June 2018.

Casella, Jean, 2015, October 21, "Off the Block," Solitary Watch, http://solitarywatch.com/2015/10/21/ off-the-block/. Retrieved 5 June 2018.

CNN, 2009, April 17. "2002 Memo: Had to Be Intent to Inflict 'Severe Pain' to Be Torture, CNN, http://www.cnn.com/2009/POLITICS/04/16/us.torture.documents/. Retrieved 5 June 2018.

Dayan, Colin. 2007. *The Story of Cruel and Unusual.* Boston. MIT Press.

Fink, Sheri and James Risen. 2017, June 20. "Psychologists Open a Window on Brutal C.I.A. Interrogations," The *New York Times*, https://www.nytimes.com/interactive/2017/06/20/us/cia-torture.html. Retrieved 5 June 2018.

Fortin, Jacey. 2017, April 26, "Report Compares Texas' Solitary Confinement Policies to Torture," The *New York Times*, https://www.nytimes.com/2017/04/26/us/texas-death-row-torture-report.html. Retrieved 5 June 2018.

Gawande, Atul. 2009, March 30, "Hellhole". The *New Yorker*, https://www.newyorker.com/magazine/2009/03/30/hellhole. Retrieved 5 June 2018.

Goode, Erica, 2015, August 3, "Solitary Confinement: Punished for Life," *The New Yorker*. Retrieved 5 June 2018.

History.com. 2009, December 4. "1991: Hostage Terry Anderson freed in Lebanon," https://www.history.com/this-day-in-history/hostage-terry-anderson-freed-in-lebanon. Retrieved 5 June 2018.

Kennedy, Merrit, 2016, February 19, "Last of 'Angola 3' Released After More Than 40 Years in Solitary Confinement," NPR, https://www.npr.org/sections/thetwo-way/2016/02/19/467406096/last-of-angola-3-released-after-more-than-40-years-in-solitary-confinement. Retrieved 5 June 2018.

Manson, Joshua. 2016, October 28. "UN Report Compare Solitary Practices in the US and Around the World," Solitary Watch, http://solitarywatch.com/2016/10/28/un-report-compares-solitary-confinement-practices-around-the-world/. Retrieved 5 June 2018.

Margulies, Joseph. 2006. *Guantánamo and the Abuse of Presidential Power*. New York: Simon & Schuster.

Office of the Inspector General. 2017, July. "Review of the Federal Bureau of Prisons' Use of Restrictive Housing for Inmates with Mental Illness," US Department of Justice. https://oig.justice.gov/reports/2017/e1705.pdf#page=1. Retrieved 5 June 2018.

Office of the Inspector General, 2017, December 11, "Concerns about ICE Detainee Treatment and Care at Detention Facilities," Homeland Security, https://www.oig.dhs.gov/sites/default/files/assets/2017-12/OIG-18-32-Dec17.pdf. Retrieved 5 June 2018.

Pilkington, Ed. 2016, February 20, "Albert Woodfox Speaks After 43 Years in Solitary Confinement: 'I Would Not Let Them Drive Me Insane," *The Guardian* (UK), https://www.theguardian.com/us-news/2016/feb/20/albert-woodfox-angola-3-first-interview-trump-confinement. Retrieved 5 June 2018.

Raemisch, Rick. 2017, October 12. "Why We Ended Long-Term Solitary Confinement in Colorado," The *New York Times*, https://www.nytimes.com/2017/10/12/opinion/solitary-confinement-colorado-prison.html. Retrieved 5 June 2018.

Reilly, Ryan J. 2017, July 12. "Federal Prisons Officials Claim Inmates Aren't Held in Solitary. DOJ Watchdog Says They Are," *Huffington Post*, https://www.huffingtonpost.com/entry/federal-prison-solitary-confinement-mental-illness_us_59664623e4b005b0fdca5f85?nf5. Retrieved 5 June 2018.

Richey, Warren. 2007, August 13, "US Terror Interrogation Went Too Far, Experts Say," *Christian Science Monitor*. Retrieved 5 June 2018.

Sacchetti, Maria. 2017, December 17. "Watchdog Report Finds Moldy Food, Mistreatment in Immigrant Detention Centers," The *Washington Post*, https://www.washingtonpost.com/local/immigration/watchdog-report-finds-moldy-food-mistreatment-in-immigrant-detention-centers/2017/12/15/c97b380a-e10d-11e7-89e8-edec16379010_story.html?utm_term=.1bc140373121. Retrieved 5 June 2018.

Solitary Watch. 2016, October 28. "UN Report Compares Solitary Confinement Practices in the U.S. and Around the World," http://solitarywatch.com/2016/10/28/un-report-compares-solitary-confinement-practices-around-the-world/. Retrieved 5 June 2018.

Sontag, Deborah, 2006, December 4. "Video Is a Window into a Terror Suspect's Isolation," The *New York Times*, http://www.nytimes.com/2006/12/04/us/04detain.html. Retrieved 5 June 2018.

Stack, Liam. 2017, March 30. "3 Men on Death Row in Louisiana Sue Over Solitary Confinement," The *New York Times*, https://www.nytimes.com/2017/03/30/us/3-men-on-death-row-in-louisiana-sue-over-solitary-confinement.htm. Retrieved 5 June 2018.

Sudworth, John. 2017, October 25. "China Lawyer Recounts Torture Under Xi's 'War on Law,' BBC News, Beijing, BBC, http://www.bbc.com/news/blogs-china-blog-41661862. Retrieved 5 June 2018.

Washington Post Editorial Board. 2017, July 15. "Solitary Confinement Is Torture. Will the Bureau of Prisons Finally Stop Using It?" The *Washington Post*, https://www.washingtonpost.com/opinions/solitary-confinement-is-torture-will-the-bureau-of-prisons-finally-stop-using-it/2017/07/15/f719de20-68c6-11e7-8eb5-cbccc2e7bfbf_story.html?utm_term=.adc722effac4. Retrieved 5 June 2018.

NOTE

1. © Springer Nature Switzerland AG 2019. Wanda Teays, "Doctors and Torture: Medicine at the Crossroads," *International Library of Ethics, Law, and the New Medicine* 80: 95–107. Used with permission.

7

Ethical Considerations for Vaccination Programs in Acute Humanitarian Emergencies[1]

Keymanthri Moodley, Kate Hardie, Michael J. Selgelid, Ronald J. Waldman, Peter Strebel, Helen Rees, and David N. Durrheim

ABSTRACT

Humanitarian emergencies result in a breakdown of critical health-care services and often make vulnerable communities dependent on external agencies for care. In resource-constrained settings, this may occur against a backdrop of extreme poverty, malnutrition, insecurity, low literacy, and poor infrastructure. Under these circumstances, providing food, water, and shelter and limiting communicable disease outbreaks become primary concerns. Where effective and safe vaccines are available to mitigate the risk of disease outbreaks, their potential deployment is a key consideration in meeting emergency health needs. Ethical considerations are crucial when deciding on vaccine deployment. Allocation of vaccines in short supply, target groups, delivery strategies, surveillance and research during acute humanitarian emergencies all involve ethical considerations that often arise from the tension between individual and common good. The chapter sets out the ethical issues that policy makers need to bear in mind when considering the deployment of mass vaccination during humanitarian emergencies, including beneficence (duty of care and the rule of rescue), nonmaleficence, autonomy and consent, and distributive and procedural justice.

INTRODUCTION

Acute humanitarian crises pose complex ethical dilemmas for policy makers, particularly in settings with inadequate health-care services, which often become dependent on external agencies for urgently needed care.[2] These ethical dilemmas are inherent in many spheres of the response activity, including measures to mitigate infectious disease transmission, which often cause outbreaks during humanitarian crises. In the initial emergency response, interventions to reduce communicable disease transmission, such as vaccination, should be deployed along with food, water, and shelter, since communicable diseases, including some that are vaccine-preventable, can spread faster and be unusually severe in the crowded, unhygienic conditions that prevail during crises. Measles, with a case-fatality rate as high as 30 percent during a humanitarian crisis, is a fitting example.[3]

Several factors need to be considered before a vaccine is deployed: the potential burden of disease; vaccine-related risks (usually minimal); the desirability of prevention as opposed to treatment; the duration of the protection conferred; cost; herd immunity in addition to individual protection; and the logistical feasibility of a large-scale vaccination program. Vaccination may be the only practical way to protect people against certain diseases, such as meningococcal meningitis and measles. Individuals who undergo medical or surgical treatment often need ongoing care; those who get vaccinated do not, yet they receive long-lasting benefits. However, the feasibility of a mass vaccination effort depends largely on available resources.

In a recent study on ethics in humanitarian health care, respondents pointed out the need for ethical guidance on issues such as vaccination during emergency situations.[4] The World Health Organization (WHO) and several humanitarian nongovernmental organizations have acknowledged this need and, in an effort to address it, WHO's Strategic Advisory Group of Experts (SAGE) on Immunization developed a framework for decision-makers on the deployment and effective use of vaccines that can save lives during emergencies.[5,6] Under the framework, countries facing crises first assess the epidemiological risk posed by a potentially dangerous vaccine-preventable disease. They then explore the feasibility of a mass vaccination campaign in light of the properties of the necessary vaccine.

The conflict between individual good and the common good is at the core of the ethical issues explored in this paper—issues pertaining to the allocation of a limited vaccine supply, the balance between benefits and harms, obtaining informed consent and research conduct. The key ethical principles that should prevail during public health emergencies are rooted in the more general ethical principles governing clinical medicine and public health. Acute humanitarian emergencies differ widely in nature, in the threats they pose, in the background conditions in which they occur, and in the type of agencies that must respond. Hence, this paper does not seek to provide specific, prescriptive guidance, but merely highlights the ethical issues that policy makers need to consider when deciding to conduct mass vaccination during any emergency response.

BENEFICENCE AND HUMAN RIGHTS

The international community and national governments have a collective duty of care to ensure that effective, affordable measures for preventing unnecessary illness and death are available to those most in need. During humanitarian emergencies, the risk of communicable disease transmission is higher than usual. According to the duty of care based on the principle of beneficence, governments must make vaccines available against the most contagious diseases. In addition to the duty of care, institutions and individuals must abide by the rule of rescue, which is "the imperative [. . .] to rescue identifiable individuals facing avoidable death."[7,8] This is influenced by the urgency of the situation, the consequences of doing nothing, the feasibility of preventing serious consequences and the sacrifice required of the responding individual or agency.[9] Humanitarian emergencies occur often enough for timely access to an assured supply of vaccine to be necessary, since certain vaccine-preventable diseases have serious outcomes, including death.[10,11] Global and local communities, including governments and nongovernmental organizations, are morally obligated to ensure this supply.

Some oppose vaccination and other measures that are not routinely offered in non-crisis settings. The underlying concern, based on the doctrines of developmental relief and sustainability, is that introducing such measures will result in aid dependency. However, the argument becomes invalid if vaccination during an acute humanitarian crisis can provide immediate protection against serious illness or death.[12] A higher standard of care is needed during public health crises because of the immediate threat to life. It is ethically reasonable for the standard of preventive care to revert to pre-existing levels after the heightened threat has subsided. After an acute emergency, some medical interventions call for ongoing care or rehabilitation. Vaccination does not, yet it provides long-lasting benefits.

Humanitarian assistance has traditionally been seen as charity, in keeping with the principle of beneficence, but owing to the growing human rights focus, it has come to be viewed as an obligation. Those who are able to help are obligated to ensure that the rights of affected individuals and populations are respected and promoted.[13] The Sphere Project's Humanitarian Charter "defines the legal responsibilities of states and parties to guarantee the right to assistance and protection."[14] The charter draws on the Universal Declaration of Human Rights, international humanitarian law (the Geneva Conventions) and the Convention relating to the Status of Refugees to establish a legal framework for humanitarian action.[15]

From a human rights perspective, vaccination equitably promotes and protects public health. Article 25 of the Universal Declaration of Human Rights states that:

> Everyone has the right to a standard of living adequate for the health and well-being of himself and his family, including food, clothing, and medical care . . . [and that] every individual and every organ of society . . . shall strive . . . by progressive measures, national and international, to secure [its] universal and effective recognition.[16]

Irrespective of the principles underlying humanitarian assistance, vaccine donations can ensure timely access to vaccines during emergencies. Although WHO and the United Nations Children's Fund (UNICEF) have agreed on five requirements for "good donations practice"—i.e., suitability, sustainability, informed key persons, supply and licensing—they acknowledge that in exceptional circumstances, including emergencies, these requirements can be overlooked.[17]

NONMALEFICENCE

All decisions made during humanitarian crises involve seeking a balance between beneficence (doing good) and nonmaleficence (avoiding or minimizing harm). Only vaccines that have proved effective and safe in routine use are likely to be considered for mass administration during the acute phase of a humanitarian crisis. Such vaccines not only protect people against specific diseases; when administered on a large scale, they confer additional benefit through herd immunity, which reduces disease transmission above specific vaccination coverage thresholds.

Vaccines are generally administered before people are exposed to the pathogen causing the targeted disease. Unnecessary vaccination entails opportunity costs and puts people at risk of side effects. The risk of contagion must justify vaccination. Four variables determine risk magnitude: the nature of the illness and attendant local epidemiological and environmental characteristics; the probability of transmission; disease severity and disease duration.[18] If a disaster occurs where vaccination coverage is already high or the risk of an outbreak is low, additional, emergency vaccination may be of minimal benefit. For example, following the earthquake in Sichuan Province in China in 2008, mass measles vaccination would have been inappropriate because a provincewide measles vaccination campaign with high coverage had just been completed.[19]

Vaccines produce benefits but can also cause individual or social harm. Side effects are an example of individual harm. These range from mild, common reactions, such as inflammation and pain at the injection site, to more severe but extremely rare events. Established vaccines, which are normally used during humanitarian emergencies, have well-known side-effect profiles, but much less is known about adverse events that can occur in ill or malnourished people during a humanitarian emergency.[20] Children in this category tend to be biologically more susceptible to vaccine-preventable diseases than others, and when their parents refuse to have them vaccinated, they may be causing them individual harm. On the other hand, vaccination is sometimes contraindicated or inappropriate. A child, for instance, can be too young to receive a certain vaccine.

Parents' refusal to get vaccinated or to vaccinate their children can cause collective harm by incrementing the pool of unprotected, susceptible individuals in a community. With herd immunity compromised, devastating disease outbreaks can occur. In these settings, individuals are morally obligated to accept vaccination to prevent harm to others.[21] Harm may result from errors of omission or commission. Failure to provide a vaccine that is indicated in a specific humanitarian emergency violates the principle of non-maleficence because it places vulnerable populations and individuals at risk of contracting a vaccine-preventable disease.

DISTRIBUTIVE JUSTICE

Distributive justice requires the fair allocation of scarce basic resources, such as shelter, food, potable water and vaccines in short supply. A small supply of vaccine could be equitably distributed through a lottery, but prioritizing particularly susceptible groups and individuals, or those most likely to spread the disease, would not be possible. Different rules govern decision-making and priority-setting during acute crises. Resource distribution during a crisis is often suboptimal because those engaged in humanitarian assistance can only do the "best they can" in the context of imperfect information, exceptional circumstances and needs far outweighing the available resources.[22]

When resources, especially staff, are scarce, decision-makers often choose among interventions—implicitly or explicitly—on the basis of cost-effectiveness because they are seeking to maximize benefits. Vaccination is highly cost effective, and, in emergencies, it can mitigate the risk of serious infectious disease. Furthermore, large numbers of people can be vaccinated quickly. Other factors to consider are how urgent and intense is the need for vaccination; how much faster can vaccination be delivered than other interventions; and how groups at high risk or with high transmission rates can be targeted in situations where other interventions, such as safe water and sanitation, cannot be rapidly deployed.

All countries, regardless of their socioeconomic status or experience with humanitarian emergencies, need to decide how to allocate resources. All societies have a shared vulnerability to emergencies, although poor societies are more severely devastated because poverty undermines resilience. When allocating resources, a balance must be sought between utility—maximizing the common good and ensuring smooth economic and social functioning—and equality and fairness. This balance is essential to garner people's trust in vaccination programmes during crises. In keeping with egalitarian considerations, resource allocation should not be discriminatory; everyone should have a fair chance of being vaccinated.[22] Furthermore, resources should be allocated with the aim of achieving "the greatest good for the greatest number." Utility can conflict with equality or fairness. You can, for example, save the most lives or avert the most DALYs (disability affected life years) by allocating vaccines to urban rather than rural areas because urban areas have greater population density,[23] but doing so systematically would be inequitable. In conflict zones, threats to the physical safety of health workers often determine which populations they can and cannot vaccinate.

Efforts to maximize utility can conflict with the egalitarian goal of helping the neediest. When limited supplies are allocated to the most vulnerable, overall health utility is sometimes sub- optimal (e.g., less aggregate well-being, fewer lives saved, and/or fewer DALYs averted). From the perspective of value pluralism, balancing utility and equality should be the goal, rather than prioritizing one or the other. When it comes to vaccination, utility is fortunately often greatest when the most socially disadvantaged groups are targeted.

The fair distribution of limited vaccine supplies was an important issue during preparations for the 2009 pandemic influenza. People in certain categories were prioritized: those at greatest risk of infection (e.g., school children and healthcare workers); those most likely to become severely ill if infected (e.g., immunosuppressed individuals and chronic disease patients); those most likely to spread infection (e.g., children and emergency service providers).[24] During humanitarian emergencies in which populations are displaced, neighbouring communities also require attention. In most circumstances, host communities and refugees should be given access to each other's services.[25] Refugee or displaced populations should not be treated as separate from the host community, and assistance programmes, including vaccination, should support everyone in the area as a whole.[26] The guiding principle should be to provide equitable access to vaccination to equalize risk. From an inclusive perspective, there is efficiency in covering two communities with all the resources available. Fair and equitable approaches result in less hostility and rivalry between the host and the displaced communities.[27]

From the point of view of utility and equity, in many cases children should be prioritized because they are generally more vulnerable than older people to vaccine-preventable diseases. In addition, saving a child's life will result in a larger reduction in disease burden because more years of healthy life are lost when a child dies.[28] Parents and caregivers often prioritize children's needs over their own. However, some communities may place greater value on the social roles of the elderly and of pregnant women and may prioritize their access to health care during emergencies.

From a utilitarian perspective, protecting frontline health workers against disease will indirectly benefit the health of the community. Under the principle of reciprocity, it is fair to prioritize the vaccination of health-care workers, who are often more exposed than others to the risk of contagion, since they are committed to caring for society. In addition, because health-care workers come into contact with susceptible individuals, they have a moral obligation to get vaccinated to avoid placing patients at risk of infection.[29]

PROCEDURAL JUSTICE

Procedural justice requires transparent decision-making with involvement of the communities affected by the decisions. To ensure procedural justice, it is very useful to have guidelines or a legal framework to follow. Guidelines are especially valuable in certain situations: when large numbers of people need to be treated or protected against disease; when delayed or suboptimal measures could lead to very poor outcomes; and when inadequate management could result in high mortality or a large-scale epidemic. Although guidelines do not have mandatory status, if they are evidence-based and contextually appropriate they should be considered normative practice and a benchmark for judging the actions of health officials and practitioners.

National legal systems should guide the implementation of vaccination programs in individual nation-states, but they seldom accommodate humanitarian emergencies. When national legislative frameworks are absent or dysfunctional, international human rights law dictates a duty of care to protect people needing assistance, and in such cases implementation should follow international health guidelines. WHO member states can legitimately follow WHO vaccination guidelines, which were developed on the strength of the evidence and which take many factors into account, including the epidemiologic and clinical features of the target disease, vaccine characteristics, costs, health system infrastructure, social impact, legal and ethical considerations, and the local context.[30,31]

Efforts to improve accountability during humanitarian emergencies have resulted in the Sphere Project, the Humanitarian Accountability Partnership, and the Active Learning Network for Accountability and Performance in Humanitarian Action.[32] All three seek to involve beneficiaries in the planning and implementation of aid programs, establish codes of conduct for responding agencies, promote technical standards, and encourage the use of performance indicators and impact assessments.

Observing appropriate rules of conduct during humanitarian crises is often difficult. In certain political contexts, health-care workers may find that following guidance from their governments or humanitarian organizations is in conflict with their commitment to promote individuals' best interests. Affected populations are often disenfranchised and unable to defend their own interests. All factors considered before the introduction of a vaccination program should be well documented and publicly available to donors, community leaders, local staff, and governments. Channels should also be established for affected communities to express their concerns directly to responding agencies.

CONSENT

Obtaining valid consent from individuals before a medical intervention is an obligation under the principle of respect for the autonomy of persons. In nonemergency circumstances, the consent process needs to be thorough and takes time. During emergencies, it has to be modified. If time permits, information on the risks and benefits of vaccination should be communicated to target populations in sufficient depth to allow individuals to make informed decisions, while bearing in mind that many will lack a basic understanding of germ theory and immunology. During emergencies, vaccination often takes place while people are too desperate for food and other basic necessities to recognize its importance. Furthermore, in some developing countries people defer to decision-makers at the expense of individual autonomy.

The amount of information provided to the public needs to be weighed against the risk of delaying action. However, any questions raised by the community should be thoroughly addressed. For example, vaccinators should be prepared to answer common questions about the diseases targeted, the benefits of vaccination, potential side effects, follow-up and alternative options. They should also know where to refer undecided individuals who have other questions, although this may not always be feasible. Visual aids and other media can be used to convey important information to the public in a time-efficient manner.

Vaccination should be voluntary unless it becomes critical to "prevent a concrete and serious harm."[33] The degree of risk to communities will determine to what extent individual rights may be restricted. Where the threat of widespread, serious infectious disease is imminent, individual liberties may be justifiably curtailed.[34] The Siracusa Principles endorsed by the

United Nations Economic and Social Council state that: "Public health may be invoked as a ground for limiting certain rights in order to allow a State to take measures dealing with a serious threat to the health of the population or individual members of the population. These measures must be specifically aimed at preventing disease or injury or providing care for the sick and injured."[35]

It may thus be permissible for those in authority to restrict individual autonomy to prevent harm to others. Although this approach has been limited to immediate or direct threat under traditional public health law, it should arguably be extended to what is "reasonably foreseeable" based on epidemiology and historical occurrence.[36] If the risk to health is extremely high, individuals should not be allowed to compromise group protection and communal rights.[37,38,39] When personal liberty is restricted to protect public health, the measures applied must be effective, the least restrictive (i.e., least liberty-infringing), proportional to the risk, equitable and non-discriminatory, minimally burdensome and in line with due process. Those whose liberty is violated should, when appropriate, be compensated, particularly if they experience vaccine-associated side effects.[40,41] In addition, individual rights should be restricted only with utmost respect for the dignity of persons.

Children are at particularly high risk of contracting communicable diseases during humanitarian crises. In most emergencies, mortality in children under the age of 5 years is generally two to three times higher than crude mortality.[42] Vaccinating children could reduce mortality in all age groups because epidemics often arise and spread among children.[43] Parents' refusal to have their children vaccinated should be respected if the risk of disease is low or the disease is mild. However, if the risk of harm to the child is high, parental authority may be overruled to protect the child's best interests.[44] In emergency settings a parent or guardian may not be available, and health-care workers should be empowered to rapidly decide whether to vaccinate a child if done in the child and community's best interests.

RESEARCH

Opportunities for health and health service research abound during humanitarian crises.[45,46] However, in resource-limited settings, medical care[47] and service delivery must always take precedence over research.[48] In disaster settings, research is often conducted by the same people who provide aid and thus "rightly takes second place to the provision of life-saving assistance."[49] If specific personnel were assigned exclusively to research, critical human resources would not be diverted away from care. Nonetheless, such personnel should only be allowed to conduct research after a local research ethics committee has determined that enough care personnel are available to meet demand.[50] Regional or international ethics review boards should be created in places without appropriate local expertise. In countries without functioning research governance structures, researchers must rely on international ethics review boards.

Research must be distinguished from disease and program surveillance.[51] Surveillance is essential for assessing vaccination coverage, informing program planning, evaluating vaccine effectiveness, and monitoring safety in the population as a whole and in certain subgroups.[52] Surveillance also allows the rapid detection of cases that may signal program failure requiring remediation. Since surveillance activities have an opportunity cost, the data collected must be analyzed and used to direct public health action.[53]

Under the principle of justice, communities where research is conducted must stand to benefit. Research protocols should be relevant, methodologically sound and explicit about the benefits and potential harms to study participants. They should also clearly explain how the findings will be delivered to study participants if they are relocated after the humanitarian crisis.[54] Research should not undermine the provision of health services and should be carried to completion.

Although most nonmedical research conducted during disasters is observational, it is subject to ethics review to ensure that individual and social benefits outweigh any risks. The level of review should be proportional to the risk associated with a specific intervention. An expedited review is admissible if the risk to participants is low, whereas a full committee review is warranted when the research involves a higher risk. If the research is urgent and very important, it can proceed without ethics committee approval, but retrospective review should be sought as soon as possible. Whenever the nature of the research to be conducted during a humanitarian emergency can be anticipated, a full review of the generic protocols should be planned and discussed in advance with local research ethics committees. Provision should be made for counselling or debriefing should participants find the research interviews traumatic or distressing.[55]

Potential research participants may have impaired ability to make decisions or provide voluntary individual informed consent following an acute humanitarian emergency, especially in "vulnerable communities," as defined by the Joint United Nations Program on HIV/AIDS. Empirical research in developing countries has shown that obtaining informed consent from study participants is not easy, even under non-emergency circumstances. Acute humanitarian crises add a layer of complexity, and decisional capacity must be carefully assessed.[56,57,58,59,60] In acute crises in which medical care is needed, patients often assume that a research intervention is known to be therapeutic or effective. During the consent process, study participants need to be made aware that they are consenting to research only, not to special or additional care.

CONCLUSION

Ethical considerations are vital to decision-making about the deployment of vaccines in acute humanitarian emergencies. Commitment to human rights and the rule of rescue place an onus on wealthy countries to ensure that life-saving vaccines are made available to the poorer countries during crises. Justice and ethics obligate those who are better off to assist those who are worse off and to allocate resources accordingly.[61] National health authorities are morally obligated to do all that they reasonably can to implement evidence-based guidelines to avert preventable harm.[62]

The allocation of a limited supply of vaccine calls for a fine balance between utility and equality and fairness. Accountability demands that decision-making be explicit, documented and open to public review.

In emergencies, the informed consent process may be reasonably modified to avoid delaying protection for vulnerable communities. Autonomy is not absolute. In situations that threaten the health and well-being of others, authorities may be required to mandate vaccination and intervene on behalf of minors against parental wishes. Finally, emergency health-care workers should be trained in ethics to improve their decision-making skills during acute humanitarian emergencies.[63]

ACKNOWLEDGMENTS

This review was prepared by WHO's Strategic Advisory Group of Experts (SAGE). SAGE's careful review and recommendations on the manuscript are gratefully acknowledged.

Competing interests: None declared.

NOTES

1. © 2013 World Health Organization. Reprinted with permission of WHO and the authors.

2. Levine C. The concept of vulnerability in disaster research. *J Trauma Stress* 2004;17:395-402. doi:10.1023/B:JOTS.0000048952.81894.f3 PMID:15633918

3. Shears P, Berry AM, Murphy R, Nabil MA. Epidemiological assessment of the health and nutrition of Ethiopian refugees in emergency camps in Sudan, 1985. *BMJ* 1987;295:314-8. doi:10.1136/bmj.295.6593.314 PMID:3115429

4. Feudtner C, Marcuse EK. Ethics and immunization policy: Promoting dialogue to sustain consensus. *Pediatrics* 2001;107:1158-64. doi:10.1542/peds.107.5.1158 PMID:11331702

5. Schwartz L, Hunt M, Sinding C, Elit L, Redwood-Campbell L, Adelson N et al. Models for humanitarian health care ethics. *Public Health Ethics* 2012;5:81-90. doi:10.1093/phe/phs005

6. SAGE Working Group on Vaccination in Humanitarian Emergencies. SAGE working group on vaccination in humanitarian emergencies: a framework for decision-making. Geneva: World Health Organization; 2012. Available from: http://www.who.int/immunization/sage/meetings/2012/november/FinalFraft_FrmwrkDocument_SWGVHE_23OctFullWEBVERSION.pdf [accessed 24 January 2013].

7. Jonsen AR. Bentham in a box: Technology assessment and health care allocation. *Law Med Health Care* 1986;14:172-4. PMID:3645228

8. Murphy L. Beneficence, law and liberty: The case of required rescue. *Georgetown Law J* 2001; 3:605-65.

9. Akabayashi A, Takimoto Y, Hayashi Y. Physician obligation to provide care during disasters: Should physicians have been required to go to Fukushima? *J Med Ethics* 2012;38:697-8. doi:10.1136/medethics-2011-100216 PMID:22543098

10. Kenny C. Disaster risk reduction in developing countries: costs, benefits and institutions. *Disasters* 2012;36:559-88. doi:10.1111/j.1467- 7717.2012.01275.x PMID:22329505

11. Hurst SA, Mezger N, Mauron A. Allocating resources in humanitarian medicine. *Public Health Ethics* 2009;2:89-99. doi:10.1093/phe/phn042

12. Bradbury M. Normalising the crisis in Africa. *Disasters* 1998;22:328-38. doi:10.1111/1467-7717.00096 PMID:9874898

13. United Nations Economic, Scientific and Cultural Organization [Internet]. Universal Declaration on Bioethics and Human Rights. Paris: UNESCO; 2005. Available from: http://www.unesco.org/new/en/social-and-human- sciences/themes/bioethics/bioethics-and-human-rights [accessed 24 January 2013].

14. Sphere Project. The Sphere Project: Humanitarian charter and minimum standards in humanitarian response. Bourton on Dunsmore: Practical Action Publishing; 2011. Available from: http://practical action.org/sphere [accessed 24 January 2013].

15. United Nations High Commissioner for Refugees. Convention and protocol relating to the status of refugees. Geneva: UNHCR; 1967. Available from: http://www.unhcr.org/3b66c2aa10.html [accessed 4 February 2013].

16. United Nations [Internet]. The Universal Declaration of Human Rights. New York: United Nations; 1948. Available from: www.un.org/en/documents/ udhr/index.shtml [accessed 24 January 2013].

17. Vaccine donations: WHO-UNICEF joint statement. Geneva: World Health Organization & United Nations Children's Fund; 2010 (WHO/IVB/10.09). Available from: http://whqlibdoc.who.int/hq/2010/WHO_IVB_10.09_eng. pdf [accessed 24 September 2012].

18. Rhodes RS, Telford GL, Hierholzer WJ, Barnes M. Bloodborne pathogen transmission from healthcare worker to patients. Legal issues and provider perspectives. *Surg Clin North Am* 1995;75:1205-17. PMID:7482145

19. Shu M, Liu Q, Wang J, Ao R, Yang C, Fang G et al. Measles vaccine adverse events reported in the mass vaccination campaign of Sichuan province, China from 2007 to 2008. *Vaccine* 2011;29:3507-10. doi:10.1016/j. vaccine.2009.10.106 PMID:19909830

20. Savy M, Edmond K, Fine PEM, Hall A, Hennig BJ, Moore SE et al. Landscape analysis of interactions between nutrition and vaccine responses in children. *J Nutr* 2009;139:2154S-218S. doi:10.3945/jn.109.105312 PMID:19793845

21. Dawson A. Vaccination ethics. In: *Public health ethics*. Cambridge: Cambridge University Press, 2011. pp. 143-53.

22. Verweij M. Moral principles for allocating scarce medical resources in an influenza pandemic. *J Bioeth Inq* 2009;6:159-69. doi:10.1007/s11673-009-9161-6

23. Ibid.

24. Selgelid MJ. Pandethics. *Public Health* 2009;123:255-9. http://dx.doi. org/10.1016/j.puhe .2008.12.005 PMID:19223051 doi:10.1016/j. puhe.2008.12.005 PMID:19223051

25. United Nations High Commissioner for Refugees. Guiding principles 2008–2012. Geneva: UNHCR; 2011. Available from: http://www.unha. org/4885959c2.htm [accessed 24 January 2013].

26. Ibid.

27. Hanquet G, editor. Medecins Sans Frontieres. Refugee health: an approach to emergency situations. Macmillan; 1997. Available from: http://www.refbooks. msf.org/MSF_Docs/En/Refugee_Health/ RH.pdf [accessed 24 January 2013].

28. Ibid.

29. van Delden JJM, Ashcroft R, Dawson A, Marckmann G, Upshur R, Verweij MF. The ethics of mandatory vaccination against influenza for health care workers. *Vaccine* 2008;26:5562-6. doi:10.1016/j .vaccine.2008.08.002 PMID:18722495

30. Draft guidelines for WHO and SAGE development of evidence-based vaccine related recommendations. Geneva: World Health Organization; 2011. Available from: http://www.who.int/immunization/ sage/1_Draft_ Guidelines_Evidence_Review_GRADING_apr_2011.pdf [accessed 24 January 2013].

31. Duclos P, Durrheim D, Reingold A, Bhutta Z, Vannice K, Rees H. Developing evidence-based vaccine recommendations and GRADE. *Vaccine* 2012;31:12-9. doi:10.1016/j.vaccine.2012.02.041

32. Humanitarian Practice Network [Internet]. Humanitarian accountability. *Humanitarian Exchange Magazine* 2011;52. Available from: http://www. odihpn.org/humanitarian-exchange-magazine/ issue-52/humanitarian- accountability [accessed 24 January 2013].

33. Verweij M, Dawson A. Ethical principles for collective immunisation programmes. *Vaccine* 2004;22:3122-6. doi:10.1016/j.vaccine.2004.01.062 PMID:15297064

34. Gostin LO. Influenza A(H1N1) and pandemic preparedness under the rule of international law. *JAMA* 2009;301:2376-8. doi:10.1001/jama.2009.849 PMID:19509384

35. United Nations Commission on Human Rights. The Siracusa principles on the limitation and derogation provisions in the International Covenant on Civil and Political Rights. Geneva: UNCHR; 1984. Available from: http://www.unha. org/refworld/docid/4672bc122.html [accessed 24 January 2013].

36. Gostin LO. The resurgent tuberculosis epidemic in the era of AIDS: Reflections on public health, law, and society. *MD Law Rev* 1995;54:1-131. PMID:11657387

37. Diekema D, Marcuse E. Ethical issues in the vaccination of children: primum non nocere today. New York: Elsevier, 1998.

38. Harris J, Holm S. Is there a moral obligation not to infect others? *BMJ* 1995;311:1215-7. doi:10.1136/bmj.311.7014.1215 PMID:7488907

39. Simons KW. Negligence. *Soc Philos Policy* 1999;16:52-93. doi:10.1017/ S0265052500002399

40. Isaacs D, Kilham H, Leask J, Tobin B. Ethical issues in immunisation. *Vaccine* 2009;27:615-8. doi:10.1016/j.vaccine.2008.11.002 PMID:19026706

41. Selgelid MJ. A moderate pluralist approach to public health policy and ethics. *Public Health Ethics* 2009;2:195-205. doi:10.1093/phe/php018

42. Toole MJ, Waldman RJ. Prevention of excess mortality in refugee and displaced populations in developing countries. *JAMA* 1990;263:3296-302. doi:10.1001/jama.1990.03440240086021 PMID:2348541

43. Galvani AP, Medlock J, Chapman GB. The ethics of influenza vaccination. *Science* 2006;313:758-60. doi:10.1126/science.313.5788.758b PMID:16906649

44. Finn A, Savulescu J. Is immunisation child protection? *Lancet* 2011;378:465-8. doi:10.1016/S0140-6736(11)60695-8 PMID:21664677

45. Collogan LK, Tuma F, Dolan-Sewell R, Borja S, Fleischman AR. Ethical issues pertaining to research in the aftermath of disaster. *J Trauma Stress* 2004;17:363-72. doi:10.1023/B:JOTS.0000048949.43570.6a PMID:15633915

46. Kilpatrick DG. The ethics of disaster research: a special section. *J Trauma Stress* 2004;17:361-2. doi:10.1023/B:J0TS.0000048961.75301.74 PMID:15633914

47. Daniels N. *Just health care.* Cambridge: Cambridge University Press; 1985.

48. World Medical Association [Internet]. WMA statement on medical ethics in the event of disasters. Ferney-Voltaire: WMA; 2006. Available from: http:// www.wma.net/en/30publications/10policies/d7/index.html [accessed 24 September 2012].

49. Ford N, Mills EJ, Zachariah R, Upshur R. Ethics of conducting research in conflict settings. *Confl Health* 2009;3:7. doi:10.1186/1752-1505-3-7 PMID:19591691

50. Siriwardhana DC. Disaster research ethics—a luxury or a necessity for developing countries? *Asian Tribune* 13 February 2007. Available from: http://www.asiantribune.com/index.php?q=node/4524 [accessed 24 January 2013].

51. Research ethics in international epidemic response. Geneva: World Health Organization; 2009. Available from: http://www.who.int/ethics/ gip_research_ethics_.pdf [accessed 24 January 2012].

52. Fottrell E, Byass P. Identifying humanitarian crises in population surveillance field sites: simple procedures and ethical imperatives. *Public Health* 2009;123:151-5. doi:10.1016/j.puhe.2008.10.032 PMID:19157467

53. Carrel M. Demographic and health surveillance: longitudinal ethical considerations. *Bull World Health Organ* 2008;86:612-6. doi:10.2471/ BLT.08.051037 PMID:18797619

54. World Medical Association [Internet]. Declaration of Helsinki: Ethical principles for medical research involving human subjects. Ferney-Voltaire: WMA; 1964. Available from: http://www.wma.net/en/20activities/10ethics/ 10helsinki/index.html [accessed 24 January 2013].

55. Wallis L, Smith W, editors. Disaster medicine. Johannesburg: Juta; 2011. pp. 9–25.

56. Abdool Karim Q, Abdool Karim SS, Coovadia MH, Susser M. Informed consent for HIV testing in a South African hospital: Is it truly informed and truly voluntary? *Am J Public Health* 1998;88:637-40. doi:10.2105/ AJPH.88.4.637 PMID:9551007

57. Joubert G, Steinberg H, van der Ryst E, Chikobvu P. Consent for Participation in the Bloemfontein Vitamin A Trial: How Informed and Voluntary? *Am J Public Health* 2003;93:582-4. doi:10.2105/AJPH.93.4.582 PMID:12660201

58. Moodley K, Pather M, Myer L. Informed consent and participant perceptions of influenza vaccine trials in South Africa. *J Med Ethics* 2005;31:727-32. doi:10.1136/jme.2004.009910 PMID:16319239

59. Molyneux CS, Peshu N, Marsh K. Understanding of informed consent in a low-income setting: three case studies from the Kenyan Coast. *Soc Sci Med* 2004;59:2547-59. doi:10.1016/j.socscimed.2004.03.037 PMID:15474208

60. Frimpong-Mansoh A. Culture and voluntary informed consent in African health care systems. *Dev World Bioeth* 2008;8:104-14. doi:10.1111/j.1471- 8847.2006.00181.x PMID:19143087

61. Rawls J. *A theory of justice.* Cambridge: Harvard University Press; 1971.

62. Emerson CI, Singer PA. Is there an ethical obligation to complete polio eradication? *Lancet* 2010;375:1340-1. doi:10.1016/S0140-6736(10)60565-X PMID:20405537

63. Hunt MR, Schwartz L, Elit L. Experience of ethics training and support for health care professionals in international aid work. *Public Health Ethics* 2012;5:91-9. doi:10.1093/phe/phr033

Part IV Discussion Topics

Wanda Teays

1. What do you believe are the most pressing health care issues we face? What should be our priorities as a society?

2. What should we do to achieve justice in health care?
   • Set out four steps that could be taken to address some of the major health inequities.

3. Udo Schüklenk asks, "What are the moral obligations of health workers to the societies that enabled their training?"
   • Share your answer to this question.

4. Given limited access to health care, should groups form their own health maintenance organizations (HMOs)? And could this be accomplished on an international scale?

5. Consider—and construct—several analogies to health care (e.g., the public school system). What sort of analogy would provide the most equitable model for a universal health care system?

6. Zenon Culverhouse examines issues of global mental health.
   • Given the range of concerns, how might we set priorities?

7. Rosemarie Tong looks at the fact that care for the elderly often falls on the children and this can be morally problematic. Equally problematic is the question of who should care for the elderly who have no children to care for them (or whose children refuse to help them).
   • Can you suggest three or four ideas for addressing this situation?

8. What are the major ethical concerns about virginity restoration surgery?

9. ICE has new rules on solitary confinement intended to limit its use. Read the following comments about enforcement of those limits, and share your response and ideas regarding how to ensure compliance. "Solitary confinement in both immigration detention and the criminal justice system is cruel, expensive, and ineffective," said Ruthie Epstein [of the American Civil Liberties Union]. "If strictly enforced throughout the ICE detention system . . . ICE's new policy could represent significant progress in curtailing this inhumane practice."

   "ICE shall take additional steps to ensure appropriate review and oversight of decisions to retain detainees in segregated housing for over 14 days," . . . Epstein stresses the concern is enforcement. (See "New ICE Directive Limiting Solitary Confinement a Good Step, But Issue Is Compliance, Say Rights Groups." (NBC Latino, September 6, 2013)

   • How can they ensure enforcement?

10. What should be done about the use of long-term solitary confinement? Look, for example, at the case of Herman Wallace, who was in solitary for 41 years—convicted of killing a prison guard, he maintained that he was innocent. (See E. Woo, "Herman Wallace Dies at 71; Ex-Inmate Held in Solitary for 41 Years," *Los Angeles Times*, October 8, 2013.)

    • What steps do you recommend?

11. How much freedom of choice should parents have in deciding whether to vaccinate their children?

    • Set out three or four reasons for and three or four against parental control over vaccinations.

12. How do we decide, and who decides, which individuals or groups have priority in access to such resources as vaccines, treatment centers, and so on?

    • What plan(s) should we put in effect now—before an epidemic or a pandemic strikes?

13. Looking at public health, a number of hospital patients were put at risk from contaminated surgical equipment used on a patient with Creutzfeldt-Jakob disease (alias "mad cow" disease). Read about the incident in New Hampshire reported on September 21, 2013:

    > Health officials have confirmed that a patient who underwent neurosurgery at a New Hampshire hospital earlier this year had Creutzfeldt-Jakob disease. The death . . . prompted authorities in two states to warn that as many as 13 patients may have been exposed to surgical equipment used during the patient's surgery, thus to the same disease.
    >
    > The now-deceased patient had undergone neurosurgery at Catholic Medical Center in Manchester. . . . By the time this diagnosis was suspected, equipment used in the patient's surgery had been used several other operations. This raised the possibility that the equipment might have been contaminated—especially since normal sterilization procedures are not enough to get rid of the disease proteins, known as prions, tied to Creutzfeldt-Jakob disease—thus potentially exposing the other patients to infection.

Eight other patients at the same Manchester hospital were being monitored for Creutzfeldt-Jakob disease. Massachusetts health authorities noted the next day that five Cape Cod Hospital patients may have been exposed to Creutzfeldt-Jakob disease too because their surgeons this summer later used the same potentially contaminated medical equipment as in the New Hampshire facility (See Greg Botelho, "Case of Creutzfeldt-Jakob Disease Confirmed in New Hampshire." CNN, September 21, 2013)

- To what degree should steps be taken to go beyond normal sterilization procedures in medical settings?
- What is an acceptable risk in such cases—though very rare—as here with Creutzfeldt-Jakob disease? Offer some ideas about what should be done to minimize or prevent such incidents as this.

14. Foster Farms, the tenth largest chicken producer in the United States, faced a public relations disaster in 2012 with an outbreak of salmonella that sickened hundreds of people. The US Department of Agriculture cited the company for unsanitary plant conditions and a dozen instances of fecal matter on carcasses. David Pierson, Diana Marcum, and Tiffany Hsu (2013) report:

> Foster Farms is an example of how salmonella has become an increasingly potent threat to consumer safety. "This is not your grandmother's salmonella anymore," said Caroline Smith DeWaal, food safety director for the Center for Science in the Public Interest. "It's a new salmonella, much more potent, and modified with the use of antibiotics on the farm." At least 278 people reportedly have been sickened in 18 states since March [2013] by a strain of Salmonella Heidelberg that has shown signs of resistance to antibiotics.
>
> Food safety advocates say virulent forms of antibiotic resistant salmonella should be handled like E. coli O157:H7, which triggers an automatic recall. ("Poultry Plants Linked to Outbreaks Won't Be Closed." (*Los Angeles Times*, October 10, 2013)

- What counts as "acceptable risk" when it comes to foodborne diseases?
- The company insists that cooking at a sufficiently high temperature will destroy the bacteria—but should that be enough to stop a recall? Share your recommendations.

15. "Because delays and shortages in producing vaccine against a pandemic are unavoidable, we need to decide in advance which groups will be the first to receive vaccine and how the government will enforce its rationing. The US national vaccine advisory committee recommended this priority for the first shots: key government leaders, medical caregivers, workers in flu vaccine and drug factories, pregnant women, and those infants, elderly and ill people who are already in the high-priority group for annual flu shots. That top tier includes about 46 million Americans." (See W. Wayt Gibbs and Christine Soares, "Preparing for a Pandemic," *Scientific American*, October 24, 2005.)

- Do you agree with this list of priorities?

16. How much is your medical privacy worth? Would you accept $50 to allow prying eyes into your medical records? Craig Klugman posted in a blog on *Bioethics.net* on August 23, 2013, that CVS pharmacies started a program early in 2013 in which "For every ten prescriptions filled, a customer can receive $5 worth of credits to be used at CVS

up to a maximum of $50 per year." That may sound good—but such loyalty means the company acquires information about your health.

- Is it worth $50 to retain privacy? Should this be a concern?
- Who is most vulnerable? What ethical questions do you foresee?

17. What sort of efforts should we be doing *now* to prepare for the ethical problems that arise in the face of the risks of a measles epidemic? Should vaccinations be a requirement?

Appendix A

Essay Questions

Alison Dundes Renteln

1. Assume that individuals who were subjected to medical experimentation in the United States and in other countries file a lawsuit against the US Public Health Service and the National Institutes of Health alleging that the government-sponsored testing violated their human rights. Select one major case study (such as . . .) and write an analytic essay explaining whether the plaintiffs would likely prevail.

2. Assume that you are the Surgeon General of the United States. It comes to your attention that an unspecified number of Muslim women seek hymen restoration surgery to avoid "honor-related" violence. The National Organization of Women and the American Medical Association advise you to issue a policy statement on behalf of the executive branch strictly prohibiting this surgery. Write a memo in which you discuss whether this operation is compatible with human rights standards and consistent with the principles of global bioethics.

3. In a liberal democracy, individuals are usually permitted the right to make their life plans. The question of whether women should have the right to decide whether to continue or terminate a pregnancy, however, is hotly contested. In what ways do basic principles of international human rights law help us resolve this matter? Consider cases we studied and the film *Vessel* in your answer.

4. What is the difference between deontological and teleological approaches to moral questions? Describe two controversies associated with the implementation of the Convention on Torture or Cruel, Inhuman, or Degrading Treatment of Punishment. How would you suggest modifying the treaty to render it more effective?

5. The World Trade Organization has devoted considerable attention to intellectual property rights and access to medicine. Discuss whether existing international standards have been implemented in a manner that successfully balances concern for both. Analyze the Doha Declaration of the TRIPS Agreement and Public Health. As part of your analysis, consider the merging trilateral cooperation involving the WTO, the World Intellectual Property Organization, and the World Health Organization. https://www.wto.org/english/tratop_e/trips_e/who_wipo_wto_e.htm.

6. Explain the relevance of the TRIPS agreement and other instruments to efforts improving access to medicine. In your essay, analyze at least two controversies in the context of evaluating the relevant instruments. What policy recommendations can you propose to harmonize these systems and address the problems these various systems seek to regulate?

7. What rights do prisoners enjoy under international law? Can states deny inmates and detainees the right to health including access to medicine, surgery, and clean water? Present a philosophical consideration of the right to health in international law and global bioethics standards. Be sure to consult Nigel Rodley's treatise *Prisoners' Rights Under International Law* (3rd ed., Oxford University Press, 2009).

8. Write an essay on the status of the human rights of transgender persons that would aid advocates of these rights. To what extent do global standards support these newly recognized rights? Analyze key cases that elucidate this question and refer to specific treaty provisions and instruments that afford insight into this matter. How, if at all, might human rights norms and jurisprudence influence domestic political debates about this issue?

9. To what extent does international human rights law afford protection to the rights of the elderly? Discuss whether the United Nations Principles for Older Persons (1991) and the proposed Convention on the Rights of Older Persons protect the aging adequately. One challenge is how best to protect choice for elderly persons with dementia. This concerns the question of legal capacity. After you analyze the scope of the protections afforded by general human rights norms and the Convention on the Rights of Persons with Disabilities regarding this right and related ones, present a series of possible solutions. What proposals can you offer to improve policies in this area?

Appendix B

Case Analysis Topics

Wanda Teays

CASES FOR ANALYSIS #1

Take your pick: answer either three cases with 700–750 words each or two cases with 1,000–1,100 words each. Think of each case in three parts: (1) your answer, (2) defense of your answer using any *one* ethicist we've studied, and (3) your reply to a different ethicist who would disagree with you.

1. How can we bring in the different voices and concerns across different groups and socioeconomic levels so global bioethics can shape policies and methodologies to address injustice in health care? And what kinds of changes should occur in universities and hospitals in terms of the training of doctors, nurses, and other caregivers?

2. Movies such as *Outbreak* and *Contagion* present the dilemmas that arise around fast-moving epidemics. One such issue is that, in many cases, there is no readily available supply of vaccines and those available are in limited supply. This leads to questions about triage.

   Answer the following:
   a. How do we decide, and who decides, which individuals or groups have priority in access to such resources as vaccines, treatment centers, and so on?
   b. What plan(s) should we put in effect now—before an epidemic or a pandemic strikes?

3. Discuss the ethical issues in medical personnel participating in coercive force-feeding by hunger strikers in prisons (e.g., those in Pelican Bay, California, in 2013) or by detainees (e.g., those held at Guantanamo Bay, Cuba).

   Answer the following:
   a. When a hunger striker may be close to death, is life-saving intervention via force-feeding morally acceptable?

4. Nurses, as well as doctors, have participated in force-feeding at Guantanamo Bay. As practiced, it has been described as brutal and painful and, even if without discomfort, violates informed consent right of refusal under patient autonomy.

    Answer the following:

    a. Besides the public stands against the participation of its members, is there something more professional organizations should be doing?

5. On its website on September 15, 2013, Amnesty International praised the Canadian government for apologizing to Canadian citizen Maher Arar. This was for Arar's torture while a victim of mistaken identity as a terrorism suspect in the war on terror. Amnesty International called for the United States to apologize as well. This has yet to happen.

    Answer the following:

    a. What should professional organizations (the AMA, WMA, etc.) do by way of a response when physician–members enable or assist in torture or "harsh interrogation"?

    b. Given medical personnel were likely participants in Arar's torture, should the WMA or the AMA also be asked to issue an apology?

6. Do you think the root of poverty and health problems links to the power differentials between economic classes—not those of North versus South? Poor people in rich countries may be at the same level of disadvantage as their counterparts in poor nations, even if they are living in a wealthier society. Picture yourself as the member of a team of advocates who are undertaking a special kind of ad campaign to address global health inequities.

    Answer the following:

    a. What are three things you'd do in your campaign to try to turn things around to improve the life expectancy of the poor?

7. Do you think it is right to restrict or even prohibit egg donation or sales? Read the following excerpt from *Science Daily* (2011), and then share your thoughts:

    > Women who have become pregnant after egg donation should be categorized as high-risk patients. Viewing patient files they found that within the past 4 years, 8 women who had received donated eggs had to be treated for pregnancy-induced hypertension. Three of these pregnancies had to be terminated prematurely because of the threat to the mother's life. The other 5 cases showed a milder course of pregnancy-induced hypertension.
    >
    > ("Egg Donation: The Way to Happy Motherhood, with Risks and Side Effects," January 25, 2011)

8. When the Environmental Protection Agency planned a two-year environmental study using infants and children up to three years old, they offered the families $970, children's clothes, and a camcorder in exchange for using pesticides in their homes.

    a. State your major concerns and then respond to this argument for using children in pesticide studies:

Linda S. Sheldon, acting administrator for the human exposure and atmospheric sciences division of the EPA's Office of Research and Development, said the agency would educate families participating in the study and inform them if their children's urine showed risky levels of pesticides. She said it was crucial for the agency to study small children because so little is known about how their bodies absorb harmful chemicals. (See Juliet Eilperin, "Study of Pesticides and Children Stirs Protests," *Washington Post*, October 30, 2004).

9. Do a study of the movie *World War Z* from the standpoint of bioethics—focus on the zombies as stricken by a virus and the ethical issues raised by the movie. Do *not* write a plot summary or use *any* review or other commentary on the movie. This is *your* analysis not anyone else's.

CASES FOR ANALYSIS #2

These cases require 1,800–2,000 words. The total word count should be listed on the cover page, along with your name and which case you selected.

Cases are listed on pages 354–55.

- Pick ONE case to study. Only one case.
- Answer each of the PARTS below.
- Set each PART out separately from one another—this is not an essay but an analysis, with the PARTs clearly marked.
- List the word count for each PART on the cover page, for example, PART ONE (102 words) and so on for each PART.
- Note the suggested allocation of words for each PART of your case study.
- You can go under or over the suggested word count for the section, but not over or under by more than 50 words, to keep the PARTs balanced.

PARTS OF YOUR CASE ANALYSIS with suggested word counts:

a. (75–125 words). PART ONE brief introduction to the topic, what you're doing in this paper, and your thesis (state your position you will be arguing here).
b. (75–125 words). PART TWO brief summary of the case, setting out key details.
c. (150–250 words). PART THREE ethical issues and concerns—recommend stating three to five.
d. (300–400 words). PART FOUR perspectives of three parties affected by the case decision (e.g., doctor, patient, family, government, insurance company, society, etc.).
e. (450–500 words). PART FIVE your argument as to what should be done. No references should be used here—just set out *your* argument.
f. (100–150 words). PART SIX ethical support—ethical theory or theorist that supports your argument.
g. (100–150 words). PART SEVEN ethical attack—ethical theory or theorist that critiques or criticizes your and your reply to that critique.
h. (150–200 words). PART EIGHT concluding statement with your reflections on the case and lessons to be learned from this case.

Select *one* of these cases:
Read *all* the choices and *pick one*.

CASE #1 12/26/2017
NIH LIFTS BAN ON RESEARCH THAT COULD MAKE DEADLY
VIRUSES EVEN WORSE
NPR
Scientists could soon resume controversial experiments on germs with the potential to cause pandemics, as government officials have decided to finally lift an unusual three-year moratorium on federal funding for the work. The research involves three viruses—influenza, SARS, and MERS—that could kill millions if they mutated in a way that let the germs spread quickly among people.

CASE #2 12/05/2017
A MAN COLLAPSED WITH "DO NOT RESUSCITATE" TATTOOED
ON HIS CHEST. DOCTORS DIDN'T KNOW WHAT TO DO.
Washington Post
Doctors in Miami faced an unusual ethical dilemma when an unconscious, deteriorating patient was brought into the emergency room with the words "Do Not Resuscitate" across his chest.

CASE #3 11/15/2017
FIRST DIGITAL PILL APPROVED TO WORRIES ABOUT BIOMEDICAL
"BIG BROTHER"
New York Times
For the first time, the Food and Drug Administration has approved a digital pill—a medication embedded with a sensor that can tell doctors whether, and when, patients take their medicine.

CASE #4 10/10/2017
NEW YORK HOSPITAL'S SECRET POLICY LED TO WOMAN BEING GIVEN
C-SECTION AGAINST HER WILL
The Guardian
A New York hospital accused of forcing a mother to undergo a caesarean section against her will used an internal policy permitting doctors to overrule a pregnant woman's medical decisions.

CASE #5 06/14/2017
DYING 5 YEAR OLD: RIGHT TO CHOOSE?
CNN

Julianna Snow is dying of an incurable disease. She's stable at the moment, but any germ that comes her way, even the common cold virus, could kill her. She's told her parents that the next time this happens, she wants to die at home instead of going to the hospital for treatment. Should her parents have let her know how grave her situation is and have asked her end-of-life wishes? Should her parents heed them? What about the doctors?

Appendix C

Bioethics Films—A Selection

DOCTORS AND PATIENTS

- *The Doctor*
- *Regarding Henry*

HUMAN RIGHTS

- *Ghosts of Abu Ghraib*
- *Taxi to the Dark Side*
- *Standard Operating Procedure*
- *Solitary Confinement* (National Geographic)
- *Rendition*
- *In the Name of the Father*
- *Human Trafficking*
- *The Stoning of Soraya M.*
- *The Killing Fields*
- *Hotel Rwanda*

PANDEMICS

- *Outbreak*
- *Contagion*
- *World War Z*
- *28 Days Later*

LIFE AND DEATH

- *The Descendants*
- *The Sea Inside*
- *Whose Life Is It Anyway?*
- *The Diving Bell and the Butterfly*
- *Amour*
- *The Farewell*
- *Dead Man Walking*
- *Dallas Buyers Club*
- *Million Dollar Baby*

VIOLENCE AND WAR

- *The Hurt Locker*
- *Polytechnique*
- *July 22*
- *Paradise Now*
- *Casualties of War*
- *Enough*
- *The Secret in Their Eyes*
- *The Accused*

ENVIRONMENTAL DISASTERS

- *Chernobyl*
- *The Wave*
- *The Impossible*
- *Silkwood*
- *Testament*
- *Erin Brockovich*

REPRODUCTIVE FREEDOM

- *Four Months Three Weeks Two Days*
- *Vera Drake*
- *Juno*
- *No Más Bebés*

ORGAN SALES AND XENOTRANSPLANTS

- *Organ Farm*
- *Brain Transplant*
- *My Sister's Keeper*
- *Dirty Pretty Things*
- *Coma*
- *The Island*

SELF-DETERMINATION

- *Eternal Sunshine of the Spotless Mind*
- *Limitless*
- *Gattaca*